The LASIK Handbook

A Case-Based Approach

EDITORS

ROBERT S. FEDER, M.D.

Chief, Cornea and External Disease Service
Associate Professor of Ophthamology
Feinberg School of Medicine
Northwestern University
Chicago, Illinois

CHRISTOPHER J. RAPUANO, M.D.

Co-Chief, Cornea Service
Co-Chief, Refractive Surgery Department
Wills Eye Hospital
Professor of Ophthamology
Jefferson Medical College of Thomas Jefferson University
Philadelphia, Pennsylvania

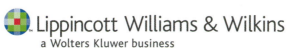
Lippincott Williams & Wilkins
a Wolters Kluwer business
Philadelphia · Baltimore · New York · London
Buenos Aires · Hong Kong · Sydney · Tokyo

Acquisitions Editor: Jonathan W. Pine, Jr.
Managing Editor: Anne E. Jacobs
Project Manager: Alicia Jackson
Senior Manufacturing Manager: Benjamin Rivera
Associate Marketing Director: Adam Glazer
Design Coordinator: Steve Druding
Cover Designer: Lou Fuiano
Production Service: GGS Book Services
Printer: RR Donnelley—China

Library of Congress Cataloging-in-Publication Data
The LASIK handbook : a case-based approach / editors, Robert S. Feder,
Christopher J. Rapuano.
  p.   ; cm.
Includes bibliographical references and index.
ISBN-13: 978-0-7817-6208-3 (alk. paper)
ISBN 0-7817-6208-1
1. LASIK (Eye surgery)—Handbooks, manuals, etc.   2. Eye—Surgery—Handbooks,
manuals, etc.   I. Feder, Robert S.   II. Rapuano, Christopher J.   III. Title.
[DNLM: 1. Keratomileusis, Laser In Situ—methods—Case Reports.
2. Keratomileusis, Laser In Situ—methods—Handbooks.   3. Cornea—surgery—Case
Reports.   4. Cornea—surgery—Handbooks. WW 39 L344 2007]
RE336.L372 2007
617.7′190598—dc22   2006009482

10 9 8 7 6 5 4 3 2 1

Dedication

This book is dedicated to the teachers who have trained us and had an impact in our careers. Most notably is Dr. Jay Krachmer, who has trained many of our nation's leaders in cornea and external disease. With his unique brand of infectious enthusiasm and clarity of thought, he demonstrated to us the importance of careful observation, the need to "think outside the box," the organizational skills needed to accomplish large projects, and the ability to motivate others to achieve beyond perceived limits. For his profound impact on our professional lives and his continued support and friendship we will always be grateful.

We also dedicate this book to the many fine residents and fellows we have trained over the years. They have stimulated us and enriched our personal and professional lives. It is an honor to contribute our experience to their training.

Contributors

Anthony Cirino, M.D.
Staff Physician
Department of Ophthalmology
Kaiser Northwest Permanente
Portland, Oregon

Robert S. Feder, M.D.
Chief, Cornea and External Disease Service
Associate Professor of Ophthalmology
Feinberg School of Medicine
Northwestern University
Chicago, Illinois

Lawrence Gans, M. D.
Assistant Professor of Clinical Ophthalmology
Department of Ophthalmology and Visual Sciences
Washington University School of Medicine
Saint Louis, Missouri

Colman Kraff, M.D.
Director, Refractive Surgery
Kraff Eye Institute
Clinical Instructor
Feinberg School of Medicine
Northwestern University
Chicago, Illinois

Marian Macsai, M.D.
Chief, Division of Ophthalmology
Evanston Northwestern Healthcare
Evanston, Illinois
Professor of Ophthalmology
Feinberg School of Medicine
Northwestern University
Chicago, Illinois

Parag Majmudar, M.D.
Associate Professor of Ophthalmology
Cornea Service, Department of Ophthalmology

Rush University Medical Center
Chicago Cornea Consultants, Ltd.
Chicago, Illinois

Christopher J. Rapuano
Co-Chief, Cornea Service
Co-Chief, Refractive Surgery Department
Wills Eye Hospital
Professor of Ophthalmology
Jefferson Medical College of
    Thomas Jefferson University
Philadelphia, Pennsylvania

Michael Rosenberg, M.D.
Associate Professor of Ophthalmology
Vice Chairman
Department of Ophthalmology
Feinberg School of Medicine
Northwestern University
Chicago, Illinois

Steven Rosenfeld, M.D.
Voluntary Associate Professor
Bascom Palmer Eye Institute
University of Miami School of Medicine
Miami, Florida

Jonathan Rubenstein, M.D.
Vice Chairman and The Deutsch Family
    Professor of Ophthalmology
Rush University Medical Center
Chicago, Illinois

Michael Vrabec, M.D., F.A.C.S.
Department of Ophthalmology
University of Wisconsin
Appleton, Wisconsin

Contents

| CHAPTER **1** | **Basic LASIK** | **3** |

Robert S. Feder, M.D. and Anthony Cirino, M.D.

CHAPTER 2 Equipment 28

Robert S. Feder, M.D., Marian Macsai, M.D., Steven Rosenfeld, M.D., Michael Vrabec, M.D., F.A.C.S., Parag Majmudar, M.D., Colman Kraff, M.D., and Jonathan Rubenstein, M.D.

CHAPTER 3 Role of Mitomycin-C in Keratorefractive Surgery 80

Parag Majmudar, M.D.

CHAPTER **8** Self-Assessment Test   254

Anthony Cirino, M.D., Robert S. Feder, M.D., Lawrence Gans, M.D., Colman Kraff, M.D., Marian Macsai, M.D., Parag Majmudar, M.D., Christopher J. Rapuano, M.D., Michael Rosenberg, M.D., Steven Rosenfeld, M.D., Jonathan Rubenstein, M.D., and Michael Vrabec, M.D., F.A.C.S.

Acknowledgments

I wish to acknowledge the special contribution of Dr. Anthony Cirino in the early development of this book. Nearly 3 years ago Tony was a second-year resident learning basic LASIK. While working through a series of cases, he and I developed the idea of creating a manual that other residents at Northwestern could use as a reference as they struggled to learn the basics of surgical planning. Eventually we did put a manual together that proved the effectiveness of a case-based approach to teaching LASIK. Tony has served as an important contributor to this book.

I would like to thank my colleagues at the Northwestern Vision Correction Associates, Drs. Surendra Basti, Paul Bryar, and Michael Rosenberg, for helping to create an atmosphere of shared learning and support, which enhances the quality of patient care. Pam Stewart, the manager of our group, assisted in the preparation of many of our cases.

Steve Dybedock, manager of the Northwestern Laser Vision Center, enthusiastically assisted in fact checking and preparing illustrations. Jonathan Shankle, our ophthalmic photographer, was responsible for many of the fine images scattered throughout the book, and Sheila Macumber, our medical illustrator, visually captured many of the ideas that are difficult to describe in words or with photography.

A special note of thanks goes to my contributors, a superior group of clinicians and teachers, who lent their time and expertise to this project and patiently put up with my steady barrage of e-mails, phone calls, and notes.

Finally, I would like to acknowledge my wonderful wife, Randi, and sons, Alex and Seth, for almost 2 years of nearly unflinching support. I used to wonder why book authors so often acknowledged their families. Now I understand and look forward to again being a fully engaged family member.
Robert S. Feder, M.D.

About two years ago Rob asked me for my thoughts on a project he was working on. As Director of the Cornea Fellowship and Co-Director of the Refractive Surgery Department at Wills Eye, he knew that I was very involved in teaching refractive surgery to residents and fellows. I was excited by the idea of collaborating on a handbook similar in concept to the Wills Manual, which I co-wrote, intended for beginning and intermediate LASIK surgeons. Although there were plenty of LASIK textbooks available, none of them started with the basics of LASIK, presented all of the important issues involved in planning and performing the procedure, and included ways to avoid and manage complications. The case presentation is an excellent way to reinforce the key teaching points. I am hopeful that those learning to perform LASIK (and who isn't still learning?) will find this book useful, educational, and interesting.

I would like to thank my loving and incredibly supportive wife, Sara, and my four children, Michael, Patrick, Daniel, and Megan, for understanding that occasionally, even when I am at home, I am at work.
Christopher J. Rapuano, M.D.

Introduction

Over the years refractive surgeons have witnessed an explosion of technological advances that have made LASIK surgery safer and more reliable for a wide range of patients. During the same period of time, experienced refractive surgeons have increasingly come to the realization that the most challenging part of LASIK surgery is planning a customized strategy for each patient. This strategy should be based on a comprehensive evaluation of psychosocial, historical, and anatomical factors. The purpose of this handbook is to help the eye surgeon develop the ability to plan a surgical strategy that will be most likely to achieve an outcome consistent with the patient's goals.

Each of the contributing authors in this book is an expert LASIK surgeon with years of experience in training others to plan and perform refractive surgery. They have each been asked to contribute because they possess a special expertise in some facet of the surgery and they have the ability to express this facet clearly and concisely. The contributions of the authors and editors reflect strategies currently used in private practice and academic centers from several regions of the country. For added balance one of our contributors is a beginning LASIK surgeon who has been successfully trained using the case-based methodology presented in this book.

The book begins with the basics of patient evaluation for surgery, including a method for presenting surgical risks without terrifying the patient. The second chapter discusses basics of corneal topography, particularly how it is used in screening refractive surgery candidates. Various lasers and microkeratome systems that are commonly used are also described in this chapter, with the addition of the nuances of technique that only experience can teach. Surgical planning incorporating the individual patient characteristics and the various technological systems will emphasize safety and reliability.

The most important part of the book is the case section, which begins at a basic level and progresses to more challenging clinical situations. The 75 cases contained in the book are subdivided into scenarios that emphasize preoperative planning, cases involving an intraoperative mishap, and others that focus on the management of postoperative complications. Some cases represent actual patient encounters, whereas others are partially fabricated to emphasize certain points. All cases are based on clinical situations the authors have encountered. It is our intention that the readers will work through these cases with pencils in hand and will develop appropriate strategies just as if the patients had been in their examination chairs. A treatment plan for managing each case is presented along with a discussion. The treatment plan will at times reflect the opinions of the case author and should not be considered the only way to manage a given patient. Several key teaching points are found at the end of each case.

Case indexes allow the reader to refer quickly to the scenarios that are most relevant to the clinical situation currently being managed. A reference index is provided for cases concerning preoperative planning. A second index identifies cases concerning only intraoperative and postoperative issues. A third index identifies cases performed with various combinations of lasers and microkeratomes. The final portion of the book is a self-test. It is a series of 50 multiple-choice questions designed to test the readers' knowledge acquired after mastering the material in the text and cases. Each question is followed by four short possible answers, there being only one correct answer. The answer is followed by a brief discussion.

It is our intention that this book will serve the function of a readily available consultant. It is our hope that our book will not sit on the shelf but will be close at hand with the pages well worn from careful study and repeated reference.

1

Basic LASIK

Robert S. Feder, M.D. and Anthony Cirino, M.D.

PATIENT EVALUATION

Careful patient evaluation is essential in order to determine whether a patient is a candidate for LASIK surgery. The criteria used to determine candidacy are divided into two parts, psychosocial and anatomical. Each will be considered individually.

Psychosocial Factors

A good candidate for LASIK surgery should be capable of understanding the risks of the procedure and that risk-free surgery does not exist. The patient must be willing and able to follow instructions before, during, and after surgery. A patient who resists listening to a discussion of the risks may be a poor candidate for surgery. If the patient is unable to understand the surgeon due to a language barrier or disability, adequate preoperative counseling and intraoperative instruction will be more difficult to achieve. The patient must be available for postoperative follow-up. Beware of the patient with the challenging schedule who may not understand the care that is required after surgery.

Managing patient expectations is one of the greatest challenges a LASIK surgeon faces. This begins with the preoperative consultation. The surgeon should avoid making grandiose statements regarding the surgical outcome or even promises about the quality of vision that will be achieved after surgery. However, patients should be told what level of visual acuity is reasonable to expect after surgery, with a subsequent enhancement procedure if needed. This can be expressed as an expected range of visual acuity that this particular patient would be expected to achieve. It is helpful to mention the surgeon's rate of enhancement for patients with similar refractive error. A preoperative patient who expects perfection after surgery is destined to be unhappy postoperatively. Do not confuse visual acuity with visual function. A patient with 20/20 Snellen acuity may be unhappy due to loss of near vision, ghosting, decreased contrast sensitivity, glare, or other problems that affect the quality of vision. Personal characteristics of the best LASIK patients include an easygoing nature, a positive outlook, a well-adjusted personality, currently using less than a full refractive error correction, and a willingness to wear glasses for reading or night driving.

Intense individuals, patients with a grim outlook, highly emotional or vitriolic patients, or highly critical patients may not be well suited to LASIK surgery.

The patient's psychosocial candidacy for the procedure should be assessed while the history is taken as well as during the examination. Input from a well-trained technician or office personnel is valuable information that should not be dismissed. However, it should not be considered a substitute for the surgeon's personal evaluation.

Anatomical Factors

In general, the most reproducible results are obtained when LASIK is performed on a healthy patient with healthy eyes. There is less risk when the orbital and lid anatomy allow adequate exposure for the microkeratome. The refractive error should preferably be well within the approved limits for the specific excimer laser being used. Patients with severe dry eye or absent corneal sensation are poor candidates for surgery. If a mechanical microkeratome is to be used and the corneal contour is abnormally steep or flat, the surgeon and the patient should be aware of the increased respective risk of buttonhole and free cap. The risk of buttonhole or free cap related to abnormal contour is of less concern when the flap is created with a femtosecond laser. The corneal thickness is a major factor in determining the amount of refractive error that can safely be treated.

Evaluation

A standardized laser refractive surgery form, designed for recording the history and examination, can assist the surgeon in documenting pertinent information in an orderly manner. The chance of inadvertent oversight in the evaluation can be reduced by using such a form. A sample preoperative form is shown in Figure 1.1. Postoperative forms are also helpful (Fig. 1.2). There is an advantage to using a form in which the results of multiple postoperative visits can be recorded on a single page. This format facilitates the ability to track postoperative findings. The sample forms shown in Figures 1.1 and 1.2 can be modified to suit the particular needs of a surgeon or practice.

History

The history should begin with a question about the patient's goals for surgery. While LASIK surgery is approved for patients at least 18 to 21 years of age, many patients will not have attained refractive stability by this age. The refractive history should contain questions about refractive stability. Ideally the refraction should be stable for at least 1 year before LASIK surgery is considered. If a glasses change of greater than 0.50 D has occurred within 1 year, the patient should be reevaluated at 6-month intervals until the measurement is stable. Patients approaching age 40 years should be questioned about their willingness to wear reading glasses. Contact lens history should be obtained. This should include

the type of lens (e.g., hard, rigid gas permeable, or soft), the duration of lens wear in years, and the typical duration of daily lens wear or use of extended wear. The use of contact lenses to obtain monovision should be noted. The contact lens prescription should be obtained. This will help the surgeon plan the proper amount of undercorrection in the nondominant eye. If the presbyopic patient has not previously used a monovision correction and is interested, a contact lens trial, undercorrecting the nondominant eye, will need to be tried at home, at work, and during leisure activities. If successful, surgical monovision may be an option.

The past ocular history should be obtained. A history of recurrent corneal erosion, corneal ulceration or other ocular infection, glaucoma or glaucoma surgery, or cataract may all have an impact on the patient's candidacy for LASIK surgery. Past medical history including diabetes, rheumatoid arthritis, pregnancy, or nursing is important. Diabetics, in addition to retinal ischemia and edema, may have poor epithelial adhesion, increasing the risk of erosion. They may also be more likely to have cataract. FDA approval has not been obtained for laser refractive surgery in patients with certain systemic diseases such as rheumatoid arthritis. If off-label use of the laser is entertained, the patient should be made aware that this is the case. Pregnant or nursing patients may have unstable refractions and it is best to delay surgery until 6 to 12 weeks after nursing has ended. Patients who become pregnant after LASIK should understand that a refractive error change may result from the pregnancy and may not be regression of the effect of refractive surgery. This should be discussed preoperatively. The change may resolve after delivery without retreatment. Patients who are immunocompromised may be at greater risk of infection.

Examination

Visual acuity at distance and near should be measured with and without correction. The best corrected visual acuity should be at least 20/20 preoperatively. If the acuity is less than 20/20, the surgeon must seek an explanation. If the acuity is reduced because of refractive amblyopia the patient may still be a candidate for surgery, provided the patient has realistic

NORTHWESTERN VISION CORRECTION ASSOCIATES
REFRACTIVE SURGERY
CONSULTATION

Name: _____   NMFF#: _____

Age: _____   Date: _____

Motivation: _____   Medications: _____

POHx: _____   Allergies: _____

PMHx: _____   Soc Hx: _____

FamHx: _____   ROS: _____

V_{SC}: V_{CC}: _____   OD: OS:

                                                     Pachymetry:

W: K: Pupil Size:

                                                     Diameter:

M: Dominance: Tension:

I have discussed the LASIK procedure with_____.

This discussion has included the visual prognosis (approximate 98% 20/40 or better, approximately_____%
20/20-20/25. We have discussed the possible need for glasses for reading and under other special conditions.
I have discussed the probability of retreatment (____). We have discussed the possible night vision problems
of glare and haloes. We have discussed complications including infection and inflammation leading to corneal
transplant, retinal detachment, flap complications of displacement, wrinkles, debris under the flap, and poor flap
construction. We have discussed temporary dry eye syndrome and the need for teardrops, medication, and/or
plugs. We have discussed CustomVue™ LASIK and I have elected to (have / not have) CustomVue™ LASIK.
We have discussed IntraLase® and I have elected to (have / not have) IntraLase® to create the flap. We have
discussed Photorefractive Keratectomy (PRK) including the issues of postoperative discomfort, potential haze,
and extended use of cortisone eye drops. The doctor has explained the risk of surgery to me and I understand it.
All my questions have been answered to my satisfaction.

Patient Signature:_____   Date:_____   Physician Signature: _____

MEASUREMENTS

Date: _____   WaveScan Done _____   Custom: _____

M: Topography Done _____   Plate: _____

C: Dilated with 1% Myd. _____   Ring: _____

K: Motility: _____   Zone: _____

SLE: Lids & Lashes: _____   Fundus   IntraLase
         Conj: _____   Disc: _____   Diameter: _____
         Cornea: _____   Vessels: _____   Thickness: _____
         AC: _____   Macula: _____
         Iris: _____   Periphery: _____   Special Instructions:
         Lens: _____

Figure 1.1

Refractive surgery preoperative consultation form.

POSTOPERATIVE REFRACTIVE SURGERY FORM

Name: _____ Age: _____ Occupation: _____

Original Procedure:	OD:_____		OS:_____		
Original Procedure	OD _____ Cyc Ref: _____		BCV: _____ K: _____		P: _____
Date:	OS _____ Cyc Ref: _____		BCV:_____ K: _____		P: _____

1st Retreat Procedure: OD: _____ OS:_____

Date of 1st Retreat:	OD _____ Cyc Ref: _____ BCV:_____ K: _____	P: _____
	OS _____ Cyc Ref: _____ BCV:_____ K: _____	P: _____

2nd Retreat Procedure:OD:_____ OS:_____

Date of 2nd Retreat:	OD _____ Cyc Ref: _____ BCV:_____ K: _____	P: _____
	OS _____ Cyc Ref: _____ BCV:_____ K: _____	P: _____

Date: _____ C/O: _____ Meds: _____

Date: _____ C/O: _____ Meds: _____

Date: _____ C/O: _____ Meds: _____

Date: _____ C/O: _____ Meds: _____

Date: _____ C/O: _____ Meds: _____

Figure 1.2

Postoperative form.

expectations for postoperative vision. Reduced preoperative visual acuity related to irregular corneal astigmatism is a contraindication to LASIK surgery.

If the patient uses contact lenses, lens wear will need to be discontinued. The surgery cannot safely be done until the refraction becomes stable. In general, refractive stability will take longer for rigid gas permeable lens users than for soft lens users. The duration of lens wear and the intensity of lens wear are also important factors affecting the time to achieve refractive stability. A rule of thumb for patients wearing soft lenses or hard lenses for 10 years would be to discontinue lens wear for 2 and 4 weeks, respectively. Longer duration of lens wear will likely require longer periods of abstinence.

For myopia the manifest refraction should not differ from the cycloplegic refraction by more than 0.50 diopter, and the axis of cylinder should not differ by more that 15 degrees. For hyperopia, the manifest and cycloplegic refractions should not differ by more than 0.75 diopter.

Keratometry values should be used to calculate the postsurgical corneal contour. If the estimate of the postsurgical corneal contour is <35.00 D, keratorefractive surgery outcome may not be ideal because the cornea may be too flat to support good visual function. To estimate the postsurgical corneal contour, the spherical equivalent of the refraction is multiplied by a conversion factor of 0.7 or 0.8. More conservative surgeons use 0.8 as the conversion factor. The product is subtracted from the average of the keratometric values. If the result is only slightly greater than 35.00 D, retreatment may leave the cornea too flat to support good visual function. This possibility would be important to discuss with a patient who has such a preoperative estimate.

Ocular dominance should be recorded. It can be determined by asking the patient to wink. Generally, patients have difficulty winking the dominant eye. Hand the patient a disposable camera and ask the patient to pretend to take a picture. The camera will be held in front of the dominant eye. Finally the patient can be asked to make the okay sign with the fingers of either hand. He or she is then asked to sight on a distant object through the circle formed with the thumb and forefinger. The hand is then brought toward the eyes and usually the hand will move toward the dominant eye. Ocular dominance is important for surgeons who like to begin a bilateral simultaneous treatment with the nondominant eye. It is also important in performing a monovision treatment. The near eye is typically the nondominant eye.

A careful external examination is required to rule out external eye disease such as acne rosacea, which can be associated with inflammatory eye disease and may require treatment before surgery. In addition, an assessment of the degree of ocular exposure is essential. The surgeon should determine if the degree of lid laxity, the orbital aperture, the prominence of the brow, the position of the globe, and palpebral fissure height are adequate to accommodate the microkeratome. As the lids are being spread apart, it is helpful to tell the patient that the sensation simulates the feeling of stretch from the lid speculum.

Significant lagophthalmos and associated exposure may be problematic postoperatively given the temporary neurotrophic status of the flap. If the eyes are dry, the patient can be reassessed 1 month after initiating treatment with tear supplements, topical cyclosporine, and/or punctal plugs. Encouraging good oral hydration is also important in patients who exercise heavily. If significant tear deficiency remains despite these measures, LASIK should be avoided. Low ambient humidity in the patient's work or home environment will be unfavorable for the borderline dry eye patient.

The pupil diameter should be measured in the dark preferably using one of the commercially available devices designed for this purpose, for example, a Colvard pupillometer (OASIS Medical, Inc., Glendora, CA). Ideally the planned treatment zone should extend beyond the edge of the dark-adapted pupil to minimize night vision symptoms. The significance of pupil size and its relationship to night vision is currently debated. The patient should also be examined for a relative afferent pupillary defect.

Motility function should be assessed to rule out a latent condition that might become symptomatic in the event of significant anisometropia postoperatively. This is especially true in the patient considering monovision treatment or a patient with a past history of strabismus surgery. A patient able to control a significant phoria may develop diplopia, if fusion is disrupted. A patient with a moderate to large-angle alternating tropia may tolerate monovision, because this individual currently fails to use the eyes together and is capable of using either eye independently. Monovision may not be suitable for a patient with a constant tropia and a strong fixation preference for one eye. Monovision would force this patient to use the deviated, nondominant eye for near vision, which might seem unnatural.

The slit-lamp examination should begin with an assessment of the lids and lashes. Inflammation in this area should be controlled prior to surgery. It is critically important to rule out the presence of corneal pathology. Contact lens–wearing patients may have peripheral corneal neovascularization, punctate keratopathy, sterile keratitis, or peripheral subepithelial fibrosis. Keratitis and punctate keratopathy may be reversible and clear after a period of time with no lens wear. Active keratitis is a contraindication to LASIK surgery. If it does not clear spontaneously, a treatment regimen should be initiated and the patient reevaluated. Subepithelial fibrosis and neovascularization are permanent changes that may impact the decision to do surgery or the planning related to proposed surgery.

Corneal diameter should be noted. Special attention to the corneal thickness is important. If the cornea is too thin for the intended treatment, LASIK surgery is contraindicated. The corneal contour should be regular. If an irregular contour is suspected on slit-limp examination, this should be confirmed using keratometry and corneal topography. LASIK surgery is most reliable when the contour is regular.

Corneal scarring within the treatment zone is a contraindication to the surgery. Scarring in the periphery with minimal thinning may be acceptable, provided the cause is not prior herpes simplex keratitis. Herpes viral infections can be reactivated by the ultraviolet radiation of the excimer laser. The presence of epithelial basement membrane dystrophy may indicate a possible defect in epithelial adhesion. Patients with this dystrophy are more likely to experience epithelial sloughing, possibly with diffuse lamellar keratitis or epithelial ingrowth. Patients with confluent guttatae may be at risk for poor flap adhesion postoperatively, if the endothelial pump functions poorly. An abnormally thick cornea, especially in the early morning, may be a sign of abnormal endothelial pump function.

All abnormalities of the anterior segment should be noted. The presence of cataract may be a contraindication to LASIK surgery. It is best to avoid LASIK surgery on the patient with a visually significant or progressive cataract. Lens-induced myopia from a nuclear cataract can be misinterpreted as LASIK regression. A patient could mistakenly believe that progressive vision loss due to cataract was due to LASIK failure. Glare from a posterior subcapsular cataract might be thought to be due to the refractive surgery.

If a small peripheral cataract is found on the presurgical examination, it is wise to follow the patient until it can be determined whether or not the cataract is progressive. The patient who decides to proceed with refractive surgery should be informed that, although the cataract may appear to be stable and not visually significant, it could unexpectedly progress and undermine the LASIK result. If cataract surgery is needed, determination of the lens implant power will be more challenging than it otherwise would be. If standard keratometry is used in biometry for a cataract patient after LASIK surgery has been done, the selected lens implant may be underpowered. The options for predicting implant power are found in the discussion of Case 58.

Intraocular pressure (IOP) should be measured preoperatively. If the cycloplegic refraction is to be done on the same day, the pressure should be measured after the refraction in order to avoid disturbing the corneal surface. If IOP is elevated, the significance should be interpreted. The pressure would, for example, be less significant if the cornea is thicker than normal and the optic nerve is normal. Significant optic nerve cupping should be evaluated with visual field evaluation. In the presence of glaucomatous field changes, the potential for nerve damage when the suction ring increases the eye pressure should be considered. In this situation alternative refractive surgery options such as a surface ablation procedure can be discussed with the patient.

The dilated fundus examination is an essential part of the preoperative evaluation. While it need not be done during an initial screening examination, it must be done prior to surgery. If significant abnormalities are found, the patient should be informed. The cycloplegic refraction on which the LASIK treatment is based should be performed before the retina is exposed to intense illumination.

The fundus examination is particularly important for the myopic patient who is at greater risk for retinal detachment. In the presence of peripheral retinal pathology, a consultation from a retinal specialist is advisable. The result of this consultation should be included in the record. Preoperative prophylactic treatment can be delivered if required. The retina surgeon should determine the timing of LASIK surgery, following any treatment. If a retinal problem were to develop postoperatively, the patient will already have a relationship with a specialist.

Diabetic retinopathy if present may impact the decision to do LASIK. Patients with evidence of significant retinal ischemia may be at risk for an ischemic event related to extreme IOP elevation. Macular edema, epiretinal membranes, and degenerative changes in the macula may all limit the postsurgical visual outcome. These issues should be discussed with the patient. It is not uncommon for previously undiagnosed retinal disease to be uncovered during the LASIK evaluation.

If the optic nerve does not appear normal, an evaluation of optic nerve function should be conducted. This evaluation would include measurement of central acuity, pupil reactivity, color vision, brightness comparison, and visual field. Obviously, some of this evaluation will already have been done before the retinal examination. Highly myopic patients often have tilted discs with peripapillary atrophy. The surgeon should rely on his or her own experience to determine if the appearance of the disc is inconsistent with the patient's refractive error.

Corneal pachymetry should be measured after the refraction has taken place to prevent surface disruption. This is a critical measurement and should be performed with an ultrasonic device. The surgeon is cautioned against relying on slit-beam–generated pachymetric maps; for example, Orbscan (Bausch & Lomb, Rochester, NY), to determine whether the cornea is thick enough for LASIK surgery. These maps provide a relative comparison of thickness at different points on the cornea but may not accurately measure the corneal thickness at any one point. Because contact lens wear can increase corneal thickness, it is more accurate to measure the thickness after the patient has been out of lenses. However, if the patient is measured just after contact lenses have been removed and the cornea is too thin for LASIK surgery, a second measurement following a period without contact lens wear will usually not improve the patient's candidacy for surgery. If the cornea is significantly thicker than 620 μm it is important to determine if abnormal endothelial function is the explanation. A correlation with the slit-lamp evaluation and possibly specular microscopy is indicated in this situation. Poor endothelial function as previously stated may lead to postoperative flap adhesion problems.

Some surgeons will measure pachymetry at different places on the cornea to be certain that the cornea is not abnormally thin inferiorly. This might occur in keratoconus or pellucid marginal degeneration.

Corneal topography must be done on every patient prior to LASIK surgery in order to avoid operating on a patient with an abnormal corneal contour. (Refer to the topography section in Chapter 2.) When the contour is abnormal preoperatively, the postoperative outcome is unpredictable.

No one index is foolproof in reducing postoperative ectasia risk. It is recommended that several indices and analyses be used to determine whether a particular patient is suitable for keratorefractive surgery.

The topographical analysis may also indicate significant irregularity, which could be contact lens induced. Serial topography performed during a period of contact lens abstinence can be used to track the corneal contour during the resolution of the irregularity and ultimately confirm that the corneal surface has become regular and stable.

Pellucid marginal degeneration (PMD) is a noninflammatory thinning disorder in which there is typically a band of inferior thinning with protrusion of the cornea superior to the thin area. Laser refractive surgery should be avoided in patients with PMD. This condition has a characteristic power map sometimes described as a "crab claw" appearance. (See the topography section in Chapter 2.)

WaveScan can be done at the same time as the topography if custom LASIK is being considered. The WaveScan is not a substitute for topography. The WaveScan will determine the degree and type of higher order aberrations. It also determines the refractive error in an objective way that can aid the surgeon when performing manifest or cycloplegic refraction. WaveScan technology can also be used postoperatively to assess the degree of higher order aberrations that may be induced after refractive surgery. The nuances of WaveScan interpretation and custom LASIK as performed with several commonly used systems will be discussed later in the text.

Discussing the Risks of Surgery

Presentation Overview

One of the greatest challenges for the beginning LASIK surgeon is to explain the actual operation and the risks of the procedure with confidence and in a manner that informs without terrifying the patient. The choice of words will make a significant difference in the patient's perception of the procedure and the surgeon. Speaking in lay language, easily understood by the patient, is key to communicating the information needed to make an informed decision. A discussion presented with enthusiasm will help as well.

The explanation of the procedure and the risks should follow the examination. If the surgeon uncovers a contraindication to LASIK surgery, this can be explained and the consultation concluded without having gone through a detailed discussion.

Explain to the patient that the discussion will cover most of the commonly asked questions. Encourage the patient to interrupt if a particular point is not clear or if there is a question, and inform the patient that there will be time at the end to ask any additional questions. Remember the goals of the dialogue are both to inform completely and to reduce anxiety. Anticipate your patient's questions and answer them before the patient has a chance to ask them. For example, if you wear glasses, anticipate that your patient will want to know why you haven't had the procedure. Have an answer prepared so you can present this information without being asked. This helps to instill confidence in the surgeon. Withholding information is improper and may increase anxiety and contribute to dissatisfaction with the surgery. Proper preoperative preparation will make the entire surgical process easier for the patient, surgeon, and staff. While many surgeons have others in the office explain the procedure and risks, there is an advantage for the surgeon to have the discussion personally. There is an opportunity to get to know this patient and determine his or her candidacy for the procedure from a psychosocial perspective. If the patient is unusually nervous, acts in an inappropriate way, seems inattentive or suspicious, or appears to have unreasonable expectations, he or she may be a poor candidate.

It is helpful to listen to one or more experienced surgeons present this material. A recording of the presentation or a typewritten script can help the beginning surgeon to prepare the first few discussions with prospective patients. Over time the surgeon will develop a talk that incorporates both the answers to questions that arise during discussion as well as portions of other doctors' presentations that seem to fit appropriately. When the presentation feels natural, the physician will appear self-assured and the patient will sense this.

Because one of the goals of the initial encounter is to instill the patient with feelings of confidence and comfort with the surgeon and staff, try to minimize the wait time in the office prior to the consultation and at every postoperative visit. During introductions ask the patient how he or she prefers to be called and ask permission to address the patient in that manner.

Sample Preoperative LASIK Patient Discussion

Here is a sample LASIK presentation with dialogue directed to the patient in italic type: "*What are you hoping LASIK surgery will do* for you?" The most common response is "to get rid of my glasses and contact lenses." The ideal response is "to become less dependent on glasses and contact lenses." Responses such as "I want to be more attractive," "I want to improve my vision beyond what I see in glasses or contact lenses," or "I don't know, I just want the surgery" are not particularly appropriate and should raise a red flag about the candidacy of the particular patient. At this point it is helpful to remind the patient that LASIK reduces the dependence on glasses and contact lenses, but that glasses may be needed for reading when you reach the middle 40s. *"Techniques such as LASIK to achieve monovision, that is, the dominant eye corrected for distance and the nondominant eye for near, can reduce the need for reading glasses."* This discussion is appropriate for patients of presbyopic age. *"Glasses may also be needed for some distance activities, such as driving at night or in the rain, but it is rare for patients to request distance glasses."*

Vision Expectations

The first question every patient wants an answer to is "How well will I see after surgery?" If the patient is a myope with ≤ −10.00 diopters of spherical error and ≤ +3.00 diopters of cylindrical, it is reasonable to expect an uncorrected visual acuity of 20/25 or better. *"Retreatment may be required to achieve this level of visual acuity. A typical retreatment rate is approximately 10%, meaning 90% of patients achieve their vision goals with one laser surgery. Retreatment rates will be higher for patients with more extreme refractive errors."* It is important to explain to the hyperopic patient that in order to successfully correct distance vision in the long run, an initial overcorrection is necessary. This will result in good near vision, but blurred distance, which may require the need for distance glasses. Over a 3- to 6-month period the distance vision will improve and the near vision may weaken.

Night Vision

"Nearsighted patients often feel they don't see as well at night. They may be aware of glare from car headlights or haloes around streetlights." If the patient does not appear to understand what glare is, dim the overhead lights and shine a light toward the patient from 2 to 3 feet away. Ask the patient if he or she sees rays of light coming from the light source. *"It is important for patients to become familiar with their night vision preoperatively so they have a basis for comparison postoperatively. Following LASIK surgery some patients will be aware of increased glare or haloes at night. This tends to occur in patients with night vision problems before surgery, in patients with large corrections (> −7.00 diopters), and/or large pupils (>7.0 mm). It is rare for a patient to feel completely disabled at night. Night vision problems can be related to blurred vision caused by residual nearsightedness or astigmatism. In this case glasses used for night driving may help. Retreatment may be a consideration. Drops used in the evening to slightly constrict the pupil (e.g., brimonidine HCl 0.15%) may also help."*

"Some patients will achieve significant improvement in night vision particularly if they are currently undercorrected." A discussion of custom LASIK as a means to reduce the risk of night vision symptoms should be included here if this is an available option. *"If you are concerned about night vision following surgery, there is a new technology that may be of interest. It is called wavefront technology and it allows us to perform custom LASIK. Light is shined into the eye and a computer analyzes the light that comes out of the eye. The computer determines your need for glasses and your higher order aberrations. These are imperfections in the visual system, which are unique to each of us and contribute to night vision problems. Custom LASIK will correct both the need for glasses and the higher order aberrations. A study reviewed by the FDA (for CustomVue LASIK with the VISX laser) showed less problem with night vision for the majority of patients treated. Not every patient is a candidate for custom LASIK and it costs more than conventional LASIK (some surgeons charge the same for custom and conventional LASIK), but if you are concerned about night vision or want the latest technology, this is it."*

Dry Eye

"Dryness affects most LASIK patients in the first 3 months following surgery. Women and patients older than 50 years are the most likely

to have these problems. Certain medications or medical conditions can contribute to this problem. Artificial teardrops help. If tear supplements are not enough, plugs can be placed in the tear drainage ducts of the lower lids to increase the amount of tear fluid on the eyes." If the patient is borderline tear deficient, the following can be added: "Sometimes these plugs are inserted prior to the surgery in order to enhance the tear fluid on the eye prior to the surgery. There is also an eyedrop that has recently become available (topical cyclosporine) that can improve a tear deficiency."

Infection

"Infection is a complication that we take very seriously. The risk around the country is approximately 1 in 2,000." If there have been no infections in your center or if your infection rate is less than 1 per 2,000, it may be helpful to tell the patient that. "We have potent antibiotics that are effective against the kind of bacteria that cause infection after LASIK. We take steps to reduce the risk of infection prior to surgery and use antibiotic drops after surgery. However, if an infection occurs and it involves the line of sight, it could have a profound impact on the visual function. Because the surgery is only done on the cornea, a scarred cornea could be replaced with clear corneal tissue. This is called a cornea transplant and is exceedingly rare following LASIK surgery."

Retinal Detachment

"Nearsighted people are at risk for a retinal detachment whether they have LASIK surgery or not. The chance increases with the degree of nearsightedness. A retinal detachment means the "movie screen" in the back of the eye becomes loose. Surgery is needed to reattach the retina. LASIK surgery may increase the chance of retinal detachment, but the overall risk is small at about 1 in 1,500. A careful examination of the retina is done prior to the surgery to be certain there is no preexisting pathology that might predispose a patient to a retinal problem."

At this point it is appropriate to summarize what has been said. "So far we have reviewed five important topics: vision expectations, night vision, dry eye, infection, and retinal detachment. Do you have any questions about this information?" If there are no questions, it is appropriate

to move on to the next part of the discussion. Additional risks of the procedure can be explained in the context of a step-by-step explanation of the procedure.

Setup for the Procedure

"Many patients take a sedative pill prior to the surgery to control anxiety. Some feel it is unnecessary. Usually both eyes are operated on at the same time, but if you prefer, it can be done one eye at a time." If the patient is of presbyopic age and the refractive error of the nondominant eye is appropriate for near vision, sequential surgery can be planned to give the patient an attempt at monovision. If unsuccessful, the second eye can be treated in a subsequent surgery. "Anesthetic drops are placed in each eye. This will keep the eyes comfortable and reduce the urge to blink. A special solution is used to clean around the eyes. One of the eyes is covered to reduce distraction. The chair is rotated to position you under the microscope. This is not a claustrophobic experience. There is nothing covering your nose or mouth, you are not restrained in any way and are given a stuffed animal to hold. Your head is supported by a form-fit cushion, which allows you to feel secure and comfortable. You look straight ahead at a series of lights, one of which is a blinking red-orange light. This is the fixation light and it is important to look at the light at all times. There may be times when it is difficult to see the light (such as when the suction ring is applied), but this will be pointed out just before it occurs. Small sticky drapes are placed on the eyelids to cover the eyelashes, additional anesthetic is applied, and an eyelid holder is inserted. It feels similar to the sensation you felt when I separated your eyelids." It is important to assess exposure and the degree of eyelid laxity during the preoperative examination by spreading the lids apart. This test serves the dual purpose of also simulating the sensation of the speculum. "The eyelid holder will prevent blinking. So there is no need to worry about an inadvertent blink."

Creation of the Flap

"At this point a ring-shaped device is placed on the surface of the eye overlying that portion where the color part of the eye meets the white part. This device will be used to raise the pressure of the eye. Have you ever had your blood pressure tested?" (Virtually every candidate for LASIK surgery will at some point have had blood pressure measured and this experience is a useful analogy for the suction ring.) *"Then you are familiar with the pressure sensation on your arm. The suction ring is similar in that it will raise the pressure in the eye. The pressure will get high enough to cause the lights to dim and go out. This is normal and necessary in order to make a perfect flap. Once the eye has reached a sufficiently high pressure the flap can be made. The flap-making device is placed on the ring. It will cause a vibration and a buzzing noise."* This describes the Hansatome (Bausch & Lomb, Rochester, NY) and other two-piece microkeratomes. *"The entire flap-making process takes approximately 30 seconds, so you will not feel the pressure sensation for very long. After the flap has been made, the pressure is released, the lights come back, and the entire apparatus is removed. The flap can then be inspected to be certain it is perfect. Rarely, 1 out of a 1,000 times, the flap is too small, too thin, off center, or incomplete, meaning it cannot be adequately lifted to expose an appropriate area for the laser treatment. In this case the flap is replaced and the vision generally returns to the preoperative level. We will then wait 6 months and try again to make a flap. The flap-making equipment is highly reliable and generally makes great flaps. I will tell you about the quality of your flap, so you don't have to wonder or worry about it."*

"An alternative way to make a flap is to use a laser. This is a newer technology that has several potential advantages over the mechanical microkeratome. The laser more precisely creates a flap of the desired thickness preserving as much cornea as possible. The potential for an abnormally thin or free flap to result is reduced quite a bit. The squared edge of the flap lays back on the cornea like a manhole cover, possibly making the flap more resistant to slipping. Finally, in the event of a loss of suction, an incomplete flap can be corrected at the time of surgery. The disadvantages are an increased cost, a 10-minute increase in surgical time, and pressure sensation for about 30 seconds longer than with the mechanical microkeratome. Finally, if it were to become necessary, the laser-created flap may be more difficult to relift a year after surgery. However, this also means that the flap is more resistant to movement in the event of an injury."*

The Laser Procedure

"At this point we are ready to do the laser portion of the procedure. The laser is not a gun as depicted in science fiction movies. It is simply ultraviolet light. It is cool and painless. Every patient worries that they will look in the wrong place and the wrong time. Our laser has a tracking device that will find the center of your pupil, and if your eye moves, the laser will follow and stay with the center target. This is similar to Air Force videos you may have seen. As long as your eye is in the tracking range, the laser will follow. If your eye moves outside the tracking zone, which occurs only rarely, the laser will not fire. The reaction time is extremely short, 30 milliseconds." (True for the VISX S3 and S4 lasers.) *"Therefore, either the laser is treating in exactly the correct place or not at all. This is a wonderful safety feature and should help to reduce fears about the laser."* Not every laser has a tracking device. It is important to be familiar with the features of the laser you will use.

The fear of a laser treatment in the wrong place is very common and needs to be addressed whether you have a tracking laser or not. If your laser does not have a tracking device, you might stress how you will monitor the patient's fixation on the target light and make certain it is in the correct location. It is helpful to provide the patient with an estimate of how long the laser portion of the procedure will take. *"When the flap is lifted, there is no sensation, but the vision may become blurred temporarily. The laser locks on the pupil center and the treatment begins. The laser makes a clicking sound. Each click is a pulse of laser energy acting to reshape the cornea. The treatment lasts less than a minute."*

After the Laser

"After the laser treatment, the flap is replaced. Fluid is used to irrigate beneath the flap to remove debris; and the alignment is checked. If all is well, the process is repeated on the fellow eye."

"Patients often ask what holds this flap in place because no stitches, glue, or staples are used in the procedure. There is a natural force that holds the flap in position, in a manner similar to the force that holds a thin slice of apple in

place on the apple. If you rub or bump the eye, the flap may become dislodged, requiring repositioning. Over 2 to 3 days surface cells will cover the edge of the flap, but it takes a year or longer for a strong bond to form between the underside of the flap and the remaining cornea. This weak bond is used to our advantage after LASIK. If, for example, there are microscopic wrinkles in the flap, similar to wrinkles in a bed sheet, this can cause ghosting or a reduction in the best possible vision. These wrinkles are called microstriae. The flap can be lifted and the wrinkles smoothed out. If there is inflammation that does not respond to drops or pills, the flap can be lifted and inflammatory material removed. If cells from the surface are caught beneath the flap they can grow into a little bump. This material can be removed after the flap is lifted."

"Most eyes respond to the laser in a predictable manner. However, if your eye responded more than expected, farsightedness might result." This is true for a myopic treatment. "Too little response and the result would be residual nearsightedness. Once the correction stabilizes at 2 to 3 months the flap could be lifted and additional laser treatment performed. Occasionally, between months 1 and 3, the result drifts back toward nearsightedness. When this regression occurs, it is usually on the order of 10% of your original correction. Retreatment for regression is also possible."

"Postoperatively the patient is examined with the slit-lamp microscope. Any abnormalities in or under the flap can be adjusted at that time. It is important not to rub the eyes after surgery and to wear eye protection that is provided. It should be used for several days both day and night. Eyedrops will be provided and should be administered four times daily. The vision will be hazy for a day or two and will gradually clear. It is normal for the eyes to feel scratchy or irritated for a couple of days. Over-the-counter pain relievers may be helpful. Patients are examined the next day, the next week, at 1 month, 3 months, 6 months, and at 1 year. The LASIK fee is all-inclusive and will cover the cost of postoperative visits, retreatment or revision, and eyedrops. If would not cover the cost of cornea transplant or retina surgery in the unlikely event that either was needed." For many surgeons a global fee covers one year of service.

Finally, it is important to discuss the surgeon's background and experience. Patients will wonder how many procedures the surgeon has performed and performs routinely. It is worth preparing a statement that is added at the end of the discussion, so that the patient will not be required to question the surgeon's qualifications to perform the surgery.

Acknowledge that this was a lot of material and express willingness to answer any questions. Tables 1.1, 1.2, and 1.3 summarize the key points of the discussion.

Table 1.1	Discussion of LASIK risks

Vision expectations 　Postoperative uncorrected vision expected 　　given patient's refraction 　Need for reading glasses 　Possible need for retreatment to achieve 　　visual goals **Night vision** 　Glare and haloes 　Custom LASIK **Dry eye** 　Possible need for tears or plugs **Retinal detachment** **Infection** **Inappropriate flap** 　Too small or thin 　Incomplete or off center	**Flap striae** 　Ghosting 　Possible need to lift flap to remove striae **Flap adherence** **Flap displacement** 　Need for eye protection **Inflammation** 　Need for drops or pills to control inflammation 　Possible need to lift flap to remove inflammatory 　　material **Ingrowth** 　Possible need to lift flap for removal **Postoperative ametropia** 　Over/undercorrection 　Regression 　Need and timing for retreatment

Table 1.2	Discussion of the LASIK procedure

Optional need for sedation
Topical anesthetic reduces the urge to blink
Simultaneous vs. sequential surgery
Prep and drape
Lid speculum prevents blinking
Fixation light
Creation of flap
  Pressure sensation
  Lights become dim and go out
  Vibration and buzzing noise

Mechanical vs. laser flap creation
Flap assessment
Lifting the flap
Laser
  Describe the type of laser
  Tracker
  Sound
Reposition the flap
Remove drape
Switch to fellow eye

Table 1.3	Postoperative information

Postoperative sensations
  Vision hazy, but improved; nap speeds vision improvement
Scratchy irritation; acetaminophen or aspirin helps
Eye protection
  Do not rub or touch the eyes for at least 1 week after surgery

Use of protective eyewear
Avoid injury during eyedrop instillation
No swimming for at least 2 weeks after surgery
Eyedrop instructions
Follow-up appointment
Physician's emergency number

SURGICAL PLANNING

Once the evaluation has been completed, the risks have been explained, and the patient has decided to proceed with LASIK, the surgeon can begin the next step, which is to develop a surgical plan. This is a crucial step in obtaining safe and predictable results. It will require an intimate knowledge of the patient's needs and expectations as well as familiarity with the equipment that will be used to perform surgery. Here lies both the challenge and satisfaction for the LASIK surgeon. The goal of this manual is to give the LASIK surgeon insight into this most important step in the surgery. The factors presented herein should be used when working the cases later on in the handbook.

The surgical plan should be developed well in advance of the scheduled surgery. Decisions made just prior to surgery may not be adequately thought out, particularly if the surgeon is relatively new to LASIK surgery. Even when the plan is developed in advance of the surgery, the data entries and calculations should be rechecked just prior to the actual surgery. Developing this habit will help avoid costly errors.

A basic set of principles will be presented here. These principles are applicable across the landscape of equipment options available. Because the planning will vary depending on the various microkeratomes and lasers used, the reader should refer to the sections that discuss the specific equipment available. As an example, Table 1.4 illustrates factors important in developing a treatment plan using the Hansatome and the VISX laser. Many of the concepts apply to other microkeratomes and lasers.

In general, the goal of the plan is to determine how best to address the following questions: What correction should be entered into the laser's computer? What is the appropriate treatment zone? What will be the maximum ablation depth? What is the appropriate flap diameter? What is the

Table 1.4	Decision making for treatment plan*
Degree of correction	FDA-approved indications for the VISX laser: Myopia: ≤ −12.00 D sphere or +5.00 D of cylinder Hyperopia: ≤ +5.00 sphere and/or +4.00 D of cylinder (≤6.00 sphere equivalent) Mixed astigmatism: astigmatism > myopic sphere with ≤6.00 D cylinder Custom myopia: ≤ −6.00 D sphere/≤3.00 D cylinder Custom hyperopia: ≤ +3.00 D sphere/≤ +2.00 D cylinder Custom mixed astigmatism: ≤5.00 D cylinder

Steep cornea
   Average K >48.50 D
   Higher risk of buttonhole
	If average keratometry reading >45.00, use 8.5-mm ring
	 Caution: Flaps cut on steep corneas tend to be large.
	 If buttonhole: replace flap, no laser, return in 6 months to
	 cut new flap; consider PTK-PRK with or without mitomycin-C

Flat cornea
   Average K <40.00 D
   Higher risk of free cap
	If K <45.00, use 9.5-mm ring
	 Caution: Flaps cut on flat corneas tend to be small. If free
	 flap or small flap: replace flap, no laser, BCL, return
	 in 6 months to cut new flap using thicker plate

Small corneal diameter	Select smaller ring diameter to avoid bleeding unless flat or large flap needed *Caution:* risk of bleeding, conjunctival or scleral extension
Large corneal diameter	Use larger 9.5-mm ring to create larger flap unless steep
Corneal vascularization	Use smaller ring to avoid bleeding
Corneal thickness	Leave >250 μm of corneal bed untouched Hansatome plates (130, 160, 180, 200 μm): flap thickness usually less than expected and even thinner on 2nd eye. If initial flap very thin, increase plate thickness on 2nd eye. *Caution:* If cornea too thin, consider PRK, although >5.00 D or 75 μm risk of haze increases. Consider using mitomycin-C or phakic IOL. If preoperative pachymetry <520 recommend intraoperative pachymetry of stromal bed; 160- or 180-μm plates most commonly used.
Ablation depth	Ablation rule of thumb example VISX 6.0-mm zone: 12 μm/diopter and 6.5-mm VISX 6.5-mm zone: 15 μm/diopter Blend zone 8.0 mm: add 8 μm for <10.00 D treatment; 11 μm for ≥10 D
Humidity	Adequate humidity: 30% to 50% *Caution:* Low humidity: cornea dehydration, ↑ ablation/pulse may cause overcorrection High humidity: ↓ ablation/pulse may cause undercorrection
Pupil size	Determine pupil size in dark with pupillometer <6.0 mm: use 6.0-mm zone

continued

Decision making for treatment plan (continued)	
	6.0–6.5 mm: use 6.5-mm zone with blend if adequate cornea ≥6.5 mm: use blend zone *Caution:* >8 mm: custom zone required; risk of haloes and glare
Surgical exposure	*Caution:* Small fissure, tight lids, deep orbit → poor flap Consider one-piece microkeratome/nasal hinge Consider microring (outer diameter 1 mm smaller) Consider stronger speculum or no speculum Consider flap creation with femtosecond laser
Dry eyes	Consider pre- or postoperative punctal plug insertion, tear supplement, topical cyclosporine *Caution:* surface disease

* This decision-making algorithm is for the VISX laser and the Hansatome.

ideal hinge position or hinge width? Once the answers to these questions have been determined, the surgeon must put this into language that the scrub technician and laser engineer can use with the available equipment at hand.

With regard to hinge width, some surgeons prefer a nasal rather than a superior hinge in a patient with a history of tear deficiency. With some equipment, the hinge width can be adjusted. A narrower hinge allows greater flap retraction, making more of the stromal bed available for treatment of a large zone.

What Correction Should Be Entered into the Laser's Computer?

Excimer laser energy delivered within the stroma as occurs in LASIK will correct more myopia than when the same amount of energy is delivered during surface ablation. Because most lasers were designed and approved for photorefractive keratectomy (PRK), a reduction factor is often needed for LASIK surgery to achieve the desired effect. More reduction is also needed as either the correction or patient age increases. Overcorrection may result if an adjustment to the correction is not made. It is important to note that some surgeons using certain lasers routinely will perform conventional (not custom) treatment without using a correction factor. This methodology may be surgeon or laser specific.

Several nomograms have been developed to appropriately adjust the correction. One example is the Bansal-Kay nomogram, which is designed for use with the VISX Star laser and only in the patient with myopia or myopic astigmatism. The reader should refer to the appropriate laser type within this book for a recommended nomogram or reduction rule to follow. Nomograms are specific to the type of correction; that is, a nomogram for myopia correction should not be used for treatment of hyperopia.

For hyperopia a different nomogram is required. There is a tendency for regression of the laser effect with a hyperopic ablation; therefore, an overcorrection may need to be added to the intended treatment to compensate for this. It is important to be familiar with the laser system being used in order to properly develop a suitable treatment plan.

What Is the Appropriate Treatment Zone?

Multiple factors contribute to the planning of the treatment zone. Pupil size, refractive error, corneal thickness, corneal diameter, corneal contour, and peripheral pathology are all important. A rule of thumb is to use the smallest zone that will accomplish the refractive treatment as safely as possible, minimizing the ablation depth when possible.

In general, the treatment zone should be larger than the maximum pupil size in the dark. This will reduce nighttime aberrations related to the treatment zone edge. For example, in a patient with a pupil of 6.0 mm, a zone of 6.5 mm or larger is desirable. One could also combine a 6.0-mm zone with a blend zone. The surgeon must be mindful that the larger the treatment zone, the deeper the ablation will be.

The greater the degree of myopic correction, the deeper the laser ablation needed to correct it. As a rule, when possible use a smaller zone when corrections are large. For example, if a patient with a large myopic correction had a pupil diameter of less than 6.0 mm, a 6.0-mm zone with or without a blend would be most appropriate. This will preserve as much cornea as possible.

In a patient with a small or flat cornea, it may be challenging to make a flap large enough to add a blend zone. These might be important factors if the same patient also had a large pupil. Treatments of hyperopia and mixed astigmatism require large treatment zones and therefore require flaps large enough to accommodate the treatment.

If the cornea is somewhat thin, a large treatment zone or custom treatment may not be possible, unless of course the refractive error is small. Surface ablation (PRK) which preserves more corneal tissue may be more appropriate than LASIK, although stromal haze becomes an issue for deeper ablations. Some surgeons have moved from LASIK to laser-assisted subepithelial keratomileusis (LASEK) in which the epithelium is brushed aside prior to the laser treatment and replaced after surgery. Haze is still a concern after large ablations. Epi-LASIK is a procedure in which a special microkeratome with a blunted blade is used to create an epithelial flap, which can be replaced after laser surgery. While Epi-LASIK is perhaps better than PRK, visual rehabilitation is slower after these procedures and there is more postoperative discomfort compared to LASIK. A patient with a large myopic correction, large pupil, and thin cornea may present the surgeon with hurdles too great for keratorefractive surgery. The best advice in this setting may be to advise against laser surgery and perhaps suggest an alternative refractive procedure. Refer to Chapter 6 for a discussion on alternatives to excimer laser surgery.

In the presence of peripheral corneal neovascularization, or peripheral pterygium or non-herpetic scar, a smaller zone, if possible, may be advantageous. This is because a smaller flap would avoid the peripheral corneal pathology.

Once the appropriate zone has been determined, the maximum ablation depth can be determined. Compromise on the ablation zone or change to a form of surface ablation may be needed once the ablation depth is calculated. For example, for large corrections a 6.5-mm zone with a blend or custom treatment may not be possible. A 6.0-mm zone with a blend may be a safer alternative.

What Will Be the Maximum Ablation Depth?

The amount of cornea ablated for each diopter of treatment is specific to each laser system. To make proper calculations, surgeons must become familiar with the conversion factor (ablation depth per diopter) unique to the laser they will be using. The treatment zone as explained earlier also affects the amount of corneal ablation per diopter of treatment. The larger the treatment zone, the more corneal tissue will be ablated. Blend zones add additional depth of ablation to a treatment. Flying spot lasers remove more tissue than variable spot or broad-beam lasers. Custom LASIK also removes more corneal tissue than conventional LASIK. The surgeon must know the laser, the type of treatment, the proposed treatment zones, and the refractive correction before calculating ablation depth. While the laser computer will calculate the maximal ablation depth prior to the actual ablation, this may be based on a nomogram-adjusted refraction and, therefore, should not be used. To determine the ablation depth, the non–nomogram-adjusted refraction should always be used. This cannot be overemphasized. Surgeons who do not adjust the treatment would use the refraction to determine ablation depth.

It is helpful to have a rule of thumb to follow for converting the spherical equivalent of the cycloplegic refraction into a corresponding ablation depth. The training course for the laser being used will usually provide the appropriate conversion factor for various treatment zones.

A myopic monovision treatment can obviously reduce the ablation depth in the near eye, because less myopic correction is required. The near eye is typically the nondominant eye. If monovision is considered for a patient, the proposed treatment plan should be tried with contact lenses preoperatively at work, at home, and at play to be certain the arrangement is acceptable. If it is not tolerated in contact lenses, the treatment will not likely be tolerated when induced surgically. If the patient being considered for monovision has an astigmatic component in the refraction, a spherical contact lens correction may not adequately simulate a myopic astigmatic laser treatment.

The ablation depth is a crucial calculation, because if the ablation is too deep relative to the patient's corneal thickness, the result will be an unstable corneal contour or ectasia. Many refractive surgeons have used 250 μm as the minimum amount of cornea that should be left untouched after the ablation has been completed. There is no proof that corneal ectasia can be prevented if this 250-μm rule is obeyed. Surgeons have experienced patients with unstable refractions or even ectasia despite their efforts to obey this rule. It is possible that the flap was actually thicker than expected and the residual stromal thickness was less than 250 μm. The ablation may be deeper than expected if the ambient humidity in the laser suite is low or if the nomogram-adjusted refraction is used to calculate ablation depth. New technologies such as the femtosecond laser allow surgeons to create flaps that are closer to the intended thickness.

It is possible that for some corneas a residual stromal thickness of 250 μm is simply not enough to maintain a stable contour. Some surgeons have adopted a 275-μm rule or even 300 μm as the minimum residual stromal thickness. Some surgeons also believe that the residual corneal thickness should not be less than 50% of the original thickness. Each surgeon must develop his or her own safety limit, but this should not be less than 250 μm.

What Is the Appropriate Flap Thickness?

As a rule of thumb with mechanical microkeratomes, thin flaps occur in patients with thin corneas, defined as a central thickness of ≤520 μm. In normal or thicker than normal corneas, the actual flap will be closer to the plate thickness. When the same blade is used on the second eye, the flap will generally be thinner. Surgeons should measure flap thickness using the method that will be discussed in detail in the procedure section to become familiar with the variance associated with corneas of different thickness and different microkeratomes. Armed with this knowledge, the surgeon can incorporate a truer estimation of the expected thickness into the treatment planning. In addition, retreatment planning is considerably easier if the actual flap thickness has been measured. Caution is advised in patients with large corrections or thin corneas, because surprises can occur with microkeratome flaps that are thicker than expected, leaving less of a residual stromal bed than expected for ablation.

The variance between the actual and intended flap thickness depends on the corneal thickness. There is generally greater variance with thinner corneas; that is, flaps made on thinner corneas are thinner. It also depends on the type of microkeratome and on the surgeon. The reader should refer to Table 2.1 for guidance on thickness variance with available microkeratomes. Some microkeratomes routinely create flaps that are slightly thicker than intended. Manual microkeratomes (see the discussion of the Moria microkeratome in Chapter 2) will create thinner flaps if the surgeon makes a faster pass. A slower pass would result in a thicker flap. The surgeon has no control over the speed of the pass if an automated microkeratome is used. The sharpness of the blade is important as well. Many surgeons use a single blade for bilateral simultaneous surgery. The sharper the blade, the deeper the cut and the thicker the resulting flap. As previously stated, if the same blade is used the flap in the second eye is usually thinner. With the femtosecond laser the variance issue appears to be less of a problem as the actual flap thickness is usually within 20 μm of the intended thickness.

What is the ideal flap thickness? Many surgeons prefer a thickness between 110 and 130 μm. Thick flaps are said to be associated with an increased incidence of microstriae due to flap edema during the procedure. Very thin flaps can be difficult to handle and may be more prone to buttonhole. They can also be more problematic during retreatment.

The scrub tech will require a particular plate to place in the mechanical microkeratome. For example, a 160-μm plate on the Hansatome will generally provide a good thickness flap for LASIK. Refer to the various sections on the microkeratomes in Chapter 2. If the cornea is quite thin, however, the resulting flap with a 160-μm flap may be thinner than desirable. If the second eye has a thin cornea, and the first flap was thinner than desired, the surgeon should consider increasing the plate thickness to 180 μm or changing the blade. The latter approach is obviously more costly.

Patients older than 50 years of age are at greater risk of corneal epithelial slip or abrasion associated with the microkeratome pass. Microkeratome manufacturers have incorporated modifications designed to reduce epithelial trauma. An example is the Zero Compression Head developed for the Hansatome. Adequate preoperative and intraoperative lubrication is helpful. Some surgeons release suction on the reverse pass to limit epithelial trauma. Diffuse lamellar keratitis is more likely to occur if an epithelial defect resulted from the microkeratome pass. A defect is usually treated with a bandage contact lens. A contact lens is usually not needed if a small epithelial slip occurs.

If an epithelial defect occurs on the first eye, modifications may be made to protect the epithelium on the second eye. The same modifications mentioned earlier can be made if the epithelium is simply loosened and shifts. If suction is released while the flap is in the microkeratome, the patient should be reminded not to move. This will avoid a sudden movement, which could result in trauma to the hinge and a free cap.

What Is the Appropriate Flap Diameter?

Flap size varies depending on the inner diameter of the ring and the steepness of the cornea. A larger inner ring diameter will allow more tissue to pass through the ring exposing it to the microkeratome. The same is true if the cornea is steep. In both cases a larger flap

will result. Therefore, when a larger flap is required, a larger inner ring diameter may be needed. However, if the corneal curvature is ≥45.00 diopters, the increased steepness of the cornea will provide the necessary boost to flap diameter even if a smaller ring is used. If average keratometry readings are ≥48.00 diopters, not only will a large flap occur, but a buttonhole is also more likely. This should not imply that buttonholes never occur if the cornea is flatter than this.

Larger flaps are essential when the treatment zone is large; for example, in hyperopic LASIK, custom LASIK, mixed astigmatism, or other large-zone ablations. A larger flap is also helpful if retreatment is likely; however, larger flaps with edges closer to the limbus increase the risk of intraoperative bleeding and may be more difficult to lift many months after surgery.

When a larger flap is required in a patient with a flat cornea with keratometry readings of <41.00 diopters, a larger ring is essential to ensure that an adequate amount of the cornea will be exposed to the microkeratome blade. A patient with a small corneal diameter, <11 mm, may present a special challenge particularly if a large treatment zone is required, because the edge of a large flap will be close to the limbus. The femtosecond laser may be advantageous in this situation because the flap diameter can be more accurately determined.

The scrub tech will require the appropriate microkeratome ring sizes for each case being done. The surgeon should refer to the information provided for several microkeratomes that is found in Chapter 2. A course on microkeratome operation may be required to use some equipment. Practice on animal eyes is helpful to gain comfort and experience with the operation of the microkeratome. Finally, observing experienced surgeons during cases is also invaluable.

THE PROCEDURE

Preoperative Medication

Not all patients require sedation for LASIK surgery. For some the idea of taking a sedative may be anxiety provoking. Unless the surgeon has a strong feeling about the need for sedation, the patient can be given the choice. Patients are usually happy about the choice they make and it gives them a feeling of control. If an oral agent is given it should be administered at least 30 minutes before the procedure, so that the effect is present during the surgery. Benzodiazepam 5 mg is usually sufficient for most patients. Remember the purpose is to allow the patient to feel "normal," not sleepy, silly, or overly anxious. Beware of the patient who has taken a minor tranquilizer at home and is requesting additional sedation. Excessive sedation can be counterproductive, resulting in a relaxed patient who is unable to maintain fixation. While it is helpful for all patients to be escorted from the laser center, a patient receiving a sedative must have an escort home.

If a patient is prone to vasovagal episodes, consideration should be given to pretreating with atropine. An intramuscular injection of 0.4 mg of atropine 30 minutes prior to surgery can prevent the symptoms of a vasovagal reaction. Patients with this history usually welcome a treatment that can prevent these unwelcome symptoms even if it does require an injection. The patient can also be reassured that while in the supine position the symptoms are less likely to occur. If a vasovagal reaction occurs, the immediate postoperative examination at the slit lamp could be challenging.

If the patient is to have PRK, consideration should be given to pretreating the patient with an oral nonsteroid anti-inflammatory agent an hour prior to surgery and for the first 2 days following surgery. This will in most cases significantly reduce postoperative discomfort.

Marking the Patient

If the patient will be treated for astigmatism or with a custom LASIK technique, marking both sides of the 90- or 180-degree meridian at the limbus and aligning the marks with the laser may improve the accuracy of the technique. This is known as *registration*. Significant cyclotorsion can occur when the patient is placed in the supine position. Without a visible mark, the treatment could potentially be delivered in an incorrect position. Before creating a flap, the registration process is performed, at which time the

head position is adjusted to align the operating microscope reticle with the limbal marks. If adjustment is needed, it is better to rotate the form-fit pillow rather than the patient's head. The patient's head is less likely to slip back into the incorrect position if only the pillow is adjusted.

The 180-degree meridian is generally easier to mark. After instillation of topical anesthetic in each eye, the slit beam is oriented in the 3 to 9 o'clock meridian, and the beam is adjusted to maximum length and narrowed to a slit. The patient is asked to focus on a distant target to avoid cyclotorsion related to convergence. A sterile skin marker is then used to identify each side of the limbus in each eye. Several applications of ink during the marking process are usually necessary to achieve a mark that lasts throughout the procedure.

At the time of this writing, iris registration technology has only recently become available. For more information on iris registration, refer to the various excimer laser sections in Chapter 2. It is anticipated that this technology will improve registration beyond what can be achieved by marking the limbus.

Prior to making the flap, marks are placed in the peripheral cornea. This will help to ensure excellent realignment after the flap is replaced. This is particularly true in the event of a free cap. The marks should be asymmetrical so a free cap cannot be placed upside down. If the intended flap will be large, the marks should be placed closer to the limbus to ensure that the flap will bisect the marks. The marks can be placed farther from the limbus if the flap will be smaller.

Setting the Oculars

Setting the oculars is important to help ensure reliable focus on the cornea during the laser procedure. The surgeon should never assume the oculars are set properly unless they have been personally checked. It is convenient to set the oculars while the patient is being prepped. One method of checking the oculars is to use the laser ablation test card as the target. The magnification should be set to the same level used for the ablation; for example, 1.6× with the VISX laser rather than the lower magnification used for flap creation. The oculars are set to the plus side by rotating them counterclockwise. While the opposite eye is closed, each ocular is rotated clockwise until the target is just in focus.

Once the oculars have been set, it is convenient to check the calibration card. The laser engineer will periodically cut plastic with the laser to ensure an accurate ablation. Unlike the YAG or argon laser, in which the laser settings are adjusted intraoperatively based on effect, excimer laser settings are adjusted preoperatively. It is also useful to check the appearance of the ablation on the calibration card for signs of irregularity. If, for example, water droplets splash up against the underside of the microscope, an uneven ablation may result. This could be detected by an examination of the ablated card.

Environmental Conditions in the Laser Suite

The laser suite conditions should be stable and consistent. They should be recorded so that you can track results and if necessary adjust them. VISX recommends that the temperature be between 60°F and 80°F and the relative humidity from 35% to 65%. Stability of conditions within these ranges is the most important aspect of monitoring room conditions, because constant changes in temperature and humidity can alter outcomes and may confound your efforts to define the need for or amount of nomogram adjustment. Environmental conditions can vary widely depending on the region of the country in which you practice as well as the season of the year. These variables need to be monitored on a daily basis and the room conditions adjusted accordingly with the appropriate humidifiers and dehumidifiers as needed.

Preoperative Checklist

To avoid errors during the procedure, the surgeon, the scrub technician, and the laser engineer should develop a checklist that is routinely followed on every case. Ideally, the checklist should be reviewed just prior to surgery. The procedure should not begin until the appropriate confirmation of the checklist has been acquired. Good communication with a staff that is trained to recognize a problem and empowered to bring a potential problem to the attention of the surgeon is critically important to accomplish safe and reliable surgery.

Microkeratome

The scrub technician and the surgeon should review the checklist designed for the microkeratome prior to the operation of the unit. This should include checking the blade for imperfections and that it is seated properly in the microkeratome head, checking that the device is assembled correctly and for the proper eye, confirming that the desired plate and ring have been selected, and briefly running the microkeratome unit to be certain the blade oscillates freely. In the case of the femtosecond laser, the scrub technician should confirm that the suction ring is intact and operational, that the cone is intact, that the applanation lens is not cracked or dirty, that the settings for flap diameter and thickness are appropriately set, that the hinge width and side cut angle are correct, and that the energy settings for the flap and the side cut are appropriate.

Excimer Laser

The laser engineer should confirm for each eye the diameter of the treatment zones, whether a blend zone is being added, and whether the correction entered into the laser is the desired one. Custom treatments should be reviewed to make certain that the appropriate wave scan has been selected and entered and that desired physician adjustments have been entered.

Prep, Drape, and Speculum Insertion

After anesthetic has been instilled, the corneas are prone to epithelial disruption; therefore, the drops should not be instilled until immediately prior to surgery. The patient should be instructed to keep the eyes closed as much as possible. The lids are prepped with povidone iodine. Plastic drapes are placed on the lashes. With the eye in downgaze the upper lid is draped. The lower lid is draped with the eye in upgaze. This helps to ensure that the lashes will be completely covered and also minimizes corneal epithelial disruption.

Many surgeons prefer to use an aspirating speculum to reduce the chance of debris collecting in the stromal interface. Speculum insertion is facilitated by inserting the upper blade with the eye in downgaze and the lower blade with the eye in upgaze. Avoid rapid separation of the speculum blades, which can cause pain and blepharospasm.

Patient Positioning

Once the chair has been reclined, the patient should be positioned in order to maximize the range of motion of the table. If the patient has a large nose, slight rotation of the head in the direction opposite the eye being treated can facilitate exposure. In other words if the right eye is being treated, the head is rotated slightly to the left to move the nose out of the field.

If the microkeratome is used to create a flap with a superior hinge, exposure inferiorly is especially important. This enables the microkeratome to clear the lower lid and speculum. Positioning the patient in a slight chin-down position can optimize inferior exposure, facilitating the microkeratome pass. This is less important with microkeratomes that create a nasal hinge.

If a superior hinge has been created, it is helpful to reflect the flap back onto the superior bulbar conjunctiva. In other words, the flap epithelium is laid down on the conjunctival epithelium. This helps to keep the flap moist and keeps the flap from wrinkling. Positioning the patient with the chin up slightly after the flap has been created will expose the superior bulbar conjunctiva, facilitating flap placement in preparation for the laser procedure.

Ring Placement

Proper ring placement will ensure that the hinge will be created in the periphery of the cornea. If the hinge position is too central, the result might be a decentered flap that does not expose enough of the corneal stroma to permit the entire area of laser treatment to be performed. To avoid this, the ring should extend just beyond the limbus in the area where the hinge will be made. For example, the ring should be placed just beyond the limbus superiorly to ensure a properly placed superior hinge. This is especially important if a large treatment area is required. If the ring is placed too far beyond the limbus, the hinge will be too peripheral. The potential consequences are bleeding from the limbal blood vessels and a decentered flap that does not expose adequate stroma opposite the hinge to allow the complete laser treatment to be performed. Good microkeratome instruction with a proctored wet lab and subsequent practice will help the beginning surgeon determine the correct placement of the ring.

It is important after correct ring positioning to apply firm posterior pressure to the ring before the suction is applied. This is true regardless of the type of microkeratome used.

Firm pressure will help avoid pseudosuction, in which the pressure is applied to the conjunctiva but not the sclera. If the eye pressure is inadequate, a small or shredded flap or a free cap may occur. Once good suction is achieved, the firm posterior pressure on the ring should be released and the ring supported lightly. This will allow the globe to "float" anteriorly and will facilitate engaging the ring with the microkeratome. Occasionally firm posterior pressure can cause the ring to abruptly slip under the speculum. If this occurs and suction is good, the ring should be gently lifted anteriorly so that the speculum will not block the microkeratome pass. Spreading the speculum wider can be helpful in this situation. Any time the surgeon lifts the ring with suction applied, care should be taken to be certain that suction has not been lost. Signs of lost suction include a pupil that becomes reactive, a patient that again sees the light, the cornea dropping posteriorly, and the presence of a sucking noise.

If the eye rolls in the nasal or temporal direction beneath the ring during the application of suction and there is a question of whether the laser treatment will fit completely under the flap, suction should be released. If the eye rolls in the temporal direction a nasal flap will result. The opposite will occur if the eye rolls in the nasal direction. Two maneuvers can help compensate for a rolling eye. First, simply increasing the posterior pressure of the ring onto the globe can reduce the movement of the eye beneath the ring while suction is being obtained. If this fails to solve the problem, placing the ring with temporal decentration for an eye that rolls in the temporal direction, or nasal decentration for an eye that rolls in the nasal direction, will often solve the problem. The eye should roll into proper position. Remember that reapplying suction several times may result in conjunctival chemosis that can lead to pseudosuction. If significant chemosis does occur it is best to wait several hours at a minimum before reapplying suction.

If a decentered flap does occur, it may still be acceptable to proceed if the ablation zone is small. Nasal decentration may still be acceptable if the treatment is centered on fixation, because most patients have a positive angle kappa. Remember, however, that a laser with a tracking device and an automatic centration device will center the ablation on the center of the pupil. The microscope reticle is a helpful guide in determining whether a laser treatment can be delivered completely under the flap. Extreme decentration can result in a flap edge at the limbus. This can be associated with hemorrhage from limbal blood vessels and blood in the interface. All blood must be cleared with a sponge to avoid an uneven ablation. Blood in the interface also increases the risk of diffuse lamellar keratitis (DLK).

In the presence of peripheral pannus or corneal neovascularization, bleeding may be avoided by creating a smaller flap. However, flap size must be adequate to accommodate the entire laser ablation. If bleeding from peripheral vessels occurs, direct pressure with a microsurgical sponge will tamponade the site of hemorrhage and usually help control it. It is preferable to control the bleeding before lifting the flap. This may reduce the chance of bleeding into the interface.

If the palpebral fissure is narrow or small or if the lids are tight, a microkeratome system, which uses a ring with a smaller outer ring diameter, can be advantageous. The use of a one-piece microkeratome has the advantage of clearing the lids more effectively; however, most of these microkeratomes when used in routine fashion create a nasal flap.

If a two-piece microkeratome is being used, the surgeon should become very familiar with its assembly prior to surgery to minimize the suction time.

If using a two-piece microkeratome in a patient with deep-set eyes, it may be difficult to lock the microkeratome on the ring. The speculum may be blocking the microkeratome from engaging the ring. Spreading the blades more fully may be helpful. Pushing the speculum posteriorly may also help provide adequate exposure. The inferior blade of the speculum may abruptly drop posterior to the orbital rim, which will enhance exposure but may be uncomfortable for the patient. Conjunctiva, lashes, and plastic drape should be cleared away from the ring with a forceps before engaging the microkeratome.

If the femtosecond laser is used to make the flap, most surgeons will create both flaps before performing the laser ablation. At this point surgeons vary with regard to immediately proceeding to the excimer laser ablation or waiting 15 to 20 minutes for the waste products within the interface to dissipate. While this waiting period may be cumbersome for the logistics of patient flow, some feel that waiting for the cornea to clear will reduce the incidence of retreatment. Others feel it makes no difference.

Flap Positioning

Various techniques are used for lifting the flap after it has been made. Some surgeons prefer to slide an instrument completely across the underside of the flap at a position 2 or 3 mm inferior to the hinge. Care must be taken using this technique not to scrape the epithelium peripheral to the flap edge, dragging it under the flap. The flap is then reflected toward the hinge and laid epithelial side down onto the bulbar conjunctiva. This keeps the flap moist and wrinkle free. The flap should be lifted slowly and carefully, because in some cases it may be adherent to the underlying stromal bed. If the flap is lifted too quickly in such cases, there is an increased risk of a torn flap hinge.

An alternative method of lifting the flap is to use a tying forceps at the edge of the flap opposite the hinge to grab the flap and lift it up, bending it back and rolling it in the direction of the hinge until the flap epithelium is completely laid over the bulbar conjunctiva. It is important not to lift the flap too high or the sides will fold under like a taco. This can lead to wrinkling or uneven flap positioning. Whatever technique is used it is important to keep the flap moist and to be gentle to avoid trauma to the flap. It is helpful to warn the patient that the vision will blur somewhat when the flap is lifted.

Flap Thickness

Mechanical microkeratomes have a fairly wide variance from intended to actual flap thickness. Thinner flaps occur in thinner corneas. If the blade is reused on the second eye, the second flap will be thinner than the first. Manual microkeratomes allow the surgeon to modify flap thickness by using a faster pass to create a thinner flap and a slower pass for a thicker flap. Automated microkeratomes have a fixed pass speed. Flaps created with the femtosecond laser have a smaller variance in thickness and are not dependent on preoperative corneal thickness or steepness.

Intraoperative pachymetry is a readily available way to determine the actual flap thickness. The surgeon should not enter the LASIK suite without having a predicted residual stromal thickness (RST) after the flap and ablation have been made. If the flap is considerably thicker than expected, the RST will be less than expected and perhaps less than is necessary for safe surgery. In this situation the laser ablation may need to be aborted to prevent ectasia. An accurate assessment of RST recorded in the chart will also be helpful if a retreatment becomes necessary.

The technique for determining flap thickness is simple. Central pachymetry is measured before the flap is made. Immediately after lifting the flap, pachymetry is again measured. The actual thickness of the flap is calculated by subtracting the measurement taken at the stromal bed from the full thickness measurement. The laser engineer should be prepared to make the necessary calculation and communicate the value to the surgeon. The surgeon, having previously written the maximum allowable flap thickness on the worksheet, will immediately know that surgery can proceed safely. Alternatively, the surgeon can simply measure the bed thickness alone. If the bed is sufficiently thick to accommodate the required ablation and still leave an adequate RST, the surgeon can proceed with the ablation.

Remember that the central corneal thickness is a variable measurement. It is thinner in the absence of contact lens wear, with increased exposure, and with decreased ambient humidity. Therefore, central pachymetry measured at the start of a case may be significantly different from the reading taken at the screening examination. Only intraoperative readings should be used for flap thickness calculation. The residual stromal tissue also thins as it becomes desiccated, so measurement and ablation should proceed without inordinate delay.

Use a probe tip dedicated to the LASIK suite. This will reduce the risk of contamination of the flap bed with fluorescein or other undesirable material that could affect the stroma or the laser treatment. Laser ablation greatly reduces the risk of bacterial contamination of the flap bed from the probe tip. The standard 20-Hz probe frequency pachymeter may not work reliably on a flap bed created with a femtosecond laser. An upgrade to a 50-Hz probe frequency unit may be required if flaps will routinely be created with the laser.

If the flap made with a mechanical microkeratome on the first eye is thinner than desired, an appropriate adjustment should be made for the second eye. This is because if the same blade is used, the second flap will likely be even thinner. The options are to use a thicker plate, a new blade, or a slower pass with a manual microkeratome.

The Laser Ablation

Before beginning the excimer laser ablation, registration of the laser reticle with the limbal marks is an important first step. This is particularly essential if the ablation involves astigmatism treatment or a custom treatment. If registration is not done, the treatment may be delivered in the wrong axis due to cyclotorsion. If the marks do not line up with the reticle, rotate the patient's headrest until good alignment is achieved.

During the LASIK procedure it is important to talk to the patient, constantly reassuring and coaching. This will help to keep the patient calm and to maintain attention on the task at hand. This is especially true during the excimer laser portion of the procedure. If there is no tracking device, the patient's attention on the fixation light is critically important. Occasionally if the patient is breathing heavily, the tracker will be unable to lock. Asking the patient to take a breath and hold it will stabilize the eye enough for the laser tracking system to lock on to the pupil. Some tracking systems require pupil dilation;

some do not. It is important to follow the guidelines set by the manufacturer and the medical monitors for the laser being used.

While laser-tracking systems have provided a significant improvement in the safety of laser refractive surgery, they are not foolproof. If, for example, a patient is slowly drifting away from fixation and the surgeon is following the eye with the joystick, the laser will continue tracking as if the patient were looking at the fixation light, resulting in an inaccurate ablation. It is also possible to have a patient looking at something other than the fixation light, despite instruction, prior to locking the tracking device on the pupil. The tracker may follow the eye even though it is not in the proper position. To avoid these problems, a quick check of the globe position before engaging the tracking device is a good habit. The scrub technician can also watch the globe position during the laser ablation.

Dimming the surrounding illumination can help the patient see the fixation light. The pupil center may vary depending on the lighting. Therefore, for custom LASIK the lighting should match the lighting during WaveScan acquisition. This will ensure that the treatment will be centered in the proper location. It is important to focus the microscope on the stromal bed just prior to the laser procedure. This can be accomplished by defocusing upward until the apex of the cornea is just out of focus. The focus is then brought downward until the view of the apex is clear. During the laser part of the procedure, it is useful to have the laser engineer or scrub technician perform a countdown at 5- to 10-second intervals. This enables the surgeon and patient to be aware of the amount of time remaining. If the patient is not holding still enough to safely continue the surgery, it is important and necessary to interrupt the laser procedure. The patient can be instructed about proper fixation. Speaking calmly and continuously to the patient can be reassuring and help the patient focus attention on the fixation light. While a tracking device is helpful, it only operates within a proscribed range. If the patient moves outside this range. the laser ablation will be interrupted.

If the treatment zone is large or the hinge is more central than desired, it is important to protect it from inadvertent ablation. Accidentally ablating the hinge and the bed would result in duplication or roughly twice the treatment in the area of the hinge. It is important to cover the hinge with a Merocel (Medtronic, Minneapolis, MN) spear or an instrument designed for this purpose.

Flap Repositioning

Following the laser ablation the flap is replaced. The goal is to have a clean interface with no folds or striae in the flap and no areas in which the flap edge is turned under. The flap can be replaced using a single or double irrigating canula. The double irrigating cannula has the advantage of combining repositioning with irrigation beneath the flap to remove debris. An example is the Viduarri irrigating cannula (Visitec no. 585216). Some surgeons irrigate beneath the flap more than once to be certain the interface is clean. A saturated nonfragmenting Merocel sponge is used to gently stroke or paint the flap from the hinge across the cornea. The alignment of the previously made corneal marks is checked. A semiwet sponge can then be used to inspect the trough at the edge of the flap, making certain the trough width is minimized and that it is symmetrical all the way around. Surgeons vary in opinion with regard to the amount of flap stroking or manipulation that is needed to reduce the risk of striae. Surgeons also vary with regard to the time allowed for the flap to dry before removing the speculum. Most wait for 1 to 3 minutes. A viscous artificial teardrop is applied to the cornea at the conclusion of the procedure.

Remove the eyelid drapes first, then the speculum. Gently lift the lower speculum blade anteriorly as the speculum is narrowed and the scrub technician pulls the lower lid inferiorly. Instruct the patient to continue fixating on the target light as the speculum is removed. This will avoid an inadvertent flap displacement. Cover the treated eye and set up for the fellow eye if bilateral surgery is being performed.

Immediate Postoperative Evaluation

After surgery is completed the patient is checked at the slit lamp. Explain to the patient that the vision should be hazy and not to worry. Assess the flap for alignment and striae as well as interface debris. The indications for flap relifting, also referred to as *refloating* the flap, immediately after surgery are significant interface debris, visible striae, poor flap alignment, or macrofolds. A low threshold for relifting a flap for any of these abnormalities is advised. It is always easier and usually more effective for the surgeon to refloat a flap immediately after surgery than after days or weeks have passed. Remember that the applied viscous tear may mask subtle striae. The scrub technician should not remove the surgical instruments until the surgeon has confirmed that the flap will not need to be refloated.

Postoperative instructions include the use of protective eyewear. The duration of eyewear use varies from 1 to 7 days. Some surgeons believe eye protection is needed only at night. The patient should be warned about eye rubbing. Prednisolone 1% and a topical fluoroquinolone should be administered and the patient instructed to use 1 drop of each four times daily for 1 week. A safe technique for drop instillation should be demonstrated to the patient. Irritation and tearing are not uncommon in the first 2 days after surgery. The patient should be warned about these symptoms and advised to use oral acetaminophen or an oral nonsteroidal anti-inflammatory agent. Instructions should be given for reaching the doctor in the event of a question or problem. The doctor or an appropriate designee should be available to receive a call. Arrangements should be made for an appointment the following day. The patient is examined at 1 day, 1 week, 1 month, 3 months, 6 months, and 1 year.

Equipment

Robert S. Feder, M.D., Marian Macsai, M.D., Steven Rosenfeld, M.D., Michael Vrabec, M.D., F.A.C.S., Parag Majmudar, M.D., Colman Kraff, M.D., and Jonathan Rubenstein, M.D.

CORNEAL TOPOGRAPHY

An in-depth discussion of corneal topography is beyond the scope of this handbook. However, a working knowledge of topography is necessary to perform LASIK safely. Topography is used as a screening tool during the preoperative evaluation to be certain the contour of the cornea is regular (see Case 26). The surgeon must not only rule out the presence of ectatic diseases such as keratoconus and pellucid marginal degeneration in an overt form, but must also be able to detect these conditions in a subclinical or subtle form. Occasionally an adult may present with mild keratoconus in an arrested form, known as forme fruste keratoconus, that does not progress. The patient may be completely asymptomatic and might never develop the clinical disease unless the cornea is weakened during LASIK surgery. The age of the patient is an important consideration. When the subclinical form is present in a young adult or teenager, one cannot be certain that the condition will not progress into a manifest ectatic disease over time. It is therefore advisable to avoid LASIK surgery in this situation.

Serial corneal topography can also be used to track the corneal contour in a contact lens–wearing patient who is avoiding lens wear in preparation for final LASIK measurements. Topography, keratometry, and refraction are all used during repeated examinations as indicators that the corneas have become stable.

Corneal topography is also an essential part of the postoperative management of the LASIK patient. Retreatment should not be performed unless the cornea has reached a stable contour, and topography can help with this determination. Topography can help evaluate a patient with postoperative vision that is less than expected. Central islands, small, steep areas in the central cornea, which may occur following treatment for myopia can be detected by topography. Postoperative corneal ectasia following keratorefractive surgery can occur even when no apparent preoperative pathology was detected. The alterations in corneal contour related to flap complications such as epithelial ingrowth, a flap buttonhole, or striae can be evaluated and monitored using topography. Comparative maps can help assess the effect of corrective surgical treatment. For all of these reasons, the topography unit is indispensable to the refractive surgeon.

The results from the more common topography units can be confounded in several important ways. For example, if the patient's fixation is off, the map will not be meaningful. If the surface of the cornea is irregular (as a result of, e.g., a dry eye or inadequate exposure), the data collection will be limited. Excessive tearing is associated with an enlarged tear meniscus that can distort the map inferiorly. Finally, some topography units will extrapolate data to fill areas for which data could not be obtained. This extrapolation can be misleading. It may be more reliable to use a unit that shows areas of data dropout as blank areas. The computer analysis used to derive color maps is based on certain physical and

2

mathematical assumptions. The data generated are only as accurate as the information captured and the accuracy of the assumptions made. Therefore, careful interpretation of the output from this equipment in the context of the particular patient is always advised.

Modern topography units generate maps that are designed to demonstrate corneal power and corneal elevation. Before interpreting a map it is important to look at the scale on which the map is based. Maps generated on different days should have the same scale in order to be meaningfully compared. The scale for an axial or power map is given in diopters. Steeper areas are red or orange and flatter areas are blue or purple. The scale for an elevation map is given in microns. This refers to the microns above or below a best-fit sphere. Cornea below the sphere is blue and above the sphere is red or orange. In some cases the elevation maps are mathematically derived rather than the result of a direct measurement.

The difference between power and elevation can be a source of confusion in interpreting maps. How can a cornea be flat and elevated at the same time? The appearance of a mesa or a flattened mountaintop is a geological structure that is flat and elevated. A similar contour abnormality on the cornea would appear blue (indicating flattening) on a power map and orange or red on an elevation map. Likewise, a spire at the bottom of a valley would appear steep on a power map, but depressed on an elevation map. Understanding the differences between power and elevation gives the surgeon a deeper understanding of the corneal contour when interpreting these maps.

Available Systems

Several types of topography units are on the market and the prices vary considerably. The most common type of unit and the most affordable is based on a corneal reflection from a Placido disk. It is generally most accurate for measuring the power of the paracentral rather than the peripheral cornea. Concentric rings are projected on to the cornea and various points on these rings are sampled, digitized, and computer analyzed. Points on adjacent rings will be spaced closer together in areas of steepening contour. The normal cornea is steepest centrally and flattens peripherally to meet the flatter scleral curve. Inferior steepening of the cornea is abnormal and may be a sign of keratoconus. The color maps that are generated correspond to the corneal power in diopters at various locations on the cornea. Typically, warmer colors indicate areas of steepening and cooler colors are areas of flattening. In addition to the videokeratoscopic view and the axial or power map, tangential maps, refractive maps, elevation maps, and difference maps can be generated.

Placido disk-only systems are limited in that they only measure the anterior surface of the cornea. These systems do not directly measure elevation. One of the pitfalls in analysis of images based on a Placido disk is the assumption that the line of sight, the corneal apex, and the center of the keratoscopic image are all in the same place. Inaccuracies in computer software analysis may result in faulty interpretation, particularly in a patient with a decentered corneal apex. The EyeSys (EyeSys Vision, Houston, TX), Humphrey Atlas (Zeiss-Humphrey, Dublin, CA), and TMS (Tomey Technology, Waltham, MA) units are examples of topography machines based on Placido disk systems.

The Orbscan (Bausch & Lomb, Rochester, NY) uses a combination of a Placido disk and a slit-scanning system. The slit beam scans the cornea from limbus to limbus, taking photographs at various intervals from a pass around the cornea. In addition to the axial or power map derived from the corneal reflection of the Placido disk, it uses the slit images to generate anterior and posterior elevation maps. The maps compare the elevation of the anterior and posterior cornea to a reference best-fit sphere. Warm colors are used to illustrate areas where the cornea is anterior or elevated compared to the reference sphere, and cool colors indicate cornea depressed compared to the reference. The scale is measured in microns. When evaluating the elevation maps, the surgeon should be mindful of the inherent inaccuracy related to comparing the aspheric cornea to a sphere.

Finally, the Orbscan generates a pachymetric map. The thickness map does not provide as accurate a measurement of corneal thickness as does ultrasonic pachymetry, but it can give a relative impression of corneal thickness over a

2

large area of the cornea. It allows the surgeon to compare the thickness of the central cornea, where the cornea should be the thinnest, with the peripheral cornea. A potential disadvantage of the Orbscan is the length of time it takes to perform a study. Eye movement, if inadequately tracked, could result in a faulty interpretation due to inaccurate data acquisition. Pachymetric data following LASIK surgery may not be as accurate as in unoperated eyes.

Pentacam (Oculus, Inc., Lynnwood, WA) is a relatively new entrant in the field of cornea topography units. The technology is based on a rotating slit-scanning device that captures images using Scheimpflug photography. Using this photographic technique, images of the entire anterior segment are recorded, enabling the unit to measure anterior and posterior corneal elevation and thickness. Curvature maps are also generated. The Pentacam can also be used to evaluate other anterior segment structures, such as the angle, iris, and lens. It, therefore, can be used in sizing a phakic intraocular lens implant. It can take up to 2 seconds to perform a study and thus must rely on a tracking device to identify and compensate for eye movements. Although this device has the potential to provide much more information than other available units, it is also substantially more expensive.

Keratoconus Detection

Topography is a key element of the LASIK evaluation because it can be used to screen for preexisting ectatic disease. Some patterns on power maps, elevation maps, and thickness maps are suggestive of keratoconus. Some topography units, particularly those based on Placido disk technology, come equipped with keratoconus detection software. No one index is foolproof in identifying keratoconus or preventing postoperative ectasia. It is recommended that several indices and analyses be used to determine whether a particular patient is suitable for keratorefractive surgery. A detailed preoperative discussion with the patient is warranted when the risk of ectasia is greater than average. Keratorefractive surgery is ill advised when the likelihood of surgically induced ectasia is high.

The pattern of inferior elevation, inferior thinning in the area of maximal protrusion, inferior steepening with superior flattening, asymmetric dumbbell, and deviation of the axis of the superior part of the dumbbell are all patterns that could be consistent with keratoconus (Fig. 2.1). Rabinowitz referred to the deviation of the superior axis as skewed radial axes and has suggested that a deviation greater than 21 degrees is an important index in screening patients for the diagnosis of keratoconus. He has suggested three additional quantitative videokeratographic indices: a central corneal power value >47.2 diopters, an inferior-superior dioptric asymmetry (I-S value) >1.2, and Sim-K astigmatism >1.5 diopters. In addition to the Rabinowitz method, the Klyce/Maeda method and the Smolek/Klyce method are other software programs designed to screen for keratoconus

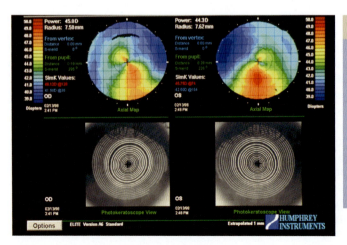

Figure 2.1

Power maps demonstrating forme fruste keratoconus OU. Note inferior steepening with superior flattening, asymmetric dumbbell, and deviation of the axis of the superior part of the dumbbell (skewed radial axes), which are all topographic findings suggestive of keratoconus. (Courtesy of Robert Feder, M.D.)

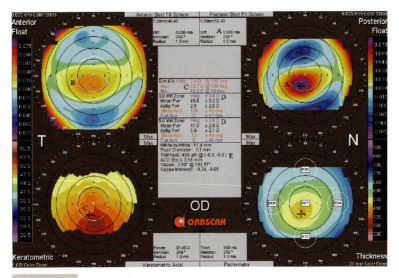

Figure 2.2

Orbscan II of a 39-year-old with 20/30 uncorrected acuity in this eye. **A:** Upper right map shows a prominent posterior float. With the cursor "+" at the apex, the posterior curve is 86 μm above the best-fit sphere. **B:** Prominent anterior float with apex in same position as the apex in the upper right map. **C:** Steep Sim-K correlates with steep power map. Also note prominent inferior steepening. **D:** Irregularity in this topographical analysis is ±3.8 and ±3.6 D at 3 and 5 mm, respectively. This is well above the accepted limits of irregularity. **E:** Thinnest part of the cornea is 486 μm. Ultrasonic pachymetry would likely measure even thinner. All of the above strongly suggests the diagnosis of keratoconus. (Courtesy of Robert Feder, M.D.)

on Placido disk-based systems. Check with the sales representative for the topography unit you use to determine what keratoconus screening software is available. Remember that these programs may not be designed to detect ectatic diseases other than keratoconus.

Another useful index found on the Bausch & Lomb Orbscan unit is the posterior elevation difference with best-fit sphere (Fig. 2.2). Rao et al. have described its use as a screening tool. The value for the posterior elevation difference is found when the cursor is placed on the highest part of the posterior elevation map. The value in the gray box to the left should ideally be <0.04 mm. A reading between 0.04 and 0.05 mm should alert the surgeon about the heightened risk of postoperative ectasia and the need to look for other corroborating evidence of preexisting ectasia. When the reading is >0.05 mm, there is often evidence in other maps of preexisting ectasia. Most surgeons advise against LASIK surgery in this situation.

Caution is also recommended when the irregularity at the 3.0-mm zone is >±1.5 D or the irregularity at the 5.0-mm zone is >±2.0 D (Fig. 2.2). Less conservative surgeons use ±2.0 and ±2.5 D, respectively. Finally, if the thinnest part of the cornea is >30 μm thinner than the central thickness, if the thinnest part of the cornea is >2.5 mm from the center, or if the peripheral cornea is not at least 20 μm thicker than the center of cornea, the postoperative ectasia risk may be increased.

Another type of analysis described by Vukich and Karpecki (P. Karpecki, O.D., *personal communication*, 4-25-05) can be performed with the Orbscan (Bausch & Lomb) topography unit using the normal band scale. This is found by going to *View* in the toolbar and selecting *Quad Map* in the drop-down menu. Then select *Normal Band*, which colors all values within a "normal range" as green. Abnormally elevated, steep, or thin areas will be depicted as orange on the otherwise green map. LASIK should probably not be done if orange areas

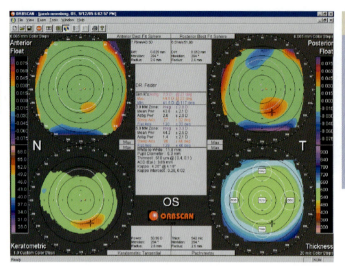

Figure 2.3

Normal band scale found by going to *View* in the toolbar, selecting *Quad Maps* in the drop-down menu, and choosing *Normal Band*. This normal band view shows orange in three of the four maps, which is one indicator suggesting against keratorefractive surgery. (Courtesy of Robert Feder, M.D.)

are seen in two or more maps. If orange is present in two maps, surface ablation would be a better option, provided the risk of ectasia has been explained. When orange is seen in three maps, the patient should probably not have corneal refractive surgery (Fig. 2.3).

Pellucid marginal degeneration (PMD) is a noninflammatory thinning disorder that presents as a band of stromal thinning 1 to 2 mm wide occurring 1 to 2 mm central to the inferior limbus usually between the 4 and 8 o'clock meridia. Corneal protrusion occurs superior to the band of thinning in contrast to keratoconus, in which protrusion occurs at the area of maximal thinning. The axial or power map in PMD typically shows against-the-rule astigmatism superiorly and with-the-rule astigmatism inferiorly resulting in a crab claw pattern. This pattern is characteristic of PMD (Fig. 2.4).

The following scenario illustrates the use of topography as a LASIK screening tool. A 30-year-old man presented for LASIK measurements after a brief screening consultation. He had reasonable expectations, understood the risks of surgery, and appeared to be an excellent candidate for surgery. The patient corrected to 20/20 with a manifest refraction of $-3.00 + 1.75 \times 30$ degrees OS. The corneal topography is shown in Figure 2.5. Notice the prominent posterior elevation with a difference from the best-fit sphere of 0.056 mm. There is also a prominent anterior elevation with the peak in the same place as

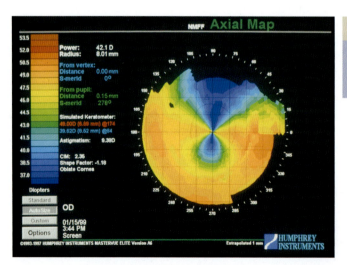

Figure 2.4

Power map of pellucid marginal degeneration. (Courtesy of Robert Grohe, O.D.)

2

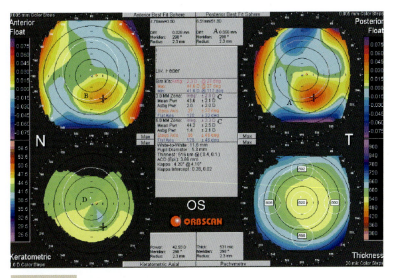

the posterior float. The irregularity at 3.0 and 5.0 mm exceeds the recommended maximum limit. The power map is quite abnormal and resembles the map in Figure 2.4, suggesting PMD. The normal band view (Fig. 2.3) shows orange in three maps. Taken together, these data should raise a large red flag that this patient should not have corneal refractive surgery.

THE MICROKERATOMES

Since the mid-1990s the instrumentation used to create a flap has become more reliable, easier to assemble, and safer to use. The number of available models has also increased dramatically. There are now one- or two-piece microkeratomes, manual or automated models, and even disposable microkeratomes. Finally, the latest innovation, the femtosecond laser, is now approved for use in the United States.

In this section, commonly used representative microkeratomes will be discussed. Included in the discussion of each device the reader will find pearls for its operation; the advantages and the disadvantages of the representative models are also presented. The

femtosecond laser will also be covered in a separate section. The material presented is designed as an adjunct to—not as a substitute for—a certification course or a user's manual. For a broader perspective readers can review the entire section or simply target the material relevant to their available equipment.

Two-Piece Microkeratome

Hansatome

This section will introduce the reader to the Hansatome, one of the more popular mechanical microkeratomes. Basic information and pearls for the operation of this instrument are provided; however a certification course must be completed prior to its use.

The Hansatome is a two-piece mechanical device designed to create a superior hinged flap as the microkeratome pivots on the slotted post of a suction ring. The motor is mounted vertically over the microkeratome head and the single-gear mechanism allows it to engage and rotate along the curved elevated gear track on the suction ring opposite the slotted pivot post. The blade, which is specifically designed for the Hansatome, oscillates within the microkeratome head at 7,500 rpm. The standard suction rings have an outer diameter of 20 mm. Microrings have the same inner diameters as the standard rings, but have an outer diameter of 19 mm. The micro-rings are useful for patients with narrow palpebral fissures or tight lids. The available inner diameters in both the standard rings and the micro-rings are 8.5 and 9.5 mm. The 8.5-mm ring is appropriate for patients with steeper corneas; that is, keratometry readings of >45.00 D, or when a smaller flap is adequate. When a larger flap is required, such as in custom treatments, large pupil treatments, hyperopia or mixed astigmatism, or when the cornea is relatively flat, the 9.5-mm ring is preferred. Patients with keratometry readings >48.00 D are at increased risk of buttonholed flaps, and patients with readings <40.00 D are at heightened risk of a free cap.

Some surgeons feel that the superior hinge is less desirable in the patient with a relative tear deficiency, because nerve bundles entering the cornea from the 3 and 9 o'clock meridia will both be severed. A nasal hinge would preserve the nerves entering the cornea from the nasal side. Other surgeons do not feel this is a significant problem, provided the surface can be stabilized preoperatively with punctal plugs, tear supplements, or topical cyclosporine. Any dry eye patient undergoing LASIK surgery should be cautioned about the added risk. All efforts should be made to enhance tear function prior to surgery. Dry eye patients whose problem cannot be significantly improved with therapy are not good candidates for LASIK surgery regardless of which microkeratome is used.

The suction ring is sufficiently thick that it can be used without a lid speculum in a patient with a narrow or small lid fissure or in a patient with a deep-set eye. The microkeratome head will be able to pass over the gear track without obstruction from the lids.

The available plates are 130, 160, 180, and 200 μm. The most commonly used plates are the 160- and 180-μm plates. The actual flap thickness is typically less than the chosen plate thickness; however, the surgeon is advised to measure the actual flap thickness using intraoperative pachymetry. This is because of the wide variance that is possible between intended and actual flap thickness. The Hansatome will usually make an even thinner flap if the patient has a thin cornea. The mean flap thickness created with the 160-mm plate is 129 μm ± 21μm and for the 180-μm plate is 136 μm ± 25μm (Table 2.1).

An early problem with the Hansatome was the relatively high incidence of epithelial loosening and defects within the newly created flap. This was particularly true in patients more than 50 years old. Since the advent of the Zero Compression Head, incidences of epithelial loosening and defects in the flap have fallen dramatically. The Zero Compression Head should be used on all patients if available. The left/right eye adapter fits between the motor and the microkeratome head. It is labeled so that only the appropriate label "R" or "L" will be visible once the unit is properly assembled.

Prior to the operation the scrub technician and surgeon should review the microkeratome checklist. The placement of the suction ring is similar to that for other microkeratomes. Refer to Chapter 1 to review this. Decision making for the Hansatome is summarized in Table 2.2.

Firm posterior pressure will help avoid pseudosuction, in which suction is applied to the conjunctiva but not the sclera. After suction has been achieved, the ring is allowed to float anteriorly and tissue that could potentially interfere with the microkeratome pass is swept aside.

Once suction has been achieved, the intraocular pressure (IOP) should be checked and a pressure >65 mmHg confirmed. The cornea is moistened with topical anesthetic. Balanced salt solution is not used, because over time the salts will interfere with the microkeratome function. The Hansatome is placed on the slotted pivot post of the ring. If the microkeratome is not aligned properly, it will not seat. Twisting the head or forcing the microkeratome down on the post will not be effective. The microkeratome should be removed, realigned properly, and then replaced. A pearl for easily aligning the microkeratome with the post is to look for landmarks on the ring and the head. On the ring of the Hansatome there is a ledge central to and just below the gear track that serves an important landmark. There is a dovetail on either side of the microkeratome head. The leading edge of the appropriate dovetail should be lined up with the inferior border of this ring ledge. This will

Table 2.1	Comparison of microkeratome models

Microkeratome	Contact Information	Standard Oscillation Speed (rpm)	Standard Translation Speed (mm/s)	Evaluated Plate Thickness (μm)	Mean Flap Thickness ±SD (μm)[1]
Amadeus	(714)247-8200 www.amo-inc.com	10,000 (4,000– 20,000)	3.0 (1.5–4.0 available)	130 140 160	147 ± 24 134 ± 15 180 ± 35
Hansatome	(800)338-2020 www.bausch.com	7,500	Preset	160 180	129 ± 21 136 ± 25
Carriazo- Barraquer	49(0)6027/508-0 www.eye-tech- solutions.com	15,000	Manual control (most common 2.5–4.0)	110 130	165 ± 27[2] 198 ± 26[2]
Moria M2	(800)441-1314 www.moria- surgical.com	15,000	(2.1 or 3.1 available)	130	146 ± 32
Nidek MK-2000	(800)223-9044 www.nidek.com	9,000	2.0	130 145 160	111 ± 19 103 ± 15 121 ± 20
Summit Krumeich- Barraquer	(800)757-9195 www.alconlabs.com	16,000	2.5	160	143 ± 23
Zyoptix XP[3]	(800)338-2020 www.bausch.com	61,000	12.0 s forward + reverse	120	116 ± 16
Becton Dickinson K-4000	(800)237-2174 www.bd.com	12,000	4.4	160	149 ± 23

[1] Solomon KD, Donnenfeld E, Sandoval, HP. Flap thickness accuracy: Comparison of 6 microkeratome models. *J Cataract Refract Surg.* 2004;30(5):964–977.

[2] 4.0 s translation speed used in the study to create these flaps.

[3] Manufacturer-supported study. Unpublished data. Dr. Hung Lee, Tan Toch Seng Hospital and National University Hospital, Singapore, 2005.

allow the microkeratome to easily drop down on the pivot post, and the leading edge of the microkeratome will drop beneath the ring ledge. With a slight manual advancement the microkeratome is fully engaged and ready for automated advancement. Proper alignment of these landmarks is illustrated in Figure 2.6.

Once the gear is engaged in the track, the forward pedal is depressed and the surgeon can let go of the microkeratome, allowing it to complete its pass. Holding the ring handle stabilizes the device. As the Hansatome is reversed, suction can be released to avoid traumatizing the corneal epithelium. The patient should be cautioned about moving the eye when suction is released and the flap is still within the device. The Hansatome and ring are then lifted off the eye as a unit.

Troubleshooting the Hansatome

Refer to general comments about microkeratome use in the basic LASIK chapter (Chapter 1). A few pearls are worth noting in case surgery fails to go as planned. If the microkeratome fails to advance at the first tooth of the gear track, before the cornea has been engaged, it is safe to reverse the device, reengage, and proceed. However, if the flap is

2

Table 2.2	Hansatome rules of thumb
Steep cornea	If K >45.00 D, use 8.5-mm ring; K >48.00 D risks buttonhole *Caution:* Flaps cut on steep corneas tend to be large. If buttonhole: replace flap, no laser, return in 6 months to cut new flap; consider PTK-PRK with or without mitomycin-C.
Flat cornea	If K <45.00 D, use 9.5-mm ring; K <40.00 D risks free cap *Caution:* Flaps cut on flat corneas tend to be small. If small free flap or small flap: replace flap, no laser, BSCL, return in 6 months to cut new flap using deeper cutting plate, or consider PTK/PRK with or without MMC.
Small corneal diameter	Select smaller ring diameter to avoid bleeding unless flat keratotomy readings or large flap needed *Caution:* risk of bleeding, conjunctival or scleral extension
Large corneal diameter	Use larger 9.5-mm ring to create larger flap unless steep keratotomy readings
Corneal vascularization	Use smaller ring to avoid bleeding
Corneal thickness	Leave >250 μm of corneal bed untouched Hansatome plates (130, 160, 180, and 200 μm): flap thickness usually less than expected and even thinner on 2nd eye. If initial flap very thin, increase plate thickness on 2nd eye or use new blade *Caution:* If preoperative pachymetry <520, recommend intraoperative pachymetry of stromal bed. 160- or 180-μm plates most commonly used.
Surgical exposure	*Caution:* small fissure, tight lids, deep orbit, poor flap Consider one-piece microkeratome/nasal hinge Consider micro-ring (outer diameter 1 mm smaller) Consider stronger speculum or no speculum Consider flap creation with femtosecond laser
Dry eyes	Consider pre- or postoperative punctal plug insertion, tear supplement, topical cyclosporine. Superior hinge may be associated with increased dryness due to more severed corneal nerves. *Caution:* Avoid LASIK if surface cannot be stabilized.

partially cut and the microkeratome becomes jammed, do not reverse and then advance. This will result in an irregular flap. If drape, lid, or speculum is blocking the Hansatome pass, clearing the track or widening the speculum may allow the pass to continue. In this case it is safe to attempt to advance the microkeratome. If the Hansatome becomes jammed and will not reverse at the end of the pass, suction can be released and the unit lifted anteriorly and inferiorly. The unit should not be disassembled until the flap has been inspected, in case a free cap has occurred and the tissue is still in or on the Hansatome.

Bausch & Lomb Zyoptix XP Microkeratome

Bausch & Lomb will soon release a new microkeratome that may replace the Hansatome. The Zyoptix XP is being developed in order to reduce the variance seen between predicted and actual flap thickness. According to the manufacturer all externally exposed gears in the translation drive will be replaced by a

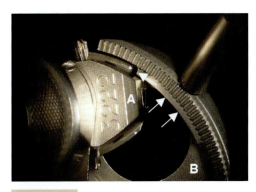

Figure 2.6

Hansatome assembly. The Hansatome **(A)** head and **(B)** ring. *Fat arrowheads* delineate the ring ledge just below the gear track. *Thin arrows* are on the dovetails of the microkeratome head. Where a thin arrow points to a fat arrow, the leading edge of the dovetail is aligned with the ring ledge. With this proper alignment the head will easily drop down on the pivot post and the dovetail will be able to pass beneath the ring ledge. (Courtesy of Robert Feder, M.D.)

"two-link" mechanism, and the suction ring will support this link mechanism. An easily changeable cutting head will be incorporated and component parts are designed for ease of assembly, interchangeability, and improved reliability. The device can be adjusted for the particular eye by flipping a lever to the right or left. A "new and improved" blade has been developed specifically for this microkeratome. Data provided by Bausch & Lomb (2005) for the 120-µm plate shows a mean flap thickness of 116.0 µm ± 16.1 µm with a range of 60 to 145 µm ($n = 50$).

Summary

In summary, the Hansatome is a convenient and reliable two-piece mechanical microkeratome that has stood the test of time. There is a relatively short learning curve for its operation, which can be reduced further by practicing in a wet-lab and by observing experienced surgeons. Certification is required prior to its use. Many variables can affect the thickness of the flaps obtained with this device. However, once a given surgeon becomes familiar with the flaps that are created by his or her hands for various situations, it can be used even more reliably. The surgeon is encouraged to routinely perform intraoperative pachymetry to be aware of the surprise thick or thin flap.

One-Piece Microkeratome (Nidek)

The Nidek Microkeratome Model MK-2000 (MK-2000) is an example of a one-piece microkeratome. The Amadeus microkeratome (AMO, Santa Ana, CA) is another example of this type of microkeratome. The MK-2000 has been approved for use in patients who have an average refractive power of the cornea >39 diopters or <48 diopters. As is the case with other available microkeratomes, the intraocular pressure must be 65 mmHg or higher in order to create a successful flap. Three different sized suction rings are available (8.5, 9.5, and 10.5 mm) and blade heads are available at 130, 160, and 180 µm. Assembly of the MK-2000 is performed prior to placement of the microkeratome in the surgical field. The blade is inspected under the microscope for any defects and rinsed free of any debris.

A unique safety feature of the MK-2000 is the wedged tip. After placement of the blade in the blade holder and oscillation of the blade holder are verified, a wedged tip is placed to secure the cover of the blade holder. This provides additional security for the blade holder. Tightening of the blade holder is done with a key, which ensures a standard corneal flap thickness. The blade holder is attached to the hand piece followed by the suction ring. Suction tubing is then connected to the hand piece. Numerous steps should be followed to ensure proper assembly, as listed in Table 2.3.

When the suction foot pedal is depressed, a long series of beeping sounds signals the building suction. The beeping sounds stop when the suction ring is sufficiently fixed to the cornea. The intraocular pressure is then verified with the handheld tonometer and a glycerin-based sterile tear solution is placed on the cornea. The forward foot pedal is depressed. The blade is advanced until it stops, the reverse pedal is depressed and the blade reverses. The suction foot pedal is depressed for a second time, the suction is released, and the unit is removed from the eye. The entire

Table 2.3	Checklist to verify proper assembly of the Nidek Microkeratome MK-2000

Verify tubing free of kinks or bends

Confirm the wedge tip is in place and tight

Depress forward foot pedal, visually confirm blade is oscillating and moving forward smoothly

Verify sound and oscillation felt in the handpiece

Visually inspect the gap between the blade and suction ring to ensure consistent width

Depress the reverse foot pedal to ensure smooth reverse movement of the blade

process takes 20 seconds or less. If suction cannot be achieved, several explanations are possible, as listed in Table 2.4.

A one-piece microkeratome system has several advantages. The most important among these is the decreased required suction time. In a two-piece mechanism, such as the Hansatome, suction is achieved prior to engaging the cutting mechanism, which must be assembled on the eye. This assembly adds to the suction time and the length of this time is dependent on the ability of the operator. However, the Hansatome may offer an advantage in the deep-set eye, because suction can be achieved with the suction ring and the eye can be displaced anteriorly or lifted up just prior to placement of the cutting mechanism. The Nidek microkeratome is easier to use than a two-piece microkeratome in patients with small palpebral fissures and tight lids. The

Table 2.4	Sources of suction failure with the Nidek Microkeratome MK-2000

Damage to the suction ring

Suction tubing not securely attached to the tube fittings

Bend or kink in the suction tubing

Residue clogging the suction tube

Clogging of the filter in the suction system

Nidek microkeratome 8.5-mm head is smaller than the Hansatome head of the same size, further facilitating placement in Asian patients and patients with smaller eyes. It has been demonstrated to have good reproducibility and can allow the surgeon to place the nasal hinge in an oblique fashion.

Numerous studies have been done to evaluate the mean flap thickness of the MK-2000. The actual mean flap thickness created with the MK-2000 is less than that stated on the plate. In a recent study, flap thickness accuracy among six microkeratome models was compared. This prospective multicenter study involved numerous surgeons. The microkeratomes studied included the AMO Amadeus, the Bausch & Lomb Hansatome, the Moria Carriazo-Barraquer, the Moria M2, the Nidek MK-2000, and the Alcon Summit Krumeich-Barraquer. Table 2.1 gives detailed information regarding numerous different microkeratomes. The contact information for each microkeratome is included along with the oscillation speed and translation speed. In most of the microkeratomes studied, the mean flap thickness was less than the actual plate thickness identified by the manufacturer. However, this was not the case for the Amadeus 130 plate, the Moria Carriazo-Barraquer 110 and 130 plates, and the Moria M2 130 plate. In each of these cases, the actual mean flap thickness was greater than that stated on the plate by the manufacturer.

Table 2.1 demonstrates the broad range of mean flap thickness and variability compared to plate thickness labeling from the manufacturer. This further emphasizes the need to be familiar with the flap thickness cut by a specific microkeratome on both the first and second eye. In all studies, it was found that when a single blade is used in a bilateral procedure, the flap cut in the second eye is thinner than the first flap. Solomon et al. further substantiated that thinner corneas are associated with thinner flaps and thicker corneas are associated with thicker flaps. They also found that first-cut eyes were associated with thicker flaps by about 6%. This study demonstrated that the Amadeus 140 and the Nidek MK-2000 had the lowest standard deviation of the most common devices. Knowing the flap thickness allows the surgeon to determine the safety of performing

LASIK by calculating the total depth of the flap cut and the laser ablation. This can also help the surgeon counsel the patient on the safety of retreatments should they be needed in the future.

Manual versus Automated Microkeratomes

Moria CB Manual Microkeratome

LASIK has developed into a reliable and reproducible procedure to correct ametropia, with the excimer laser machines capable of cutting incredibly precise patterns on the cornea. In contrast, the microkeratomes have demonstrated variability in the flap thickness they create between cases, between eyes in the same patient, and between microkeratome heads. Furthermore, the microkeratome heads are notoriously mislabeled by most companies, with the flap thickness created being only marginally related to the number on the microkeratome head.

Moria has developed several excellent microkeratomes with both manual and automated translation systems. The manual Moria Corriazo-Barraquer (Moria CB) microkeratome was one of the first pivoting microkeratomes allowing for superior-hinged LASIK flaps. It allows one to control the flap size according to the nomogram for suction ring selection, and flap thickness according to selection of the appropriate precalibrated microkeratome head.

The Moria CB microkeratome has several advantages over some of its competitors. The low-profile, small-diameter suction ring can fit in patients with small lid fissures. The microkeratome head fits in a protected dovetail groove, rather than having exposed gears. Thus, once the head is engaged in its groove, nothing can jam the gears or prevent the full excursion of the head in creating the flap. The preassembled blades can only be inserted one way—the correct way—in the microkeratome head, thus preventing improper insertion. The blade oscillates at 15,000 rpm, creating a smoother stromal bed than many of its competitors. Setup is fast and simple, and the same for both eyes, thus eliminating another potential source of error.

Certain safety features complement this unit. There is little risk for confusion with the foot pedals, because there is one pedal for vacuum and one for blade oscillation. The vacuum unit contains two pumps. One pump acts as the backup and will take over instantaneously if the first pump fails. The machine operates only when disconnected from the power supply or the electrical outlet. A rechargeable battery backup provides the power for normal operation of the microkeratome; hence, there is no problem with loss of external power, as may occur with a power outage. Like most microkeratomes, a Barraquer applanation tonometer is included for checking the IOP after applying the vacuum ring, but before beginning the microkeratome pass, to ensure adequate suction.

The Moria CB microkeratome provides flexibility in designing the flap. The location of the flap hinge can be varied for the full 360 degrees simply by placement of the suction ring. The hinge will be located in the quadrant where the suction ring post is located.

One can select a flap diameter by varying the suction ring size (-1, 0, $+1$, $+2$, or H). The higher the ring number, the thicker the ring. A thicker ring allows less corneal tissue to protrude and be cut by the microkeratome, once adequate suction has been obtained. The steeper the cornea, the more tissue would naturally protrude through the ring; therefore, a higher suction ring size would be selected to compensate for this. Refer to the Moria nomogram, which relates corneal steepness to the suction ring size, given in Table 2.5. The H-ring is designed for hyperopia and creates a flap diameter greater than 10 mm, which can be useful for hyperopic LASIK where the ablation zone may approach 10 mm and an adequate stromal bed is necessary. An applanation lens with diameter markings can be temporarily placed on the cornea prior to the microkeratome pass in order to predict the flap diameter.

The flap thickness can be varied by selection of the appropriate sized microkeratome head. The higher the head number, the thicker the associated plate, and the thicker the flap will be. In addition, the flap thickness can be affected by the translation speed of the microkeratome pass. The faster the pass, the thinner

Table 2.5	Moria CB microkeratome nomogram

Desired Flap Diameter (mm)	$K \leq 39\,D$	$39\,D < K \leq 41\,D$	$41\,D < K \leq 43\,D$	$43\,D < K \leq 46\,D$	$46\,D < K$
8.0	0	+1	+2		
8.5	−1	0	+1	+2	
9.0		−1	0	+1	+2
9.5	H		−1	0	+1
10.0		H		−1	0
10.5			H		−1
11.0				H	

Notes: For corneas <11.0 mm in diameter, optical zone size will increase by 0.25 mm; for corneas greater than 11.5 in diameter, optical zone size will decrease by 0.25 mm.
Verify optical zone with applanator lens; be aware of the large flap diameters created with the H ring. These are suggested combinations only. Appropriate ring selections may vary with individual patients.

the flap that is created. In contrast to an automated microkeratome, the speed of the pass can be modulated with this manual device. Culbertson studied the effect of translation speed on flap thickness and the results are summarized in Table 2.6. Flap thickness is also affected by the sharpness of the microkeratome blade. Studies have shown that flaps in the first eye treated are usually thicker than flaps in the second eye. The blade is sharper for the first eye, and cuts a thicker flap, or conversely, a duller blade cuts a thinner flap. Finally, flap thickness will vary depending on whether the cornea is thin or thick preoperatively. Using the 130-μm head, Culbertson (Culbertson et al., 2002 ISRS meeting, *unpublished data*) demonstrated that corneas thicker than 620 μm had a mean flap thickness of 190 μm, whereas corneas thinner than 480 μm had a mean thickness of 126 μm.

The Moria CB microkeratome has a unique low-vacuum setting, which provides additional options in selected cases. After creation of the flap using the standard high-vacuum setting, it is reset to a low vacuum, allowing the suction ring to remain attached to the globe at a much safer level of IOP. The ring can be used to control the globe position and allow alignment of the axis of astigmatism, or hold the globe steady in a poorly cooperative patient or one with nystagmus. The low-vacuum setting can also be used to control limbal bleeding in cases with large flaps.

The Moria CB microkeratome also has several disadvantages. The microkeratome heads are labeled as 110, 130, or 150 μm, but in actuality the flaps cut are commonly thicker. The 110-μm head cuts about a 140-μm flap, the 130-μm head cuts about a 160-μm flap, and the 150-μm head cuts about

Table 2.6	Effect of translation speed on flap thickness for the Moria CB with a 130-μm head

	Speed of Translation (s)	Mean Flap Thickness (μm)	Range of Flap Thickness (μm)
Regular pass	2.5−3.8	158	109−201
Fast pass	1.5	132	110−145
Slow pass	5.9	174	162−193

Source: From Culbertson et al., 2002, ISRS meeting, *unpublished data* for 130 eyes from 65 patients, with permission.

a 180-μm flap. This is in contrast to the Hansatome heads, which usually create flaps thinner than the label on the head (e.g., the 160-μm head cuts around a 130-μm flap). For a comparison of the Moria CB to other commonly used microkeratomes, refer to Table 2.1. Several recent studies have demonstrated that the 130-μm head cuts with a great deal of variability with flap thicknesses ranging from 109 to 201 μm. When one is trying to calculate the residual stromal thickness (RST) during the preoperative evaluation, one must assume some consistent flap thickness in the calculations. If the flap thickness truly varies to such a great extent, it is difficult to be certain that there will be adequate RST. Several studies have shown that most CB microkeratome heads create relatively consistent flap thicknesses, even though there is such variability between similarly labeled heads, so it is important to create a unique nomogram with mean flap thickness for each individual microkeratome head.

The ability to vary the translation speed with the manual CB microkeratome is an advantage when trying to modify the flap thickness from the expected thickness. However, it can be difficult to control for the variability in translation speed from case to case because manual operation cannot be as consistent as an automated machine.

Another disadvantage of the Moria CB microkeratome is its high profile—its suction tubing and wires extend vertically from the top of the microkeratome and come very close to the microscope optics on the VISX S4 excimer laser.

Moria M2 Automated Microkeratome

The Moria M2 automated microkeratome has a compact, ergonomic design and offers options for altering the flap thickness, flap diameter, and hinge chord length. It offers many of the same advantages as the manually operated CB microkeratome, with the added benefit of automated translation for a more consistent microkeratome pass.

The advantages of the Moria M2 automated microkeratome include the low profile, which easily fits underneath the microscope on the laser. The small-diameter suction rings can fit in patients with small lid fissures and deep orbits. There are no gears. The M2 loads easily on its mounting post and is secured in place using a locking ring, rather than a dovetail design.

One particularly attractive feature for many surgeons is the ability to work with both hands once suction is applied. One hand can be used to stabilize the suction ring and the other to clear the speculum and lid out of the way.

The Moria M2 microkeratome possesses two motors, one for blade oscillation and one for translation of the cutting head. The blade oscillates at 15,000 rpm creating very smooth stromal beds. The translation motor is equally powerful and generates smooth cuts within 4 seconds without any deterioration in cutting quality or speed, even when working with irregular corneas. Having two motors also allows for reverse translation without blade oscillation.

Like the CB microkeratome, the Moria M2 also utilizes two vacuum pumps, so the backup pump will automatically and instantaneously take over if the first pump fails. The M2 utilizes the same vacuum unit as the CB, thus it also offers a low-vacuum setting for axis alignment of the globe, control of the globe during laser ablation, and the ability to decrease limbal bleeding with larger flaps.

A customized keratectomy is possible through control of flap thickness, flap diameter, hinge width, and hinge location. The flap thickness is controlled by selection of the microkeratome head. The 110 head cuts about 140 μm, while the 130 head cuts about 160 μm. Refer to Table 2.1 to compare the M2 with other microkeratomes. The automatic translation provides two constant and reproducible translation speeds, the slower 3.1-second pass and the faster 2.1-second pass. The option of greatly varying translation speed to affect flap thickness, which is possible with a manual microkeratome, is less versatile with this device.

The flap diameter can be varied by selection of the appropriate suction ring size (−1, 0, +1, +2) (Table 2.7). The higher the ring number, the thicker the ring base, the less the cornea will protrude and be applanated, and thus the smaller the diameter of the flap created. Three different stop positions enable the surgeon to modify the hinge size and the size of the bed for ablation. The ability to customize hinge size may be particularly helpful

summary of the advantages and disadvantages of the femtosecond laser.)

Because the creation of an adequately sized flap with the laser is less dependent on corneal curvature than with mechanical microkeratomes, patients who would be at higher risk of a small free cap or buttonhole on the basis of curvature may be femtosecond laser candidates. Flat or steep, LASIK patients should have a regular corneal contour. In addition, the laser can be used to create more consistent, thinner flaps than can be made with blade microkeratomes. This conclusion is based on an unpublished consecutive series of 100 Intralase flaps in which the variance from attempted to achieved flap thickness was on average 20 μm. This is in contrast to the Amadeus microkeratome in which a variance of flap thickness of more than 40 μm was experienced. The tighter variance between expected and actual flap thickness may allow patients with relatively thin corneas or highly myopic patients to undergo the procedure. Intraoperative pachymetry is still essential prior to excimer ablation to ensure adequate RST. Finally, patients with smaller corneas can be treated with less risk of invading the sclera, because of the ability to better adjust flap diameter.

The surgeon has control of many of the parameters of the flap, the most important being thickness, diameter, hinge location, hinge angle, and side cut angle. The power of each spot can be adjusted and must be specifically set for each individual laser. The spot separation and line separation can also be adjusted. Once power settings and spot separation are at desirable levels, they are usually not adjusted for each patient.

Most refractive surgeons agree that the femtosecond laser can create a LASIK flap more safely than with a microkeratome. The risk of epithelial defects and free caps is far less than with a blade microkeratome. The ability to alter flap parameters just prior to the laser ablation of the cornea has reduced other complicated situations such as inadequate centration and hemorrhage from inadvertent cutting of limbal vessels.

The eye pressure is not elevated as greatly with the IntraLase suction ring so, in theory, there is less potential for optic nerve damage.

This advantage should be tempered by the fact that the Intralase suction ring must be in place for a longer duration, usually 60 to 90 seconds. Most blade microkeratomes create thinner flaps on the second eye when the same blade is used for both eyes. They also create thinner flaps in thinner corneas and thicker flaps in thicker corneas. This is not the case with the femtosecond laser. The 60- to 70-degree angle on the side cut theoretically may make the flap more resistant to displacement soon after surgery. The flap is definitely more resistant to displacement 1 year after surgery; in fact, it may be difficult to lift the flap for retreatment.

Technique

As with any surgical procedure, there is a learning curve associated with using the IntraLase. With some practice, the techniques involved are easy to master. It is certainly easier for the scrub technician to operate the laser and handle the disposables than to assemble and maintain a blade microkeratome.

Some surgeons recommend pretreating patients with topical steroids for several days prior to surgery to reduce the postoperative risk of diffuse lamellar keratitis (DLK). However, if DLK is a problem, paying careful attention to reducing power settings for the flap and the edge is essential. A small dose of a minor tranquilizer (e.g., 5 mg of diazepam) is given preoperatively to reduce anxiety. A drop of chilled naphazoline instilled preoperatively will reduce the risk of associated subconjunctival hemorrhage caused by the suction ring. This is strongly recommended and should be done on every case.

The patient is placed in the supine position on a laser chair with a three-axis adjustment, if possible. The chair and the laser should be centered to allow for the full range of motion that might be necessary for a successful ablation. Surgeons vary with regard to which eye is routinely treated first, the dominant, the nondominant, or the same eye each time. The fellow eye is covered to avoid diplopia or confusion by the patient in terms of which light to observe. Sterile, chilled buffered proparacaine is applied to the cornea. Some surgeons instill a drop of topical fluoroquinolone or a drop of prednisolone 1%. The lashes are also draped to aid in exposure

2

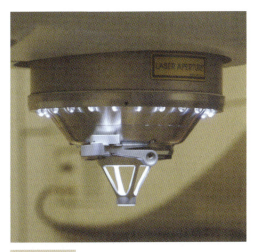

Figure 2.7

IntraLase with cone attached. (Courtesy of Robert Feder, M.D.)

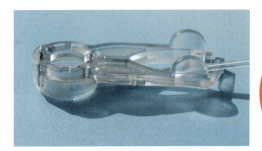

Figure 2.8

IntraLase suction ring. (Courtesy of Robert Feder, M.D.)

and lessen the chance of contamination, although the risk of contamination is extremely low and some surgeons do not drape the lashes until the flap is lifted. The suction ring can be inserted and used without lid speculae.

The laser cone (Fig. 2.7) is examined and the applanating lens should be inspected under the laser microscope to identify any debris or faults that could adversely affect the ablation of the cornea. The patient is then brought underneath the laser microscope and the head is adjusted to allow for equal exposure of the superior and inferior bulbar conjunctiva. The ideal amount of chin elevation is sometimes achieved by instructing the patient to make a fist and place it under the chin. Some surgeons find it useful to mark the pupil center. A 3-mm optical zone marker can be used for this purpose; however, if too much dye is placed on the marker, a circular pattern may be etched into the stromal bed.

The suction ring (Fig. 2.8) is a manually operated, syringe-controlled device. The increase in IOP associated with its use is generally less than the pressure achieved with the pump-controlled suction devices used with microkeratomes. It is inspected to make sure it is in good working order. The ring is placed on the eye and centered on the pupil. Hash marks on the ring are useful in confirming

good pupil centration. It is difficult to compensate for inadequate ring centration during the docking process, so it pays to complete this step properly. Slight superior decentration ensures that the hinge will be located peripherally and will not affect the docking process adversely. Suction is applied by releasing the depressed syringe. It is important to observe the eye during this process in order to detect globe rotation, which can occur during suction application. The consequence of undetected rotation would be a decentered flap. If globe rotation occurs, suction should be released and the ring reapplied to compensate for an expected rotation. Once the ring has been successfully applied, it is helpful to rotate the patient's head and adjust the chin height so that the iris plane is parallel with the floor and the patient's nose will not interfere with the successful docking of the laser applanating lens through the ring to the cornea. It is also important to be certain there is no pool of tears or anesthetic within the ring prior to the docking procedure. Fluid within the ring can interfere with proper applanation and result in an uneven ablation. A sponge can be used to remove fluid if detected.

The surgeon gently squeezes the handle on the suction ring, which increases the diameter of the ring aperture. This allows the ring to accommodate the applanating lens as the lens is slowly lowered down along the Z-axis during the docking procedure (Fig. 2.9). Observing the video display during the docking process will help confirm that centration is

2

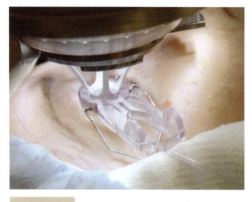

Figure 2.9

Docking of IntraLase cone with suction ring positioned on the eye. (Courtesy of Robert Feder, M.D.)

the pupil to dilate widely, so some surgeons prefer not to use the pupil as a reference.

If the applanation pressure is light, dark areas may be seen within the normally white ablation pattern. This does not seem to cause a detectable irregularity of the ablation or difficulty lifting the flap. In addition to the flap, the laser creates a pocket near the hinge to allow the waste materials, namely carbon dioxide and water, to vent. However, if the applanation pressure is excessive, the waste material will accumulate, creating an opacified bubble layer (OBL) (Fig. 2.10A). Some surgeons have experienced difficulty lifting the flap in areas of OBL. Extensive OBL also may interfere with the laser-tracking device. Some

ideal. Newer rings have a self-locking mechanism to allow for easy passage. As the cornea is applanated, the ring needs to stay parallel to the eye to avoid a break in suction. Likewise, the diameter of the flap may be reduced if the ring does not remain parallel. It is helpful to carefully support the ring by the handle as the lens is entering the ring. Once the cornea is properly applanated, the ring is gently lifted up and the handle is released. This reduces the ring aperture, allowing it to securely grip the lens in position. If the centration is not perfect or if some excessive meniscus is detected, a subtle tilt of the ring as the handle is released can help. If applanation or centration is poor, the handle should again be squeezed to release the lens and the lens should be elevated and the docking process repeated. It is possible for epithelial defects to occur if there is excessive manipulation of the lens on the cornea. The FEMTEC laser has a curved patient interface that does not applanate the cornea.

Complete applanation of the cornea must be achieved with the Intralase, or an incomplete flap or side cut may occur. A small meniscus of nonapplanated cornea outside the flap is desirable. After successful applanation, the outline of the flap will appear on the viewing monitor of the laser. Slight decentration can be corrected using the arrow keys on the laser keyboard; however, the diameter of the flap will be decreased as the degree of adjustment increases. It is not uncommon for

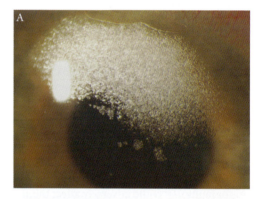

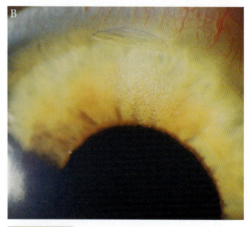

Figure 2.10

A: Opacified bubble layer noted immediately after creating a flap with the femtosecond laser. **B:** OBL dissipates after 20 to 30 minutes. (Courtesy of Robert Feder, M.D.)

surgeons will brush OBL to the periphery; others will laser directly through the opacity. Opinions vary with regard to whether the excimer treatment should occur immediately following the creation of the flap or, alternatively, after a waiting period has allowed the waste products within the cornea to dissipate (Fig. 2.10B).

The 30-kHz laser ablation takes about 30 seconds and can be observed through the microscope or on the video display, ensuring there is no loss of suction during the treatment and that the ablation is complete. After successful creation of the side cut, the suction ring is released. The second eye is treated in an identical manner. If loss of suction occurs, the laser should be stopped immediately by releasing the laser foot pedal. Because the suction ring is a manual device, independent from the laser, a loss of suction will not stop the ablation. A loss of applanation and movement of the eye are easily identifiable signs of a suction break. Loss of suction during flap creation can occur either when the raster pattern is being created or when the side cut is made. Assuming suction can be regained, the surgeon can retreat immediately, at the same depth. If this occurs it is important to use the same applanating lens to ensure that ablation will occur at the same depth. This is a significant advantage of the Intralase over the blade microkeratome.

Another advantage of the Intralase is the flexibility of hinge width and placement. The superior hinge may be associated with less flap displacement. Side cut angle, flap diameter, and the energy settings for both the flap and the side cut can be adjusted. It is worthwhile to initially follow the manufacturer's recommendations given during the installation and certification process. Adjustments and modifications can be done incrementally at a later time.

Prior to lifting the flap reference marks are placed in order to aid in flap realignment following the excimer ablation. Lifting the flap requires care and patience. The patient is positioned under the excimer laser, the eyelids are draped, and the speculum inserted. A Sinsky hook or Lehman IntraLase spatula with a semisharp edge (Asico AE 28275) (Fig. 2.11) is used to start the lift, for about a millimeter under the flap and for about

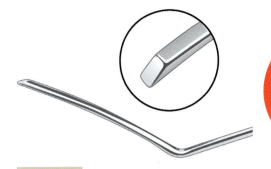

Figure 2.11

Lehman Intralase spatula with a semisharp edge.

1 clock hour. There may be some variance in the side cut, especially if it was near an area of nonablated tissue. This may result in the side cut not being complete. In this case an alternate area should be chosen to start the lift. The surgeon must watch to ensure that he or she is in fact in the lamellar plane and not simply lifting up an edge of epithelium. If the surgeon finds inconsistent or incomplete side cuts on several consecutive cases, the side cut energy should be increased by 0.1 or 0.2 mJ. Increased side cut energy may be associated with increased postoperative inflammation.

An alternative way to begin the flap lift is to score the side cut incision for a few millimeters on either side of the hinge. The spatula is inserted from the scored incision on one side across the flap, sweeping peripherally to ensure the interface is connected with the pocket superiorly, and the flap is dissected all the way to the hinge (Fig. 2.12A). The spatula then exits through the scored area on the other side.

The blunt spatula is then used to separate the flap from the underlying stroma (Figs. 2.12B and C). With the 15-kHz laser, there can be significant variation in the ease of dissection within different areas of the same cornea and from patient to patient. The 30-kHz laser is fast enough to allow a larger number of smaller spots, which greatly facilitates flap dissection. With the standard laser some surgeons find that younger patients and patients with brown irides may have flaps that are more difficult to lift. The spatula should be swept from the superior hinge in the inferior direction with no more than a third to half of

2

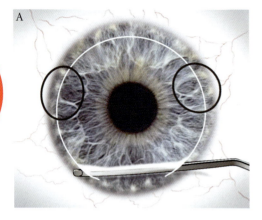

A

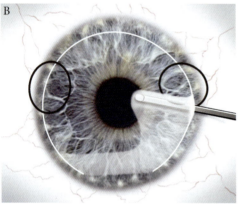

B

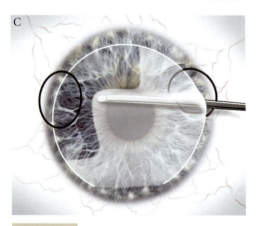

C

Figure 2.12

Flap lift technique following femtosecond laser application. **A:** After scoring the flap edge near the hinge on either side, a spatula is passed across the flap. **B:** The interface is separated by starting at the superior hinge and sweeping inferiorly. **C:** Dissecting one third of the flap at a time reduces the risk of tearing the hinge.

the flap being dissected at a time. Following the contour of the cornea, that is, uphill superiorly and downhill inferiorly, is a pearl that helps to simplify the dissection. Being overly aggressive, for example, trying to lift the flap in one broad sweep, may result in a tear in the flap or a free cap. If an area is difficult to lift, multiple small sweeps can dissect the peripheral aspect of the area until ultimately the entire portion of the flap has been separated. It is important to avoid excessive force. If a second laser pass was performed after an incomplete ablation, it may be better to start the dissection inferiorly. This will help establish the flap separation at the correct depth.

If a tear in the flap edge occurs, a bandage lens should be placed on the cornea until the epithelium has healed. In addition, a buttonhole in the flap may also occur during dissection if a small area of stroma is not ablated. Buttonholes may also occur in areas of previous corneal foreign body scars. In these cases the scar may represent a thinner area of stroma that has been filled in by an epithelial plug. During creation of the raster pattern, if one observes what appears to be a micro suction break with a small bubble, great care must be taken when lifting the flap in this area.

If the flap edge is near the limbus, an OBL pattern may be seen in the nonablated cornea; this is generally of little consequence. Venting of waste materials peripherally is actually advantageous because the interface is protected and these materials will not impact the excimer ablation. Hemorrhage from lasering through peripheral neovascularization is much less of a problem with the IntraLase than with blade microkeratomes. The laser effect seems to effectively control the bleeding. Another consequence of a peripheral flap edge is the movement of a gas bubble into the anterior chamber. This rare event is likely due to waste gas entering the eye through the canal of Schlemm and the trabecular meshwork. Depending on the size of the bubbles and the type of laser, tracking the pupil may be difficult. The bubbles will dissipate over several hours and the problem will not be of consequence.

After the flap is completely retracted, the remainder of the treatment proceeds in the usual fashion. In general, the flaps created with the 15- or 30-kHz lasers are quite smooth. After surgery the corneas should be checked for flap alignment, striae, and interface debris. If any of these are detected, the problem should be immediately corrected. Postoperatively, the care of the eye is essentially the same as in blade LASIK, although occasionally there is a phenomenon known as side cut haze, which may require several weeks of additional topical steroid treatment.

A superior hinge is an ideal location for flaps. On the first day postoperative visit flap slips with a nasal hinge occur, and a temporal hinge appears to offer questionable advantage in terms of reducing the incidence of post-LASIK dry eyes. Using the IntraLase to make the corneal flap exposes the patient to the same short-term and long-term risks that go with traditional LASIK.

Further Considerations of the Femtosecond Laser

The advantages and disadvantages of this laser are summarized in Table 2.9. The use of the IntraLase for flap creation involves acquiring the skills for docking and flap dissection. The learning curve is no steeper than that for a traditional microkeratome. Discussion and observation with experienced surgeons can be quite helpful in making a smooth transition to the femtosecond laser.

Diffuse lamellar keratitis is a greater postoperative risk with IntraLase than with blade microkeratomes, particularly during a surgeon's initial cases. This often occurs near the flap edge and is often related to excessive laser energy for the raster ablation and side cut. When the energies are appropriately adjusted, the incidence of DLK decreases dramatically. Some surgeons pretreat with topical steroid drops or alternatively use topical steroids more aggressively in the postoperative period.

The IntraLase procedure is more costly than creating a flap with a blade microkeratome. There is the cost of the laser as well as the cost of the single-use applanating lens and suction ring. Case duration is also increased significantly. This is particularly true if the excimer procedure does not immediately follow the IntraLase procedure. With experience the duration of the average case decreases.

The incidences of free cap, inadequately small flap, marked decentration, and buttonhole are much reduced with the IntraLase. Microstriae still occur and are relatively easy to treat provided there is early intervention.

There have been scattered case reports of delayed photosensitivity weeks after an uneventful treatment. Patient's visual acuity remains good, slit-lamp appearance of the flap remains normal, and the condition generally responds to a short course of topical steroids. This syndrome has been referred to as GAPP (good acuity plus photosensitivity) or TLS (transient light sensitivity).

Centration on the visual axis may on occasion be less than ideal, but it is quite rare to abort a case because of a severely decentered flap. Bleeding from the flap edge is less of a problem than with a blade microkeratome and usually does not prevent treatment. These cases might benefit from a slightly longer course of steroids postoperatively.

Incomplete ablation can occur with loss of suction or if there is an undetected fluid meniscus. In general the ablation can be repeated once suction is restored, provided the same applanating lens is used. If the side cut is not complete in an area, Vannas scissors or a Beaver blade should be available in the laser suite to complete the flap.

Finally, after many months IntraLase flaps can be more difficult to lift than a microkeratome flap. Certainly, some flaps will lift more easily than others and there are some even a few months after surgery that are difficult to lift. But this is a challenge that should be explained to the patient preoperatively. Despite these potential shortcomings, the femtosecond laser for flap creation represents a significant advance in the safety of LASIK surgery and has the potential to widen the patient selection criteria.

THE EXCIMER LASERS

From the early days of photorefractive surgery excimer laser systems have undergone continuous improvement. Active tracking and more sophisticated laser delivery systems have enabled surgeons to employ customized treatments based on wavefront technology. Although it is beyond the scope of this handbook to cover every laser available, four representative laser systems are presented. A contributing author with a wealth of experience using a particular laser will discuss that laser system. If available, both conventional and custom treatments on each system are reviewed. The emphasis is to provide the reader with clinical pearls based on experience rather than to recreate a user's manual or a substitute for a certification course. This is an educational supplement meant to provide basic information and assistance to the reader in preparation for the LASIK case section of the handbook. Readers can learn about each of the laser systems or focus on the material relevant to the available equipment.

The Bausch & Lomb Technolas Platform

The Bausch & Lomb Technolas system is capable of conventional LASIK with the PlanoScan software, as well as wavefront-guided LASIK using the Technolas 217z Zyoptix System for personalized laser vision correction. The FDA-approved treatment ranges are listed in Table 2.10. This can be found on page 55.

PlanoScan for Conventional LASIK

A key feature of the conventional PlanoScan software is its customizable optical zone, with an additional blend zone that extends the diameter of the central optical zone by a total of 3 mm. Unlike the VISX system, which allows the user the option of selecting either a small zone (6.0 mm) or a large zone (6.5 mm) with an optional blend zone (only the final −1.00 D of treatment is applied to the 8-mm optical zone), the blend on the Technolas PlanoScan system is automatically built-in, and it extends the radius of the treatment by 1.5 mm (or the overall diameter by 3 mm). For this reason, unwanted nighttime visual symptoms with conventional PlanoScan are minimal. The incidence of subjective night vision symptoms with this system compares favorably with custom treatments using other excimer lasers. Typically, a 6.0-mm optical zone provides a total ablation of 9.0 × 9.0 mm for spherical corrections, and even larger ablations for cylindrical corrections, in which the Technolas maintains the minor axis of the ellipse and

extends the major axis. This is in contrast to other systems, which decrease the minor axis to create the elliptical ablation. The enlarged optical zone does come at the expense of a deeper ablation, so caution must be used when performing LASIK in patients with large corrections or relatively thin corneas. In general, the ablation depth for the Technolas laser is approximately 15 μm/diopter at a 6.0-mm optical zone, and ranges from 10 μm/diopter at a 4.5-mm optical zone to 25 μm/diopter at a 7.0-mm optical zone.

The Technolas PlanoScan platform can provide refractive accuracy without nomogram adjustment provided the operating room conditions are stable and the surgeon monitors surgical outcomes to verify results are consistent with intended corrections. In general, treat younger patients based on the manifest refraction, provided that the cycloplegic refraction is within 0.50 D. If the cycloplegic refraction is significantly different from the manifest, then a postcycloplegic refraction is recommended. For patients who are older than 40 years of age, treat using the cycloplegic refraction, especially if there is a difference of 0.50 D or greater from the manifest refraction. For patients between 21 and 30 years of age, aim for a target postoperative refraction of +0.50 D. Of course, this plan depends greatly on surgical technique and operating room conditions. In cases of unusually low humidity or prolonged ablation times, overcorrections may occur.

Custom LASIK Introduction

The Technolas 217z Zyoptix System for personalized laser vision correction consists of three components: (1) the Zywave Diagnostic Workstation, incorporating the Orbscan IIz and Zywave II, (2) the Zylink software, and (3) the Technolas 217z excimer laser. Wavefront-guided, "custom" treatments may be performed for myopic corrections up to −7.00 D sphere and astigmatic corrections up to −3.00 D with a spherical equivalent ≤ −7.50 D at the spectacle plane. The Zyoptix system is not currently approved for treatment of mixed astigmatism, hyperopia, or hyperopic astigmatism. For corrections beyond the approved range, the conventional PlanoScan software may provide an option.

The Zywave II aberrometer is indicated for measuring, recording, analyzing, and displaying visual aberrations; for example, myopia, hyperopia, astigmatism, coma, and spherical aberration. It assists in prescribing refractive corrections, for example, by exporting wavefront data and other types of patient-specific data to a compatible refractive laser indicated for wavefront-guided treatments. The Zywave II aberrometer measures the complete optical system with the use of an advanced wavefront sensor based on the Hartmann-Shack principle. The surgeon receives highly detailed wavefront information about the way in which light reflected from the patient's eye is unevenly scattered, thereby affecting the quality of vision.

The Hartmann-Shack Principle

The Zywave II projects low-intensity HeNe infrared light into the eye (Fig. 2.13A) and captures the diffuse reflection from the retina. The reflected light is focused by a Lenslet array and displayed by a CCD camera (Fig. 2.13B). The captured image is known as the *centroid picture*. An aberrated eye will show the white dots with different intensities and patterns, indicating deviation of the wavefront (Fig. 2.13C). The deviations are calculated based on the image captured by the CCD camera, and the actual wavefront pattern is shown graphically in color-coded maps (Figs. 2.14A and B).

Wavefront-Guided Treatment

It is important that patients discontinue contact lens wear prior to the Zywave evaluation. Soft contact lenses should be discontinued for at least 2 weeks and rigid lenses for at least 3–4 weeks until refraction and topography are normal and stable. In planning custom or wavefront-guided Zyoptix treatments, it is important that the pupil size at the time of wavefront measurement be at least as large as the planned optical zone size. In this situation, the undilated Zywave examination can be used for calculating the Zyoptix treatment. However, in many cases, pharmacological dilation of the pupil will be required to meet this requirement. This is in sharp contrast to the VISX WaveScan system in which pharmacological

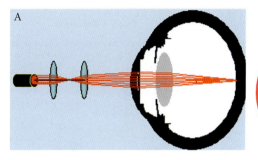

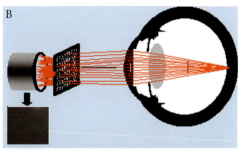

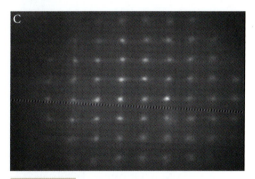

Figure 2.13

Hartmann-Shack principle. **A:** Low-intensity HeNe infrared light is projected into the eye and captures the diffuse reflection from the retina. **B:** The reflected light is focused by a Lenslet array and displayed by a CCD camera. **C:** An aberrated eye will show the white dots with different intensities and patterns indicating wavefront aberration. (Courtesy Bausch & Lomb.)

dilation to achieve wavefront data should be avoided. When capturing the Zywave measurement, pharmacological dilations should be performed using a standardized protocol, so that it produces a round and centered pupil relative to the undilated pupil. Cycloplegia is not required, and should actually be avoided. The recommended regimen is to instill phenylephrine 2.5% and capture the

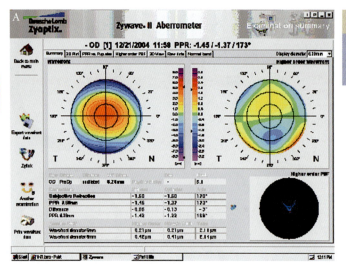

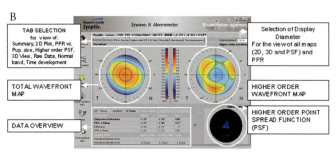

Figure 2.14

A, B: Zywave II aberrometer color-coded maps. (Courtesy Bausch & Lomb.)

wavefront within 10 to 15 minutes in order to minimize the effect of cycloplegia on the wavefront examination. Of course, factors such as patient age, iris color, and undilated mesopic pupil size will impact the dilation regimen. It is important to use the same lighting conditions for each Zywave examination, preferably in the dark, in order to obtain maximal dilation. A minimum of one undilated examination and one dilated examination should be performed if the conditions for treatment based on the undilated examination are not satisfied. If patients are being treated on the same day as the Zywave examination, and need to be dilated, a minimum waiting time of 4 hours is recommended, and the pupil should be ≤7 mm in diameter.

Once the Zywave wavefront measurements and Orbscan data have been collected, the Zylink software is then used to adjust the data based on the surgeon's preference. The subjective refraction (manifest or cycloplegic) should be compared with the predicted phoropter refraction (PPR). The PPR is an estimate of the wavefront, and is not used for treatment. The treatment is based directly on the wavefront. If the difference between the subjective refraction and the PPR is greater than or equal to 0.75 D (sphere), 0.5 D (cylinder), or 15 degrees (axis), the Zywave will give a warning (exclamation point adjacent to the refraction in the Zywave printout). This is for informational purposes only; the software will still allow the user to perform the ablation. In the Zylink software, the surgeon can select an adjustment factor, based on an individual nomogram. The initial nomogram adjustment for new Zyoptix users is to decrease the spherical component by 10% (i.e., enter 90% in the "Sph %" field in the Zylink software). The cylindrical component cannot be adjusted.

Each surgeon should carefully examine his own results, and individualize the nomogram. Bausch & Lomb will assist with the collection and analysis of the first 20 cases with 1 to 3 months of follow-up. Within the

Zylink software, the surgeon also must select the optical zone for the Zyoptix treatment. The ideal optical zone size is selected based on the patient's mesopic pupil. Bausch & Lomb recommends that the optical zone be 0.2 to 0.5 mm larger than the mesopic pupil size, or a minimum of 6.0 mm, whichever is larger. Corneal thickness or maximum allowable optic zone size in the Zyoptix software may constrain this recommendation. If the surgeon wishes to use a fixed optical zone for all Zyoptix patients, a 6.5-mm optical zone may be used, based on the clinical results reported from the Zyoptix FDA study.

An important component to any wavefront-guided ablation is the ability to place the laser pulses precisely in the location desired. This is accomplished by registration, in which points in the laser correspond to the same points on the eye, and by the use of a tracking system. While active cyclotorsional tracking is currently unavailable, cyclotorsional registration is available on the VISX STAR S4. It enables the laser to make a single rotational adjustment prior to the ablation. Currently, Bausch & Lomb does not have iris registration software. Until that technology is made available, it is important to mark the 3 and 9 o'clock limbus in the upright position (marking the patient was described on page 21), and then position the patient's head so that the 180° meridian corresponds to the horizontal axis of the reticle visible through the right ocular of the microscope.

The reticle itself must be aligned with the laser appropriately, and the surgeon performs that quite easily prior to the beginning of the Zyoptix case. First, the pupillary diameter (PD) on the microscope must be set to the surgeon's preference. This is critical because changing the PD on the microscope will cause rotation of the reticle. Once the oculars are set, pressing the F5 button on the keyboard will cause the tracking light, the center of the three light switches on the console, to move from the center of the reticle to a position that is horizontal to the center.

Toggling the F5 button will cause the light to alternate positions. The imaginary axis formed by the alternating light is the true 180-degree meridian, and the reticle in the right ocular of the microscope should be rotated so that its horizontal reference line matches the true horizontal axis of the laser.

When F5 is pressed the red light will move to the 9 o'clock position. The imaginary line between the primary and secondary positions of the red dot should correspond to the alignment of the reticle. If the reticle is not so aligned, the ocular may be rotated in order to accomplish this.

The second component of accurate registration is the ability to track the eye movements so that each laser pulse is placed precisely at the correct location on the cornea. The Technolas 217 active eye tracker consists of an infrared imaging camera system capturing the geometric center of the undilated pupil at a sampling rate of 120 Hz plus a scanning system to respond and compensate to any pupil movement found by the camera within 2.4 ms. The active tracking range is defined as a deviation of 1.5 mm from original fixation. Within this active range the laser adjusts the excimer pulses to the intended location according to the pupil position; however, if the eye moves outside this range, the laser will interrupt the treatment. To account for very fast eye movements (e.g., sudden loss of fixation), a dynamic tracking module recognizes the speed of eye movements by calculating positional changes of the center of the pupil between pictures captured by the eye tracker's video camera system. If the eye speed exceeds a clinically significant value, the eye tracker software simply interrupts the pulsing until the eye stabilizes again. In the Bausch & Lomb system, the surgeon defines the treatment center according to pupil reference, always having full visual control throughout the entire treatment, and this should be done prior to each ablation. This is accomplished by manually adjusting the treatment center using the keypad. The surgeon can also modify the treatment center at any time, although this is usually unnecessary once the treatment has begun.

For more information on the Bausch & Lomb Zyoptix platform, contact information can be found on page 268.

VISX STAR S4 Platform

The VISX STAR S4 laser platform with ActiveTrak can be used to perform conventional LASIK as well as custom surgery. CustomVue LASIK with this laser requires the use of the WaveScan, a separate device used to acquire and analyze wavefront images and allow the surgeon to design an appropriate custom treatment profile. These data are then transferred to the laser. Conventional and custom treatment will each be discussed.

Conventional LASIK

The purpose of this section is to discuss conventional LASIK with the VISX STAR S4 laser. Generic comments using the excimer laser to perform LASIK surgery are found in the basic LASIK chapter (Chapter 1).

The VISX laser is one of the most widely used excimer lasers in the United States. A number of hardware and software technologies that have become available since 1998 have made the system safer and easier to operate than it used to be. These include Active-Trak 3-D eye tracking, variable spot scanning, autocentering, CustomVue, and iris registration. The ActiveTrak 3-D eye tracking system available on the STAR S4 laser platform tracks eye movements with an undilated pupil within a zone of 2.0 mm in the Z-axis and 1.5 mm in the X-Y-axis. Eye movement outside this tracking zone will be sensed within 30 ms and the surgeon will be unable to fire the laser. When proper fixation is reestablished, the tracking system will resume tracking with the same reference point and laser treatment can continue from the point of interruption.

Variable spot scanning (VSS) is also available on the VISX STAR S4 system. VSS, as the name suggests, represents a change from the older broad-beam laser delivery system to variable laser spot size delivery with the spot diameter varying from 2 to 6 mm. The advantage of this innovation is a smoother treatment, possibly reducing the incidence of haze after surface ablation. It also allows the laser to smoothly integrate a blend zone extending the ablation zone out to 8.0 mm. This is useful for treatments in patients with large pupils. The use of the blend zone feature requires at least 1 D of treatment at the corneal plane, a well-centered flap large enough to accommodate the treatment, and a cornea that is thick enough to accommodate

the added ablation depth. The added ablation depth is 8 μm for treatments up to 10 D and 11 μm for treatments beyond 10 D. Three additional advantages are that the VSS does not ablate as deeply as a typical flying spot laser and the treatment time is not as lengthy as the flying spot laser with a single sized small spot. Finally, the VSS keeps the corneal temperature constant. This is important because the laser will ablate more tissue as the tissue temperature increases.

The VISX STAR S4 laser pulse repetition rate can be adjusted from 1.5 to 10 Hz for conventional treatment and from 6 to 20 Hz for custom treatment. The repetition rate for the custom treatment is variable and is set by the laser. Currently the S4 platform is required for custom treatment.

The autocentering feature on the STAR S4 laser automatically finds the geometric center of the undilated pupil, so it is unnecessary for the surgeon to find the pupil center prior to engaging the tracking device. The pupil center can vary under different lighting conditions. It is therefore important to keep the lighting as low as possible at the time of autocentering and engaging the active tracking system so that the center of the pupil during treatment will be the same as the pupil center during refraction or WaveScan.

The FDA has recently approved iris registration (IR). This supplants the need for mechanically marking the patient prior to a custom laser treatment, but cannot be used for conventional LASIK. This will be discussed in greater detail in the next section on LASIK with the VISX CustomVue.

One of the major advantages of the VISX STAR S4 laser is the wide range of refractive errors approved by the FDA. Table 2.10 shows a comparison of the FDA-approved treatments for various lasers. Unlike many available laser systems, the VISX has been approved for conventional treatment of myopia and hyperopia with and without astigmatism as well as mixed astigmatism. Approved patient treatment extends from +5.00 to −14.00 D with up to +3.00 D of astigmatism for hyperopia (spherical equivalent < +6.00 D) and +5.00 D of astigmatism for myopia. The mixed astigmatism

Table 2.10	Several FDA-approved LASIK lasers			
	Myopia	Hyperopia	Mixed	Wavefront Guided
Bausch & Lomb Technolas 217A, Technolas 217z Zyoptix	−1.0 to −12.0 D MRSE with or without <−3.0 D of astigmatism	+1.0 to +4.0 D with ≤ +2.0 of hyperopic astigmatism	N/A	Myopia with sphere ≤−7.0 D and astigmatism ≤−3.0 D and MRSE ≤−7.5 D at the spectacle plane
VISX STAR S4 and WaveScan wavefront system	≤ −14.0 D with or without astigmatism of −0.5 to −5.0 D	+0.5 to +5.0 D with or without astigmatism ≤ +3.0 D SphEq <+6.0 D	≤ 6.0 D cylinder; plus cylinder is greater than myopic sphere of opposite sign	Myopia ≤ −11.0 D with ≤3.0 D astigmatism Hyperopia ≤+3.0 D with ≤+2.0 D astigmatism Mixed astigmatism ≤5.0 D astigmatism
Alcon LADAR Vision	Up to −9.0 D with or without astigmatism from −0.5 to −3.0 D	< 6.0 D with or without astigmatism < −6.0 D	Same as hyperopia	Myopia ≤−8.0 D with or without astigmatism <0.5 D Myopic astigmatism from −0.5 to −4.0 D
Nidek EC-5000	−0.75 to −14.0 D with or without astigmatism ≤ 4.0 D	N/A	N/A	N/A

treatment is approved for up to +6.00 D of astigmatism, as long as the myopic sphere is less than the cylinder and the two are of opposite signs; that is, treatment in plus cylinder form. The laser is also approved for custom treatment of all of the these situations. The range of available treatment is only slightly smaller for custom than conventional treatment. Conventional treatment at the upper limits of the approved range is less reliable than at lower levels of refractive error. Most surgeons will explore alternatives to LASIK at the extremes of refractive error (see Chapter 6 for a discussion of alternatives to LASIK).

Treatment Zones

The treatment zones available for conventional LASIK using the VISX STAR S4 laser for the correction of myopia are 6.0 and 6.5 mm. As stated earlier the blend zone will extend the treatment zone to a diameter of 8.0 mm. Hyperopic treatment requires a treatment zone of 9.0 mm with the deepest part of the ablation occurring at 5.0 mm, that is, 2.5 mm from the center of the ablation. Mixed astigmatism treatment also requires an ablation zone of 9.0 mm. When planning these treatments, the flap must be of adequate size and centration to accommodate the entire treatment zone.

Nomogram Adjustment

Several nomograms are available for treatment of myopia and myopia with astigmatism. Some surgeons use rules of thumb rather than a nomogram specifying the adjustment for specific corrections and/or decade of age. Because a starting place is necessary, nomograms for myopia and for hyperopia are provided. When beginning to plan treatments, the reader is encouraged to seek out the advice of experienced colleagues who use the VISX laser in the specific laser suite that will be used. Advice from faculty at a VISX certification course or from the medical directors at the company is also of value.

2

Myopia

Because ablation within the corneal stroma using the VISX laser to correct myopia results in a greater refractive effect, an adjustment to the intended treatment is needed to prevent an over-correction from occurring. The nomogram-adjusted treatment is what will be entered into the laser. The Bansal-Kay nomogram was designed only for treatment of myopia with the VISX STAR S2 laser system, but continues to be effective for conventional myopia treatment with the S4 laser system. In this nomogram the percentage reduction increases with age and the amount of correction in the spherical equivalent. The correction is applied to the spherical component only. The astigmatism component is left unadjusted. This nomogram is a useful starting point; however, surgeons should always carefully evaluate postoperative data from many cases and adjust their preferred nomogram accordingly.

Use of the Bansal-Kay nomogram (Table 2.11) requires five steps:

Step 1: Calculate the spherical equivalent from the cycloplegic refraction. For corrections with >7 D of myopia, the vertex distance of the cycloplegic refraction should be noted. The VISX STAR S4 laser uses 12.5 mm as the default vertex distance and converts this to the refraction at the corneal plane. The correct vertex distance should be entered in patients with high myopia.

Step 2: Find the appropriate reduction percentage on the nomogram by locating the correct diopter range in the left-hand column and the correct patient age range in the top row.

Step 3: Multiply the spherical equivalent by the selected reduction percentage to obtain the appropriate diopter reduction.

Step 4: Reduce the sphere in the cyclo-plegic refraction by the calculated diopter reduction.

Step 5: This final refraction is given to the laser engineer to log into the laser computer.

Table 2.11 Bansal-Kay LASIK myopia nomogram for VISX STAR laser

Diopters	Age 18−20	21−25	26−30	31−35	36−40	41−45	46−55	56 and older
0−1	4	4	4	5	6	7	7	8
1−2	4	4	4	5	6	7	7	8
2−3	4	4	5	5	7	8	8	8
3−4	5	5	5	6	7	8	8	8
4−5	5	5	6	6	8	8	8	9
5−6	5	5	6	6	8	9	9	10
6−7	6	6	7	7	9	10	10	11
7−8	7	7	7	8	9	10	11	12
8−9	8	8	8	8	10	11	12	12
9−10	9	9	9	9	11	11	13	13
10−11	10	10	10	10	12	13	14	14
11−12	11	11	12	12	13	13	15	15

Notes: Multiply percent by spherical equivalent and subtract from the sphere in the cycloplegic refraction.
Nomogram target = plano, adjust to undercorrect.
Individual results will vary with each laser, surgeon, humidity, and altitude.
Some data have been extrapolated.
Recommend starting laser ablation within 15 s of lifting flap.

Source: From Dr. Jay Bansal, unpublished data, with permission.

Example. Patient A is 26 years old and has a cycloplegic refraction of $-3.50 + 1.00 \times 90$ and, therefore, a spherical equivalent of -3.00 D. Based on the nomogram (Table 2.11) a 5% correction is necessary to achieve the desired LASIK result.

5% $\times$ -3.00 (spherical equivalent) $= 0.15$ (the sphere in the cycloplegic refraction is reduced by this amount)

$-3.50 + 1.00 \times 90$

$+0.15$

_____

$-3.35 + 1.00 \times 90$ (Enter this into the VISX system.)

An alternative rule of thumb used at Wills Eye Hospital involves three steps. Step 1, convert the intended correction to minus cylinder form; Step 2, reduce the sphere by 10% for patients under age 50 years and 15% for those older than age 50; and Step 3, reduce the cylinder 5% to 10% for refractive astigmatism <1.5 D and 10% to 15% for >1.5 D.

Hyperopia

For conventional treatment of hyperopia with or without astigmatism using the VISX STAR S4 laser, the manifest refraction should not differ from the cycloplegic refraction by more than 0.75 D. With the VISX laser, regression of the ablation effect is expected to occur over a 3- to 6-month period. Therefore, enhancement should not be considered until the surgeon is certain the correction has stabilized. Because of this anticipated regression a compensatory nomogram-adjusted boost to the spherical portion of the treatment is required. This will usually induce myopia in the short run and patients should be warned about this possibility preoperatively. Hyperopic patients of presbyopic age or older will usually appreciate the improved unaided near vision that occurs in the short run.

Similar to the myopia nomogram the percentage adjustment increases with increased spherical equivalent and age. In contrast, however, the nomogram adjustment is added to the sphere portion of the treatment. The astigmatism correction is left unadjusted.

Example. Patient B is 56 years old and has a cycloplegic refraction of $+2.50 + 1.00 \times 90$ and, therefore, a spherical equivalent of $+3.00$ D. Based on the hyperopic nomogram (Table 2.12), a 30% addition is necessary to achieve the desired corrected value needed for LASIK.

30% $\times$ $+3.00$ D (spherical equivalent) $= 0.90$ (the sphere in the cycloplegic refraction is increased by this amount)

$+2.50 + 1.00 \times 90$

$+0.90$

_____

$+3.40 + 1.00 \times 90$ (Enter this into the VISX system.)

This hyperopic nomogram was originally designed for the VISX STAR S2 laser. It still has utility for use with the STAR S4 laser; however, individual surgeons need to modify the nomogram based on an analysis of postoperative results from many cases. The laser suite conditions (e.g., temperature and humidity) and the particular VISX laser can affect the surgical outcome.

Mixed Astigmatism

The mixed astigmatism treatment on the VISX STAR S4 laser is not a nomogram-adjusted treatment. In other words the desired treatment can be entered directly into the laser computer. Surgeons differ with regard to whether they enter the cycloplegic refraction or modify the manifest refraction retaining the astigmatism amount and axis, but reducing the sphere to be consistent with the cycloplegic refraction. The FDA-approved mixed astigmatism profile for conventional and custom ablation is a distinct advantage of the VISX laser, because other laser systems do not have such approval, requiring off-label multicard treatments to achieve the desired result.

Ablation Depth Calculation

Myopia. To calculate the ablation depth the non–nomogram-adjusted refraction is used. This cannot be overemphasized. Ablation depth rules of thumb for the VISX laser are 12 μm/diopter of spherical equivalent for myopia correction with a 6.0-mm treatment zone and 15 μm/diopter for a 6.5-mm treatment

Table 2.12	VISX laser nomogram for primary and secondary hyperopia

| | Preoperative Manifest SE | | | Secondary Hyperopia | |
Age (y)	0–2 D (%)	2–4 D (%)	4–6 D (%)	Post-RK (%)	Post-LASIK (%)
20–29	0	+10	+20	−4	−14
30–39	+10	+18	+25	−2	−10
40–49	+17	+23	+28	−1	−4
50–59	+30	+30	+30	0	+4
60–69	+35	+32	+31	+2	+8

Notes: Table indicates the percent of the preoperative manifest spherical equivalent (SE) that is added to or subtracted from the spherical component of the correction. The full cylinder is entered into the laser. For example, a +2.00 +2.50 × 90 degrees refraction in a 33-year-old with primary hyperopia would be adjusted as follows: +3.25 D (SE) × 0.18 = 0.59, which results in a treatment of +2.59 +2.50 × 90 degrees.

The nomogram was derived from a regression analysis for trends by Drs. Lindstrom, Hardten, and associates, using a Hansatome and the VISX S2 Smoothscan at 10 Hz. Actual results were included for age groups when there were enough patients to influence the results of the regression analysis.

Source: Lindstrom RL, Linebarger EJ, Hardten DR, Houtman DM, Samuelson TW. Early results of hyperopic and astigmatic laser in situ kertomilleusis in eyes with secondary hyperopia. Adapted from *Opthalmology*, 2000:107; 1862, with permission.

zone. The addition of an astigmatic component to a myopic treatment will make the spherical equivalent less than the sphere. Therefore, the resultant ablation depth will be less when astigmatism is being treated in addition to myopia. The addition of an 8.0-mm blend zone adds 8 μm to the maximum ablation depth for treatments of less than 10 diopters and 11 μm for treatments greater than 10 diopters.

The following example will illustrate how to calculate the ablation depth for a refraction of −3.50 + 1.25 × 120 degrees using the rules of thumb. The first step would be to decide on the appropriate treatment zone. If the zone were 6.5 mm with an 8.0-mm blend zone, the ablation depth/diopter conversion factor would be 15 μm/diopter. Multiply the spherical equivalent by the conversion factor. The blend zone treatment would add an additional 8 μm of treatment. In this case the spherical equivalent would be 3.50 − 1.25/2 = 2.88 diopters. Simply multiply 2.88 diopters × 15 μm/diopter = 43.2 μm. Add an additional 8 μm for the blend zone for a total of 51.2 μm or roughly 51 μm for the ablation. Remember this is for myopia treatment on the VISX laser only; other lasers may ablate more or less per diopter of treatment.

An alternative method for calculating the ablation depth with the VISX laser is to use the appropriate ablation depth tables for the 6.0 mm zones (Table 2.13) and 6.5-mm zones (Table 2.14). These tables were generated by entering the various non–nomogram-adjusted corrections for the given zone into the laser. These tables continue to have utility despite being generated on an earlier version of the laser; however, changes in laser delivery can influence the ablation depth. Similar tables can easily be created as newer generations of lasers are developed. Most important is to avoid using the nomogram-adjusted treatment to calculate ablation depth, which would undervalue the true ablation depth.

The tables are used in the following manner. After deciding which zone to use, look for the appropriate spherical power in the left column and the amount of cylinder on the top row. If the astigmatic power in the cycloplegic refraction is in between two values, simply extrapolate between the values.

For example, if you were calculating the ablation depth for a refraction of −3.50 + 1.25 × 120 degrees for a 6.5-mm treatment zone with a blend zone to 8.0 mm, look at the 6.5-mm table for −3.50 D. The ablation depth for −3.50 D is 54 μm. Added astigmatism correction will lessen the ablation depth. The ablation depth for a hypothetical refraction of −3.50 + 1.00 × 120 degrees is reduced to 39 μm. At a refraction of −3.50 + 2.00 × 120 degrees the ablation depth shown on the table is decreased to 33 μm. Because 1.25 is one quarter of the way

Table 2.13 Ablation depth myopia treatment with VISX STAR S4 6.0-mm zone

Depth of ablation for 6.0-mm treatment zone (μm)

Platform: VISX S4
Plus Cylinder
Date: 9/15/05

		Plus Cylinder					
		0.00	1.00	2.00	3.00	4.00	5.00
Sphere	−1.00	13	7	9	18	28	38
	−1.25	17	7	11	16	26	36
	−1.50	20	10	13	14	23	33
	−1.75	23	13	15	15	21	31
	−2.00	26	15	14	18	18	28
	−2.25	29	16	14	20	20	26
	−2.50	33	20	14	22	22	23
	−2.75	36	23	18	24	24	24
	−3.00	39	26	21	21	26	26
	−3.25	42	29	23	21	28	28
	−3.50	45	33	25	20	30	30
	−3.75	48	36	27	23	32	32
	−4.00	51	39	30	26	27	34
	−4.25	54	42	32	28	27	36
	−4.50	57	45	34	30	27	38
	−4.75	60	48	35	33	27	40
	−5.00	63	51	39	35	31	34
	−5.25	66	54	42	37	33	33
	−5.50	69	57	45	39	35	33
	−5.75	71	60	48	41	38	33
	−6.00	74	63	51	43	40	36
	−6.25	77	66	54	46	42	38
	−6.50	80	69	57	48	44	40
	−6.75	80	71	60	50	46	42
	−7.00	85	74	63	51	48	45
	−7.25	87	77	66	54	50	47
	−7.50	89	80	69	57	53	49
	−7.75	92	80	71	60	55	51
	−8.00	94	85	74	63	57	53
	−8.25	96	87	77	66	59	55
	−8.50	98	89	80	69	61	57
	−8.75	101	92	80	71	63	59
	−9.00	103	94	85	74	65	61
	−9.25	105	96	87	77	65	63
	−9.50	107	98	89	80	69	65
	−9.75	110	101	92	80	71	67
	−10.00	112	103	94	85	74	69
	−10.25	114	105	96	87	77	71
	−10.50	116	107	98	89	80	73
	−10.75	118	110	101	92	80	75
	−11.00	120	112	103	94	85	77
	−11.25	122	114	105	96	87	79
	−11.50	124	116	107	98	89	80
	−11.75	124	118	110	101	92	80
	−12.00	128	120	112	103	94	84

2

| Table 2.14 | Ablation depth for myopia treatment with VISX STAR S4 6.5-mm zone |

Depth of ablation for 6.5-mm treatment zone (μm)

Platform: VISX S4
Date: 9/15/05

		Plus Cylinder					
		0.00	**1.00**	**2.00**	**3.00**	**4.00**	**5.00**
Sphere	−1.00	16	9	NA	NA	NA	NA
	−1.25	20	9	NA	NA	NA	NA
	−1.50	24	13	NA	NA	NA	NA
	−1.75	28	16	NA	NA	NA	NA
	−2.00	31	19	18	NA	NA	NA
	−2.25	35	22	17	NA	NA	NA
	−2.50	39	23	17	NA	NA	NA
	−2.75	43	28	23	NA	NA	NA
	−3.00	46	31	26	26	NA	NA
	−3.25	50	35	28	26	NA	NA
	−3.50	54	39	31	26	NA	NA
	−3.75	57	43	34	29	NA	NA
	−4.00	61	46	37	32	34	NA
	−4.25	65	50	39	35	34	NA
	−4.50	68	54	42	38	34	NA
	−4.75	72	57	45	40	34	NA
	−5.00	75	61	46	43	39	42
	−5.25	79	65	50	46	41	42
	−5.50	82	68	54	49	44	42
	−5.75	86	72	57	51	47	41
	−6.00	89	75	61	54	49	45
	−6.25	92	79	65	57	52	47
	−6.50	96	82	68	59	55	50
	−6.75	96	86	72	62	57	53
	−7.00	100	89	75	64	60	56
	−7.25	103	92	79	67	63	58
	−7.50	105	96	82	68	65	61
	−7.75	107	96	86	72	68	63
	−8.00	110	100	89	75	70	66
	−8.25	112	103	92	79	73	69
	−8.50	114	105	96	82	75	71
	−8.75	116	107	96	86	78	74
	−9.00	119	110	100	89	80	76
	−9.25	121	112	103	92	83	79
	−9.50	123	114	105	96	85	81
	−9.75	125	116	107	96	87	84
	−10.00	127	119	110	100	89	86
	−10.25	130	121	112	103	92	88
	−10.50	132	123	114	105	96	91
	−10.75	134	125	116	107	96	93
	−11.00	136	127	119	110	100	95
	−11.25	138	130	121	112	103	98
	−11.50	140	132	123	114	105	100
	−11.75	140	134	125	116	107	101
	−12.00	144	136	127	119	110	104

from 1.00 to 2.00 D, reduce the ablation by one quarter the difference of the depth for 1.00 and 2.00 D of astigmatism. The appropriate reduction in this case would be 8 × 0.25 or 2. The ablation depth would be 39 μm − 2 μm = 37 μm. An additional 8 μm must be added because of the blend zone for a total ablation depth of 45 μm. This is similar to the 51-μm depth estimated by the conversion factor method. It is always safer to choose the greater of the two estimates to determine if the RST will be adequate.

The standard hyperopic treatment with the VISX laser is a 9.0-mm zone with a maximum ablation depth of 8 μm/diopter of spherical equivalent occurring at a 5-mm ring around the treatment center. The maximum ablation depth is therefore in an area of the cornea that is usually thicker than the center. Hyperopia treatments are usually less of a challenge regarding ablation depth than the myopia treatments. Since in hyperopia the nomogram-adjusted refraction is greater than the preadjusted refraction, the greater value should be used for ablation depth calculations.

In mixed astigmatism on the VISX laser there is no nomogram adjustment. Therefore, the expected ablation depth can be taken from the laser computer prior to surgery and used to determine if the cornea is of adequate thickness.

Summary

The VISX S4 laser provides effective treatment for a wide array of refractive errors. It is FDA approved for more types of treatment than any of the more commonly used lasers. The system is easy to operate for the surgeon and the laser engineer. VSS provides a smooth treatment that is tissue sparing. The blend zone allows treatment of patients with large pupils. The autocentering and ActiveTrak 3-D eye tracking features of the VISX STAR S4 increase LASIK safety and accuracy, particularly for the patient with poor fixation or for patients requiring lengthy treatments. Iris registration is available for custom treatments, but not for conventional treatments, requiring surgeons to continue to mark patients prior to astigmatism treatment.

CustomVue/WaveScan

With the advent of wavefront technology and custom laser ablation, LASIK surgeons have had to acquire new skills and rethink their approach to patient education, patient selection, and treatment planning. Prior to the development of these capabilities, refractive surgeons treated only spherocylindrical corrections with varying optical zones. With the availability of CustomVue with the VISX STAR S4 VSS platform, the refractive surgeon can offer the patient a potentially more precise customized treatment. Whether the patient is at greater risk for nighttime vision problems or has a complex mixed astigmatic refractive error with significant higher order aberrations, the surgeon can plan and offer an appropriate treatment. This section will discuss the use of CustomVue and WaveScan, the VISX device used to acquire wavefront data. Hopefully, after reviewing this section, the reader will have a more complete understanding of the critical issues needed to perform CustomVue treatments.

Prior to starting custom treatments, completion of the online VISX CustomVue training course is required. This course reviews the basic hardware and software, as well as the patient data needed to perform treatments.

Approved Range of CustomVue LASIK Treatments

The VISX STAR S4 laser with CustomVue is FDA approved for one of the widest ranges of custom correction of the available laser systems (Table 2.11). Wavefront-guided LASIK with the VISX STAR S4 is approved for patients with myopia up to −11 D [maximum wavefront refraction (WR) sphere −11.75 D] with or without astigmatism up to 3.00 D (maximum WR cylinder 3.75 D), as long as the spherical equivalent does not exceed −11.75 D [manifest refraction (MR) or WR]. Mixed astigmatism, from 1.00 to 5.00 diopters of cylinder, can now be treated with CustomVue.

Wavefront-guided LASIK is approved for patients with hyperopia and uses a 6.0-mm optical zone and a 9.0-mm treatment zone for the reduction or elimination of hyperopia and hyperopic astigmatism up to +3.00 D sphere (maximum WR sphere + 3.75 D) with cylinder

≤2.00 D (maximum WR cylinder +2.75 D), up to a maximum manifest refraction spherical equivalent of +3.00 (maximum WR spherical equivalent +3.75 D).

Although not FDA approved, the treatment cards for hyperopia allow treatment beyond this range. Caution is advised in this territory until sufficient experience with CustomVue treatment of hyperopia has been acquired. In higher treatments of this sort, the surgeon must remain mindful of the final estimated keratometric value. High hyperopic corrections in patients with a preoperative keratometry above 45.00 D can result in corneas above 50.00 D postoperatively and this could have an adverse impact on BSCVA.

Advantages and Disadvantages

In addition to its wide potential treatment range, several other important benefits are observed when using the VISX CustomVue system. It offers improved visual function at night compared with conventional treatment. This is especially important for patients who have these complaints prior to surgery, for patients with higher degrees of myopia who are within the approved range of treatment, and possibly important for patients with large pupils. Patients should understand that custom treatment does not guarantee the absence of glare and haloes after surgery. In contrast to the Alcon system, the surgery is performed without pupil dilation. CustomVue LASIK not only reduces higher order aberrations, but also may induce fewer new aberrations. Because of the customized nature of the treatment, visual function even during the day may be improved beyond the previous best-corrected acuity, although it is difficult to predict which patients will achieve this higher function.

Incorporating the refraction acquired from the WaveScan unit into the preoperative patient examination, the so-called wavefront-adjusted manifest refraction (WAMR) can at times result in greater visual acuity than that achieved through retinoscopy and more typical refraction techniques. Greater flexibility exists for modifying treatment zones to accommodate patients with large pupils. An illustration would be the patient with a low myopic correction and large pupil. With conventional treatment on the VISX STAR S4 at least −1.00 D at the

corneal plane is needed to add a blend zone. This is not the case with the custom treatment. Finally in the event a retreatment for a patient with excessive higher order aberrations (HOAs) is necessary, a PreVue lens can be cut based on the WaveScan, which allows the patient to determine the value of the retreatment preoperatively both during the day and at night.

Surgeons vary with regard to which patients should be offered CustomVue LASIK. Some will offer the treatment to all patients who are candidates for the procedure. Others prefer to restrict the procedure only to selected patients, for example, those with large pupils, large degrees of higher order aberration, and so forth.

The disadvantages of the CustomVue treatment must include the increased cost to the patient and to the surgeon. Additional skills are needed to acquire and use the data generated by the WaveScan unit to plan surgery. This will involve more technician time and surgeon time. The approved range of custom surgery is less than for conventional LASIK on the VISX STAR S4. This is especially true for custom retreatment. Not all patients are candidates for the procedure. If there is poor agreement between the wavefront refraction and the manifest refraction, the treatment cannot be done. While there is flexibility to adjust the sphere, neither the axis nor power of the cylindrical correction can be modified. The flexibility in sphere adjustment is not great enough to accommodate a monovision treatment, so true monovision cannot be performed using CustomVue. The ablation depth is greater for a custom procedure than the equivalent conventional treatment, preventing custom LASIK in some patients with thin corneas. This technology will raise patient expectations and in the event that results do not match expectations there is the potential for an unhappy patient.

The advantages and disadvantages of CustomVue with the WaveScan analysis are listed in Table 2.15.

The WaveScan

The WaveScan unit is the VISX wavefront device used to capture the high-quality images that are necessary to create a custom treatment. The recent WaveScan software upgrade

Table 2.15	Advantages and disadvantages of VISX CustomVue with WaveScan analysis

Advantages	Disadvantages
Greatest approved treatment range	Increased cost for WaveScan and VISX STAR S4 upgrade
Greater likelihood of improved night vision	Increased cost for the patient
Potential for improved BSCVA using wavefront-adjusted manifest refraction.	Increased technician time
Ability to adjust power of the sphere and add a nomogram adjustment if results dictate	Increased surgeon time
Flexibility to adjust treatment zones even for low corrections out to a maximum of 9.0 mm	Need to acquire new skills
	Inability to adjust cylinder power or axis
	Unable to treat monovision
No need to dilate intraoperatively	Deeper ablation than conventional
Ability to cut a PreVue lens	Increased patient expectations

2

(Version 3.5, June 7, 2004) changed the method of ablation calculation from Zernike polynomial to Fourier analysis. The Fourier analysis utilizes data over the entire pupil, up to 6.0 mm, in incremental 0.1-mm steps. This method reproduces the complex shapes generated by CustomVue software with greater fidelity than when Zernike shapes were used. In addition to changing the way the ablation profile is calculated, it also includes a 4.5% boost over the prior treatment software.

The WaveScan unit can be used as an adjunct for refracting a potential conventional LASIK patient, particularly if a patient cannot be refracted to 20/20. It can also be used to evaluate postoperative LASIK patients, who have complaints despite seemingly excellent visual acuity. The WaveScan data can also be printed to facilitate the comparison of pre- and postoperative higher order aberrations. However, it is primarily used to plan custom LASIK.

The WaveScan is not a screening tool to rule out keratoconus nor is it a substitute for corneal topography. Corneal topography must be used as an independent evaluation to identify patients with ectatic disease, forme fruste disease, or patients at risk for postoperative ectasia. (Refer to the earlier section on corneal topography, page 28.) The presence or type of HOAs does not dictate whether or not a patient is a candidate for a CustomVue treatment. Even

patients with high root mean square (rms) values and a high percent of HOAs can have CustomVue surgery, provided other previously discussed criteria for LASIK have been met. The rms value is a mathematical representation of the total higher order aberrations in the eye. No clinical correlation has been established between preoperative HOAs and postoperative results. Conversely, patients with a low degree of HOAs may still benefit from custom surgery, since CustomVue is less likely to induce new HOAs.

Some possible ablation profiles generated by the WaveScan software cannot actually be treated with the laser, because the treatment may exceed the approved range. This must be evaluated carefully prior to surgery. The newer version of the WaveScan software will indicate whether or not the treatment is within range and is supported by available treatment cards.

There are a number of screens in the software with which you need to become familiar. It is important for the surgeon to take an active role in picking the treatments and adjusting the design screen for each patient as surgery is planned. Once the treatment has been selected and designed, the plan is calculated and downloaded for data transfer to the STAR S4 VSS laser. A printout of the treatment plan is produced for the chart and the data are uploaded to the VISX S4 VSS laser.

WaveScan Acquisition

Acquiring comprehensive and reliable clinical patient data preoperatively is essential to obtaining excellent surgical outcomes. Most of the preoperative assessment for custom LASIK is similar to what is required for conventional LASIK. Wavefront data acquisition is a clear departure from the conventional patient evaluation. The following describes the essentials of WaveScan acquisition.

The WaveScan unit should be calibrated daily when it is booted. This is a fast and simple process. The joystick operates much like a slit lamp. Just align the white dots with the horizontal line of the cross and the blue circle with the pupil margin. Use the autofocus button and joystick to focus the white dots and optimize focus.

Be sure the patient is positioned correctly at the instrument and verify the head position between each image. If the pupil does not naturally dilate to 5.0 mm, then a CustomVue treatment is not recommended. Do not dilate patients to acquire a treatment profile. The VISX treatment algorithms are based on the natural pupil and intentional pharmacologic alteration, either topical or systemic, may alter the quality of the results. This may require that the patient sit for a while in a darkened room. It is important that the patient does not accommodate while being imaged. To aid younger patients and ease accommodation, instruct them to look "through" the target not to stare "at" the target. Getting several good-quality WaveScan images with a large enough pupil can be difficult at times, especially with older patients.

Always take at least three good-quality images per eye, trying to get all four check marks green. If the system does not recognize the image as acceptable (e.g., pupil <5 mm), it will not automatically save it, but it can be saved manually. However, it is not recommended to use such profiles for treatment, because the data can be unreliable. The system will create a treatment profile (designated by a "T"); transfer this profile to the laser using a floppy disk and print a copy for the patient record. The laser sometimes cannot read "recycled" diskettes, even if confirmed on the WaveScan; therefore, always use new diskettes of the highest quality or the USB stick provided

by VISX. If using diskettes, upload them to the laser in advance of surgery to confirm that the treatment profile is available. Because of the larger image file, IR treatments must be downloaded and transferred to the laser using the USB memory stick.

Some additional basic guidelines include the following:

- Set the vertex on the WaveScan to 12.5 mm.
- Set the convention to minus or plus notation, depending on the convention with which you are more comfortable.
- For myopic patients, verify that the sphere does not exceed -11.75 D, the cylinder does not exceed -3.75 D, and the spherical equivalent is ≤ -11.75 D. These are the FDA limits, beyond which no treatment option is currently available.
- For hyperopic patients, the spherical equivalent does not exceed $+3.00$ D and verify the cylinder does not exceed $+2.00$ D. Treatment is possible beyond these ranges, but is considered off label.
- Obtain at least three undilated WaveScan captures with at least a 5-mm and preferably a 6-mm pupil.
- Check the quality of the images. There should be at least three out of four green checks in the quality box.

Patients within the range of approved refractive error that have been successfully captured on the WaveScan (pupil diameter ≥ 5.0 mm), must also have sufficient corneal thickness, regular topography, and good correlation with the refraction in order to be treated with the CustomVue system.

Treatment Planning

The second step in preparing to perform a CustomVue treatment is the design of the ablation shape for each individual eye. The VISX instruction and training protocols recommend use of the Automated Exam Selection Mode, which requires a minimum of three quality WaveScan measurements. This is a good way to start incorporating CustomVue into a refractive practice. This mode will signal a warning if one or more of the selected exams exceed the following criteria:

- One or more examinations have a <5.0-mm pupil size.

- Two or more exams have spherical equivalent values differing by >1.0 D.
- The selected exam has a higher order rms that differs from the average by more than 0.07 μm.

The surgeon always has the option of ignoring the warning and proceeding with the treatment.

An alternative method can be considered as one becomes more comfortable with the instrumentation and more confident with the clinical outcomes. Set the "treat" setting to a single exam and select the WaveScan refraction (WR) that most closely correlates with the manifest refraction (MR) and cycloplegic refraction (CR). This also allows one to check image quality and evaluate the pupil image. Individually checking and selecting the WaveScan ensures that only high-quality measurements are used for treatment. As IR becomes the standard for CustomVue treatments, the ability to check image quality and pupil image will become more important. Occasionally the manifest and wavefront refractions are consistent and accurate, but the image of the eye will illustrate that the eyelid is covering a portion of the pupil. In this circumstance that particular WaveScan should be disregarded and another selected. Sometimes, more images will need to be captured to ensure good quality. During evaluation of the images, do not let preoperative higher order rms values determine eligibility for treatment, because these are subtle features that vary greatly among individuals. The FDA clinical trials did not base any inclusion or exclusion criteria on HOAs or rms values. Instead, look for correlation between the WR, MR, and CR using the criteria in Table 2.16. In general, the WR cylindrical power and axis are very accurate. If the differences between MR/CR and WR sphere exceed the guidelines, then:

- Repeat both. WR may be more minus if the patient is accommodating.
- Check the BSCVA using the WR (WAMR).
- Check the CR.

If the MR and WR deviate greater than allowed by these guidelines, then the patient may not be suited for a wavefront-guided treatment.

When beginning CustomVue treatments, use the full WaveScan refraction with no nomogram adjustment. The newer Fourier analysis is very accurate and minimal nomogram adjustment is needed. It is still important for surgeons to monitor individual results because of the variations in outcome that result from technique, environmental conditions due to the season and geography, and WaveScan and laser variability. It is helpful for surgeons to keep records of cases and results 1-month postoperatively to revisit the adjustment question. It will take several dozen cases to get enough data on which to base a nomogram adjustment for treatment.

The design screen offers the surgeon two options for treatment adjustments. The surgeon has the ability to adjust the amount of spherical correction ±0.75 D. Additionally, a second option for adjustment on the design screen is the percent nomogram adjustment. This can be adjusted ±10%. The nomogram adjustment makes the change to the entire treatment, sphere, cylinder, and HOAs. Once the surgeon starts to analyze the outcomes, then these two methods allow sufficient flexibility to fine-tune the treatments to improve postoperative results. When it is time to

Table 2.16	Allowable difference between WR, MR, and CR	
	Myopia	Hyperopia
MR and CR	<0.75 D	<0.75 D
MR and WR (WR minus MR)	−0.50 to +0.75 D	<0.75 D
CR and WR	−0.50 to +0.75 D	<0.75 D
For cylinder >0.50 D	<15 degrees	<15 degrees

incorporate an adjustment, use the design screen and be sure to check that the proper vertex distance is entered. Use only new, non-recycled diskettes to download treatment or the VISX USB stick, because the laser may not recognize the ablation profile. Before surgery always check the diskettes or USB stick on the laser to be sure the laser will read the profile.

The default ablation diameter for CustomVue treatments is 8.0 mm with an optical zone of 6.0 mm. For hyperopia the optical zone is 5.0 mm with an ablation diameter of 9.0 mm. If possible, keep the ablation zone diameter slightly larger than the measured mesopic pupil size. Enlarge the ablation zone beyond the default zone setting, if needed. This does not increase the amount of tissue removed during the ablation, but rather increases the diameter of the smoothed edge. The maximum ablation diameter is 9.0 mm. Some experienced refractive surgeons simply enlarge the ablation diameter to 9.0 mm on all myopic treatments. When doing this, one must consider the diameter of the flap that will be created and attempt not to ablate cornea outside the stromal bed. Enlarging the ablation zone is probably an important step that helps minimize complaints of nighttime glare and haloes. The surgeon should personally make this adjustment on all patients without relying on a technician. This forces the surgeon to look at the selected scan and ensures that the quality of the WaveScan images is good and appropriate for each patient to be treated.

Patient Preparation

The third step in the process is to prepare for surgery using proper alignment and orientation techniques to ensure fidelity in transmitting the custom shape to the cornea. In the absence of the iris registration (IR) upgrade, use a sterile marking pen to mark the limbus at 3 and 9 o'clock, as described in the chapter on basic LASIK. This will allow the surgeon to adjust for cyclorotation of the eye, which can occur when the patient is positioned under the laser.

The FDA has recently approved IR; however, some surgeons still mark the patient in case the IR fails to capture. Because it relates the laser to the WaveScan, IR is available only for custom treatments. The fully automated IR system will signal the surgeon if the orientation of the eye or head under the laser is different than during WaveScan acquisition or if the pupil center has shifted. The laser can then compensate for this movement. IR is not an active tracking system. The IR system and the appropriate laser compensation are set prior to the ablation and remain fixed until changed by the surgeon. If the eye continues to move, the laser would need to be reset to compensate for this movement. If the eye were to move again, the surgeon would need to stop and reregister. During the VISX clinical trials the IR system was found to be convenient and reliable, as well as user friendly.

Because it uses iris features to recognize the patient's eye, it also serves as a double check of identity and helps prevent treatment to the wrong eye or patient. Tracking and alignment are even more important for wavefront-guided treatments because the ablations always contain unique features that are not symmetrical, unlike spherocylindrical ablation profiles.

Treatment

Most experienced refractive surgeons feel that different microkeratomes will not have significant impact on the results of CustomVue treatment provided that surgeons are consistent with their technique. Remember, as mentioned earlier in the text, that CustomVue treatments will remove more tissue per diopter, so residual bed depth will become more of an issue. The surgeon needs to know the range of flap thicknesses that his or her particular microkeratome will produce. Always check the central pachymetry of the stromal bed to confirm that sufficient RST is present. If the clinical situation requires a thinner flap, the femtosecond laser may be a more desirable option. Some surgeons prefer to wait for a significant opacified bubble layer to dissipate before proceeding with the custom ablation. This has not been well studied and remains controversial.

Align the limbal marks with the reticle hash marks or, if available on your system, engage IR; focus the microscope on the surface of the stromal bed; and center the reticle over the pupil. The pupil centroid through a small pupil is located in a different position than through a dilated pupil. Before engaging the ActiveTrak with automatic centering, reduce the room illumination and the microscope illumination also, if possible, so that the custom treatment will be centered at the same location as the WaveScan. Once centered and tracking is engaged, depress the laser pedal to begin treatment. CustomVue treatments should never be performed without the ActiveTrak engaged. The speed of laser treatment is variable; therefore, the surgeon should not be alarmed by the change in the sound of the laser compared with conventional treatment.

Summary
Careful attention to details and acquisition of reliable data will result in the best possible outcomes. It is important for the surgeon to understand the WaveScan system so that necessary guidance can be provided to staff and potential errors recognized and prevented.

The VISX STAR S4 with CustomVue currently has the widest range of approvals for conventional and wavefront-guided treatments and has many features that make it a user-friendly system. Calibration is fast and simple to perform. The user software interface is intuitive. Also, if your laser suite has sufficient room, a femtosecond laser can be in the same room allowing the surgeon to use the same chair. The autocentering and tracking features are extremely versatile and robust under most lighting and pupillary conditions. Use the minimum lighting that allows the ActiveTrak to autocenter and track the pupil in order to match the lighting conditions during WaveScan acquisition and CustomVue treatment. This better aligns treatment centration.

New iris recognition technology should also provide surgeons with greater comfort when treating eyes with greater amounts of cylinder and HOAs. Once the surgeon becomes more experienced and has gathered sufficient data, the $\pm 10\%$ nomogram adjustment and the ± 0.75 D physician adjustment can be used to develop individual nomo-

grams. These are very helpful for fine-tuning results for individual patient needs. This laser platform is upgradeable, serviceable, and reliable. The field service, training materials, and customer care center at VISX are also helpful. Contact information for VISX can be found on page 268.

The LADARVision System
The LADARVision System is comprised of either the LADARVision 4000 laser or the new LADAR 6000 and the LADARWave aberrometer. The two devices were designed to work together to perform CustomCornea, Alcon's wavefront-guided customized procedure.

Alcon's LADARVision 4000 excimer laser system was originally approved for conventional correction of myopia, but was designed from the outset to provide the capability for wavefront-guided customized correction. Like many of the newest excimer laser systems on the market (e.g., Bausch & Lomb, WaveLight), Alcon's LADARVision 4000 is considered a scanning-spot laser. However, the LADARVision laser offers a "flying small-spot" 0.8-mm Gaussian-shaped laser spot that is delivered through a high-speed scanning system. The move to small flying small-spot technology was driven by the desire to perform customized or wavefront-guided refractive surgery; and a beam size of 1.0 mm is deemed necessary to correct fourth-order Zernike aberrations. These flying spot lasers are different than their earlier counterparts, which utilize large "broad-beam" technology. Flying spot lasers require sophisticated eye tracking and beam scanning technology to ensure optimized beam placement.

Because of the small beam, flying spot lasers require a beam scanning mechanism to deliver the complicated shot sequence that produces the ablation profile. It is important that each shot be accurately placed, so consideration of eye movement is critical and an accurate eye tracker is vital to realizing the potential of the flying spot laser system. The LADARVision lasers employ a tracking device that uses the same laser radar technology originally developed to help NASA spacecraft rendezvous and dock with satellites during service calls. This technology, called LAser raDAR, is used to track the movement of the eye 4,000 times per second, 15 times faster than other excimer laser systems used today, providing a space-stabilized image to the laser and to the computer monitor. The capability of a space-stabilized image, which essentially holds the eye in place on the monitor for optimal control and accuracy, is unique to the LADARVision System.

The human eye moves 100 times per second, and, without a sophisticated tracking system to lock onto the eye and remain fixed on its movements, the laser used to reshape the cornea during LASIK could become misaligned and deliver an undesired outcome. The LADARVision laser is the only laser eye surgery system that uses this innovative laser radar tracking technology. All other LASIK systems use slower, video-based tracking systems, which require surgeons to occasionally stop the LASIK procedure when the video-based system is unable to keep pace with the eye's movements.

System Setup and Surgical Planning

Operation of the system was designed so that the surgical process is straightforward. Each surgery day a performance test is carried out to ensure that the system is operating within specifications. In addition, a calibration sequence before each patient's surgery measures beam location and energy levels to optimize the shot pattern generated for the ablation. A user-friendly interface guides the user through these routine steps.

As with all laser systems, the refractive surgeon should be prepared to track clinical outcomes with reasonable consistency. Such factors as the laser suite environment (temperature and humidity) and patient demographics may subtly alter the operation of the excimer laser in your clinic. Past clinical outcomes should be used to monitor trends such as undercorrection or overcorrection of sphere and/or cylinder. The development of a nomogram is a well-established method to compensate for site-specific effects. There are no particular laser-specific considerations regarding the Alcon LADARVision laser and surgical planning and/or outcomes tracking. With conventional surgery, the surgeon can use a personally developed nomogram to modify the sphere and cylinder to adjust for the aforementioned site-specific effects. We have not found the need for routine use of a nomogram adjustment for conventional LASIK or PRK with the Alcon LADAR-Vision laser. This is in contrast with the VISX STAR S4, in which reduction in treatment is widely used for LASIK surgery. With the LADARVision laser, the measured manifest or cycloplegic refraction is entered into the laser's computer without adjustment. We have not found a need to adjust our plan based on patient age, degree of refractive error, or corneal power. However, within the approved operating range for conventional LASIK, modification of the sphere and cylinder can allow the surgeon the options for off-label uses such as monovision or other nonplano correction, to accommodate the specific needs of the patient.

With the CustomCornea wavefront-guided correction, the spherical component of the correction can be modified by ± 0.75 D. If a surgeon has developed a nomogram, the LADARWave aberrometer will allow the input of the nomogram into a surgery planning software tool that resides on the LADARWave aberrometer computer. This planning tool, called Custom Surgery Planning Software (CSPS), offers ablation depth profiling, nomogram and patient-specific offset management, and comprehensive surgery summary data. When a wavefront is measured and processed with the CSPS, the appropriate nomogram-adjusted offset will be provided. The ability to add an additional offset to the proposed treatment is always available, as long as the final result is a spherical equivalent value within ± 0.75 D of the wavefront spherical equivalent. The CSPS nomogram handles the spherical component of the refraction only. The available treatment ranges for conventional and CustomCornea treatments with the Alcon platform are shown in Table 2.17. These treatment ranges accommodate most LASIK candidates. Patients with degrees of myopia, hyperopia, and astigmatism outside of these ranges are usually excluded from LASIK based on poor predictability secondary to their extreme refractive errors, corneal thinness, or extremely flat or steep keratometry measurements.

Table 2.17	Alcon LADARVision and CustomCornea FDA-approved treatment ranges		
	Conventional		CustomCornea
	Myopia	Hyperopia and Mixed Astigmatism	Myopia
Max sphere	< −9.00 D	< +6.00 D	≤ −8.00 D
Cylinder	≤ −3.00 D	< −6.00 D	≤ −4.00 D
Spherical equivalent	≤ −10.00 D	+6.00 to −3.00 D	≤ −8.00 D

One of the additional requirements for surgical planning with the Alcon LADARWave is the need to perform pupillary dilation, because the eye tracking system requires a fixed pupil size between 7 and 11 mm. A large pupil is important to ensure capture of a majority of the aberrations in the optical system. If the pupil is not dilated, then the peripheral aberrations, often the suggested reason for night vision difficulties, will not be measured, or subsequently treated. This is another point of contrast between the Alcon and VISX systems. Remember that for VISX WaveScan data acquisition, pharmacological pupillary dilation should not be done; and CustomVue treatment is also performed without dilation. If you are moving from a system that used a video-based tracker that did not require dilation, you will be required to modify your preoperative workup to provide the necessary time for dilation. Some patients may not be able to initially be dilated sufficiently for adequate tracking of the pupil. Usually, dimming the room lights and instilling topical 10% phenylephrine allows most of these patients to dilate sufficiently. The lens implant in a pseudophakic patient may confound the tracker, which mistakenly captures the IOL optic rather than the true pupil diameter. In the pseudophakic patient the 11-mm white calibration target can be used for initial test tracking. This will help the device find the pupil when tracking just before the treatment. For tracking at the time of treatment, the device looks for that 11-mm-diameter circle first and then contracts from outside to inside thus capturing the wider diameter of the pupil prior to encountering the smaller diameter of the IOL optic.

Minimal operational changes may need to be implemented within the office to accommodate preoperative pupil dilation. Advance planning aids in minimizing the impact on the surgical schedule.

The preoperative evaluation, other than wavefront acquisition, has been summarized in the chapter on basic LASIK. Based on the complete examination, a surgical plan is developed. The surgical plan is based on a combination of the manifest and cycloplegic refraction. The dominant eye generally is treated on the MR without adjustment, and treatment of the nondominant eye is generally on the CR without adjustment. The magnitude and axis of astigmatism are influenced by the corneal maps and keratometry. The laser treatment diameter can be adjusted from 5.0 to 8.0 mm based on mesopic pupil size. A complete written plan is brought to the laser room. Other surgeons using this laser system may use different treatment planning methods. The certification course, consultation with other experienced surgeons using the laser, and personal experience all help a surgeon develop a preferred method for treatment planning.

Conventional LASIK Surgery

The initial step in conventional surgery is to enter relevant patient data into the surgery database. The laser treatment screen illustrates the intended treatment, optical zone size, the depth of ablation, and duration of treatment. Centration photos for one or both of the patient's undilated eyes are then collected. The limbus and the daytime pupil, on which the ablation is centered, are identified on the photographic images using circular reticles; and their positions as they relate to each other are recorded. These landmarks are important references for the ablation pattern. Usually, the centration photos are taken at the time of the initial patient evaluation. These photos are stored in the laser hard drive and recalled at the time of treatment.

On the day of surgery, the treatment plan is entered into the computer in minus cylinder form. The patient's pupil is then dilated. If the patient has astigmatism, a mark is made at the 6 o'clock limbus with the patient sitting up and looking with both eyes in primary gaze at a distance target. Once the patient lies down, the pupil is test tracked and corneal thickness is measured. The surgeon then compensates for cyclotorsion of the eye by adding additional corneal marks centered on the 6 o'clock limbal mark as a point of reference. These additional marks are then extended past the limbus at 3 and 9 o'clock to help align the astigmatism axis on the treatment screen. The flap is then cut and the corneal bed thickness is measured with pachymetry to calculate corneal flap thickness. The tracker is then engaged and the limbal ring and horizontal astigmatic reference mark are placed in alignment with the 3 and 9 o'clock limbal marks. The ablation can then be performed. The flap is replaced and irrigated after ablation.

Conventional correction with the LADARVision System has a number of important features:

- An unavailable algorithm obviates the need to consider multipass surgery for mixed astigmatism or hyperopia cases.
- Optical zone sizes for conventional surgery can be modified based on pupil size, and expected ablation depths will be displayed to help plan surgery.
- An effluent removal system reduces unwanted plume effects from the laser. A software hinge mask can be employed to protect the LASIK flap, eliminating the need to use sponges or other apparatus during the procedure that could adversely affect the outcome.

Unique to the Alcon LADARVision platform are the following:

- The optical zone size specified for myopia or hyperopia with astigmatism will be the effective optical zone. The user-defined blend zone is outside of this optic zone. This is in contrast to some systems that blend inside their defined optical zone, reducing the size of the effective optical zone.
- During surgery, the monitor displays a space-stabilized image with the tracker data overlaid so that fixation and tracking can be confirmed throughout the surgery.
- The hinge mask feature mentioned earlier allows the surgeon to ensure that laser shots are not delivered at the flap hinge in LASIK cases.
- The automatic centration and registration system ensures the ablation is applied at the daytime line of sight with the proper orientation. This is important for conventional surgery and critical for wavefront-guided customized surgery.

The main operating screen for the LADARVision platform shows the space-stabilized image, with the hinge mask and the limbal and horizontal alignment tools seen on the eye. It also shows the real-time image of the patient's eye.

LADARVision System Pearls

We have found that our laser does not need any nomogram adjustment. We do not adjust our treatment plan based on age, gender, corneal contour (provided it is regular), or thickness. We avoid treating myopic patients that will end up with a cornea flatter than 35 D. We also avoid hyperopic patients in which treatment may result in a cornea steeper than 48 D. Patients with mesopic pupils that are equal to 8 mm or less can be treated. Patients with pupils larger than 8 mm must be warned that the maximum ablation zone is 8.0 mm; therefore, they have an increased possibility of glare and haloes. The laser is quite effective for treating astigmatism, especially mixed astigmatism in which it uses a cross cylinder ablation profile to minimize tissue loss.

CustomCornea with the LADARVision System and Laser Wave Aberrometer Technology

LADARWave Aberrometer Technology

The Alcon LADARWave aberrometer is the wavefront measuring device that measures, creates and provides the ablation profile for CustomCornea wavefront-guided surgery. It is based on Hartmann-Shack principles (see page 51). Several proprietary technologies increase the accuracy and reliability of the LADARWave unit. When measuring wavefront scans, a number of factors should be considered, particularly if the wavefront is to be used as the basis for refractive surgery. The most important aspects are discussed next.

1. Accommodation. Accommodation-induced myopia is unavoidable in younger patients. If unaccounted for, it may seriously compromise the planned wavefront-guided correction. To avoid this, the LADARWave system incorporates the use of a fixation target with an adjustable focal distance. A wavefront measurement is made to estimate the refractive error of the patient and then the fixation target is adjusted accordingly. Additional real-time wavefront measurements are then taken, calculating the defocus (sphere) term each time. To the patient, the fixation target is "moved" to represent a distant focal point until consecutive defocus terms are similar, then the target is moved slightly beyond this point. This process is equivalent to "fogging" at the phoropter and ensures that the patient is not accommodating. The LADARWave unit utilizes automatic fogging to ensure the accurate wavefront images are captured regardless of a patient's ability to control accommodation.

2. Dynamic Range. The issue of dynamic range is related to how much aberration a wavefront device can measure. There are two components of dynamic range. The first is the range of patients with nominal aberrations that can be measured. The second is the severity of aberration that can be measured in a given eye. Typically, there is a trade-off relationship when using Hartmann-Shack technology; that is, a reduction in accuracy for an increase in range, and vice versa.

The LADARWave aberrometer has a large dynamic range because the basic Hartmann-Shack principles have been augmented with some unique technology. Proportional array spacing improves the resolution of the Shack-Hartmann image without sacrificing range. This gives the LADARWave unit a large dynamic range and a great ability to measure highly aberrated eyes.

3. Dilation. It is well known that the aberrations in the periphery of the cornea are greater than those in the paraxial region. If one is using a 6.5-mm optical zone, the aberrations should be calculated to the edge of that zone to provide optimal correction. Because a natural pupil of that size is less common even in dim light, the LADARWave aberrometer requires pupillary dilation to ensure an accurate wavefront is captured over the entire intended treatment zone. The wavefront images from the dilated pupil will not be the same as those for an undilated pupil, because the undilated pupil wavefront will not take into account all of the peripheral aberrations. Appropriate compensation for the change in wavefront location eliminates this concern during surgery. This compensation is only possible if the wavefront is registered to some fixed feature of the eye, as described next.

4. Auto-Registration. The wavefront measured with an aberrometer is very sensitive to relative position, so it is vital that the location of the wavefront measurement be recorded with each wavefront captured. This is important not only at the time of image capture, but even more importantly, at the time of surgery. The LADARWave aberrometer requires that each patient have a centration photograph taken for each eye undilated and under controlled lighting conditions. The center of the undilated pupil is referenced to the limbus of the eye. This process is called *centration* and is now automated on the system to save time and increase accuracy. After centration, the eye is dilated to capture the necessary five wavefront images. Each of the calculated wavefronts is then automatically referenced to the limbus using the centration point to establish relative position. This is the only way to ensure that averaging wavefronts derived from multiple images is not affected by small changes in eye position between readings. This

cross-shaped illumination, which appear as arcs, and a horizontal line are set to intersect over the center of the pupil with the joystick. Once centered, the tracking system, which tracks the pupil is activated.

The Nidek EC-5000 permits the surgeon to adjust the transition zone diameter. This allows a smoother transition of the refractive power from the center to the periphery than would occur with a single ablation zone. In our recent study, the use of a peripheral transition zone 1.0 mm larger than the pupil under scotopic conditions resulted in a low incidence of postoperative glare and haloes and did not adversely affect the uncorrected visual acuity postoperatively. A 6.5-mm optical zone was used with a transition zone 1.0 mm larger than the scotopic pupil (7.0-, 7.5-, 8.0-, 8.5-, or 9.0-mm transition zones) (Table 2.18).

The original look-up tables and nomograms supplied by Nidek and available in the certification course were designed for use with a 5.5-mm optical zone and a 7.0-mm transitional zone. Examination of Table 2.19 reveals the ablation depth of three different myopic corrections (-3.00, -5.00, and -7.00 D) at different optical zone/transitional zone settings. This table includes the actual numbers taken from the laser and is made available to demonstrate the effect of changing the optical/transitional zones. Examination of these ablation depths reveals that a significantly greater amount of tissue is removed depending on the expansion of the optical and transitional zones; as such, the development of a customized nomogram is required. Any nomogram needs to be customized for each individual surgeon, laser, and laser suite.

The effects of temperature, humidity, and individual surgeon factors cannot be overemphasized. Each surgeon must individually validate the customized nomogram presented in this section. Note also that if the Nidek laser is being run on the 2.25e system software, further customization may be required. Following this nomogram, the authors demonstrated that LASIK did not adversely affect patients' postoperative visual acuity nor did it lead to a higher incidence of complications or side effects. Patients having LASIK by this nomogram reported an equivalent or lower incidence of glare and haloes than in other published reports for the Nidek and other excimer lasers.

| **Table 2.18** | NIDEK EC-5000 excimer laser myopic astigmatism nomogram for a 6.5-mm optical zone increasing the treatment zone by 1.0 mm larger than the scotopic pupil |

Use the Nidek LASIK look-up table (provided by Nidek) as a base.
Begin with negative cylinder refraction.
Look up the spherical and/or cylinder treatment on Nidek nomogram.
For cylinder ablation, treat the full cylinder up to 1.25 D, and follow the Nidek LASIK look-up table for more than 1.25 D cylinder regardless of the treatment zone.
Measure the pupil preoperatively after dark adaptation with the Colvard pupilometer.
Set the treatment zone at least 1.0 mm greater than the maximum pupil size.
Reduce the spherical component of the treatment that is identified on the Nidek LASIK look-up table according to the table below.
Reduce the spherical component by the recommended amount and treat the cylinder as recommended above.
Enter new spherical treatment and cylinder treatment into Nidek EC-5000 excimer laser.

Optical Zone (mm)	Treatment Zone (mm)	% Reduction in Sphere
6.5	7.5	12
6.5	8.0	17
6.5	8.5	22
6.5	9.0	27

Table 2.19 Myopic correction ablation depth using the Nidek EC-5000 (total ablation depth in μm)

Optical Zone/ Transitional Zone	−3.00 D (μm)	−5.00 D (μm)	−7.00 D (μm)
5.5/7.0	42.1	68.3	93.0
6.5/7.5	55.2	89.3	121.0
6.5/8.0	59.8	96.7	131.5
6.5/8.5	64.5	104.4	141.9
6.5/9.0	69.5	112.4	152.8

Hyperopic and hyperopic astigmatism are not yet currently FDA approved for treatment in the United States. The studies are ongoing, with data demonstrating substantial equivalence to other lasers. In Europe, the treatment of hyperopia and presbyopia are currently in use. The limited FDA-approved range is a distinct disadvantage of the Nidek laser. However, surgeons are using off-label software in the United States, and this software is available outside the United States where FDA regulations do not apply. FDA regulations apply to the laser itself. Off-label use is frequently considered a scope of medicine issue that is not regulated by the FDA; however, off-label use must be disclosed to the patient and the discussion well documented in the chart. Other lasers are available that are FDA approved to treat both hyperopia and mixed astigmatism; however, good randomized controlled prospective comparative trials are not currently available.

Numerous alternatives are available to treat astigmatism. In a negative cylinder excimer ablation, the laser flattens the steepest meridian to correct the astigmatism. This induces less flattening in the flattest meridian through a coupling effect and results in an excess hyperopic shift in the spherical equivalent. If a negative cylinder ablation is used to treat mixed and simple myopic astigmatism, the excess hyperopic shift needs to be compensated with a spherical hyperopic ablation. Chayet and colleagues designed a bitoric ablation pattern for the Nidek EC-5000 to treat mixed and simple myopic astigmatism that balances a negative cylinder ablation with a positive cylinder ablation. By avoiding a spherical ablation, bitoric laser treatments result in less tissue removal. A modification of this bitoric system was introduced by Vinciguerra.

The Nidek EC-5000 laser is not yet approved for the treatment of mixed astigmatism. However if the laser has access to off-label hyperopic software, then a multistage, multizone treatment can be utilized for the treatment of mixed astigmatism off label. One such nomogram is presented in Table 2.20. This bitoric ablation pattern for mixed and simple myopic astigmatism balances a negative cylinder ablation with a positive cylinder ablation. This bitoric laser treatment results in less tissue removal but requires adjustment of the spherical treatment to compensate for the hyperopic shift. Examples of how this nomogram is used follow. (Refer to Table 2.20 as you read these examples.)

Example 1:

Patient refraction: $-4.00 - 6.00 \times 180$

Spherical equivalent: -7.00

Negative cylinder $\times 0.35 = A$

$-6.00 \times 0.35 = -2.10$

Spherical equivalent $- A = B$

$-7.00 - (-2.10) = -4.90$

$B \times 0.85 = C$

$-4.90 \times 0.85 = -4.165$

Treatment 1: Plano -3.00×180
5.5 mm/7.5 mm (OZ/TZ)

Treatment 2: Plano $+3.00 \times 90$
5.5 mm/9.0 mm (OZ/TZ)

Treatment 3: -4.165 sphere
6.5 mm/7.5 mm (OZ/TZ)

where OZ is the optical zone and TZ is the transition zone

Table 2.20	Multistage, multizone nomogram for the Nidek EC-5000 excimer laser

Always begin with negative cylinder refraction.

Treatment 1

Plano − 1/2 cylinder power at the axis of negative cylinder refraction (6.5-mm optical zone/7.5-mm transition zone)

Treatment 2

Plano + 1/2 cylinder power at the axis positive cylinder refraction (5.5-mm optical zone/9.0-mm transition zone)

Treatment 3

Negative cylinder × 0.35 = A (A is the induced hyperopic shift)

Spherical equivalent − A = B. If B is hyperopic, skip next step and enter B as Treatment 3; if B is myopic, continue to next step (C).

B × 0.85 = C (B or C is sphere treatment)

Example 2:

Patient refraction: +1.00 − 2.00 × 180

Spherical equivalent: Plano

Negative cylinder × 0.35 = A

   −2.00 × 0.35 = −0.70

Spherical equivalent − A = B

   Plano − (−0.70) = +0.70

Treatment 3 is A, +0.70, because it is the induced hyperopic shift

Treatment 1: Plano −1.00 × 180

   5.5 mm/7.5 mm (OZ/TZ)

Treatment 2: Plano +1.00 × 90

   5.5 mm/9.0 mm (OZ/TZ)

Treatment 3: +0.70 sphere

   6.5 mm/7.5 mm (OZ/TZ)

An unpublished study of this nomogram on 32 eyes of 22 patients resulted in an uncorrected visual acuity of 20/40 in 100% of patients and 20/20 in 57% of patients at the 6-month postoperative mark. A best-corrected visual acuity of 20/20 was achieved in 100% of patients and mild overcorrection in the spherical equivalent (0.50 to 1.00) was found in 43% of eyes. A multistage, multizone LASIK nomogram for mixed astigmatism can effectively and safely correct refractive errors with good visual acuity outcomes; however, refining and customizing the nomogram is required to avoid overcorrection of the spherical equivalent. The nomogram provided in Table 2.20 is intended solely as a starting point for surgeons wishing to use the Nidek EC-5000 to create their own multistage, multizone LASIK nomogram for mixed and simple myopic astigmatism.

The Nidek EC-5000CX is the current FlexScan–equipped version of the original Nidek EC-5000 laser. The Nidek EC-5000CX is not currently FDA approved for use in the United States. A 2,000-Hz eye tracker has been approved for use in the United States. This tracker system constantly monitors the position of the patient's undilated pupil and is not affected by instruments passing in and out of the surgical field. It is both an active and passive tracking system that does not require dilation of the pupil or pretracking imaging of the patient's eyes. This eye tracker can be used to detect cyclotorsion.

An additional development has been the introduction of the OPD-Scan Refractive Power/Cornea Analyzer, the ARK-1000. This tool provides a refractive power map, wavefront map, corneal topography, autorefractor, and keratometer in one. It utilizes the principle of skiascopic phase difference for refractive map measurement. The corneal topography employs Placido disk technology. The unique wavefront system measures 1,440 data points in 0.4 second, mapping both regular and irregular astigmatism. This system generates a target refractive map, a Zernike graph, an HOA map, and a wavefront total aberration map. The FinalFit software, which is currently available outside the United States, converts the OPD-Scan's refractive, wavefront, and topography data into custom ablation algorithms for use by the Nidek EC-5000CX excimer laser system. This new upgraded excimer laser offers a smoother ablation surface with less ablation depth per diopter than previous software and a smoother transition zone. Customized ablations are possible when these two systems are combined.

Contact information for Nidek, Inc. can be found on page 268.

SUGGESTED READINGS

1. Buratto L, Brint S, Ferrari M. Surgical instruments. In: Buratto L, Brint SF, eds. *LASIK: principles and techniques.* Thorofare, NJ: Slack Inc; 1998:44.

2. Flanagan GW, Binder PS. Precision of flap measurements for laser *in situ* keratomileusis in 4428 eyes. *J Refract Surg.* 2003;19:113–123.

3. Huang D. Physics of customized corneal ablation. In: Krueger R, Applegate RA, MacRae SM, eds. *Wavefront customized visual correction.* Thorofare, NJ: Slack Inc; 2004:179.

4. Lindstrom RL, Linebarger EJ, Hardten DR, et al., Early results of hyperopic and astigmatic laser *in situ* keratomileusis in eyes with secondary hyperopia. *Ophthalmology.* 2000;107:1858–1863.

5. Macsai MS et al. Effect of expanding the treatment zone of the Nidek EC-5000 laser on laser *in situ* keratomileusis outcomes. *J Cataract Refract Surg.* 2004;30:2336–2343.

6. Muallem MS, Yoo SY, Romano AC, et al. Corneal flap thickness in laser *in situ* keratomileusis using the Moria M2 microkeratome. *J Cataract Refract Surg.* 2004;30:1902–1908.

7. Pop M, Payette Y. Risk factors for night vision complaints after LASIK for myopia. *Ophthalmology.* 2004;111:3–10.

8. Rabinowitz YS. Videokeratographic indices to aid in screening for keratoconus. *J Refract Surg.* 1995; 11:371–379.

9. Rao SN, Raviv T, Majmudar PA, et al. Role of Orbscan II in screening keratoconus suspects before refractive corneal surgery. *Ophthalmology* 2002;109:1642–1646.

10. Rueda L et al. Laser *in situ* keratomileusis for mixed and simple myopic astigmatism with the Nidek EC-5000 laser. *J Refract Surg.* 2002;18:234–238.

11. Sarkisian KA, Petrov AA. Experience with the Nidek MK-2000 microkeratome in 1,220 cases. *J Refract Surg.* 2001;17(Suppl 2):S252–S254.

12. Solomon KD et al. Flap thickness accuracy: comparison of 6 microkeratome models. *J Cataract Refract Surg.* 2004;30:964–977.

13. Stein RM. Automated microkeratome makes flap creation simple, safe. Ophthalmology Times. January 1, 2003.

14. U.S. Food and Drug Administration. LADARvision excimer laser system for photorefractive keratectomy (PRK), Report No. P970043/S1, Washington, DC: Author; September 24, 1999.

15. Vinciguerra P, Camesasca FI, Torres IM. One-year results of custom laser epithelial keratomileusis with the Nidek system. *J Refract Surg.* 2004;20(Suppl 5): S699–S704.

16. Vinciguerra P, Camesasca FI, Urso R. Reduction of spherical aberration with the Nidek NAVEX customized ablation system. *J Refract Surg.* 2003; 19(Suppl 2):S195–S201.

Role of Mitomycin-C in Keratorefractive Surgery

Parag Majmudar, M.D.

Mitomycin-C (MMC) is an antibiotic derived from *Streptomyces caespitosus,* and its cross-linking properties enable it to bind to DNA and prevent replication. For that reason, this alkylating agent was originally used as a systemic chemotherapeutic agent. In a manner similar to the way in which MMC prevents replication of neoplastic cells, it can also prevent fibroblastic proliferation as well. This property was recognized to be beneficial in prolonging the success of glaucoma filtration surgery, and its use in this capacity is commonplace. In addition, MMC also has proven to be helpful in the management of corneal intraepithelial neoplasia and pterygium. Recently, however, the use of MMC has become a popular topic for discussion in the context of refractive corneal surgery as a modulator of wound healing following excimer laser surface ablation.

A well-recognized, but perhaps poorly understood, complication of corneal surface ablation with the excimer laser is the development of corneal haze. Its incidence has fortunately diminished with the advent of sophisticated excimer laser technology. The improved technology has allowed for a more homogeneous distribution of laser energy, which may result in smoother ablations on the corneal stroma and may prevent activation of stromal keratocytes, which deposit ground substance and abnormal collagen causing clinically significant haze. Nonetheless, corneal haze is still seen following surface excimer laser procedures. Despite the promise of laser-assisted subepithelial keratectomy (LASEK), haze can be seen following this procedure as well.

In 1991 Talamo et al. described an animal model of photorefractive keratectomy (PRK) haze and analyzed the effects of MMC on haze prevention. Their results showed that eyes treated with MMC developed significantly less corneal haze. Our group described the first human series of eyes to receive treatment with MMC for post-PRK corneal haze. In those early cases, recurrent corneal haze resulted in severe visual disability and patients were contemplating corneal transplantation. We postulated that the antiproliferative effect of MMC on the activated stromal keratocytes might prevent further haze formation, and developed the protocol for the treatment of corneal haze following surface excimer laser ablation, which is widely accepted today.

Because MMC was successful in preventing recurrence of existing haze, the protocol was expanded for prophylactic use in patients predisposed to the development of corneal haze following primary surface ablation for high myopia, and surface ablation over irregular LASIK flaps, such as buttonholes. Although this application of MMC remains controversial, there is evidence that it can be safe and effective.

TREATMENT OF EXISTING CORNEAL HAZE WITH MITOMYCIN-C

The technique of superficial keratectomy with MMC for existing corneal haze is described in this section. It is important to note that MMC in no way eradicates corneal haze; rather MMC prevents the stromal keratocytes from depositing additional scar. Therefore, it is imperative that the scar be completely removed. Two methods are used to remove scar tissue: mechanical debridement using a 64 Beaver blade or a diamond-dusted burr, like that used for pterygium removal and excimer laser phototherapeutic keratectomy (PTK). Both methods may work equally well. In either case, multiple intraoperative trips to the slit lamp may be required in order to gauge the efficacy of the keratectomy and also to determine the end point. When using PTK, care must be taken to vary the distribution of pulses throughout the corneal surface in order to prevent unwanted hyperopic shifts.

Once the scar has been removed, it is of the utmost importance to follow the protocol for MMC application meticulously in order to prevent potential complications. This begins with procurement of the medication. Significant deviation from the concentration and duration of exposure can lead to vision-threatening adverse events. Our protocol is to have MMC 0.02% (0.2 mg/mL) prepared by an independent compounding pharmacy in order to minimize errors in dilution. A common area of confusion is the unit of measure for the MMC, 0.02% is equivalent to 0.2 mg/mL, but there have been anecdotal case reports of 0.2% being used. This is 10 times the suggested concentration and results in severe endothelial toxicity.

Once the MMC has been correctly prepared, 1-mL aliquots may be frozen for several weeks until ready for use. The MMC is thawed prior to surgery and placed in an empty disposable contact lens well. Proper application of MMC to the corneal surface is best achieved by using a "corneal light shield" (Mentor or Solan), a 6- to 8-mm circular Merocel sponge, which is commonly used in the operating room to shield the retina from microscope phototoxicity during corneal surgery. The advantage of the corneal light shield over a Merocel spear is that the sponge achieves better contact with the corneal surface and, more importantly, prevents excess MMC from coming into contact with the limbus. Limiting the spread of MMC is critical in reducing potential postoperative complications. The corneal light shield is placed in the MMC solution at the beginning of the case and is left in the solution until needed.

During application of MMC, care should be taken to ensure that the sponge is wet but not dripping with MMC. The sponge is placed on the central cornea, and the surgeon must meticulously monitor the surface to prevent MMC from coming into contact with the limbus and conjunctiva. The duration of exposure is exactly 2 minutes. After the allotted exposure time, the MMC-soaked sponge is carefully removed and discarded, a cellulose sponge is used to remove any excess MMC left on the cornea, and the surface of the eye is vigorously irrigated with 30 mL of balanced salt solution. These steps remove excess MMC from the corneal stroma, and will also help to minimize potential complications.

Typical postkeratorefractive surgery medications are administered—topical antibiotics, corticosteroids, and nonsteroidal antiinflammatory agents—and a therapeutic bandage contact lens is placed. The cornea is carefully monitored for reepithelialization, which typically occurs in 3 to 5 days. The patient should be forewarned that visual recovery may be slow, and that the final refractive error is difficult to predict. The possibility of the future need for refractive treatment should be explained.

PROPHYLACTIC TREATMENT WITH MITOMYCIN-C

Mitomycin-C may be used selectively in primary surface ablation cases, in order to prevent the development of corneal haze in predisposed patients. The definition of the high-risk patient following surface ablation has evolved, especially after the introduction of the newer generation excimer lasers. Early in the PRK experience, it was felt that the threshold for developing haze was a surface ablation to correct more than 6.00 D of myopia. Patients were often counseled that in ablations greater than −6.00 D, the risk of haze was significant. However, assigning a haze potential to a particular dioptric level of correction appears arbitrary. This became very evident with the introduction of the flying spot lasers, which not only removed more tissue per diopter of correction, but also gave surgeons the ability to expand the treatment zone. Munnerlyn's formula, $S = d^2 \times D/3$, where S is ablation depth, d is ablation diameter, and D is correction in diopters, dictates that with expanded optical zones, the depth of ablation is directly correlated with the square of the ablation diameter. Patients began to develop haze following surface ablation for as little as −4.00 D of myopia if a larger optical zone, such as 8 mm, was selected. Intuitively, the potential for haze is correlated with the total amount of energy delivered to the cornea, and this in turn is directly related to the depth of ablation.

Our definition of high risk has changed to incorporate the total depth of ablation, not just the dioptric level. Because a −6.00-D myopic ablation with a first-generation broad-beam laser with a 6-mm optical zone equates to a depth of ablation of 72 μm, our criteria for the use of prophylactic MMC is 75 μm of excimer ablation, regardless of the actual dioptric correction.

An important issue in the prophylactic use of MMC is potential overcorrection following surface ablation. This effect may be due to inhibition by MMC of the compensatory wound healing following surface ablation procedures. This may result in persistent hyperopia and, therefore, we currently use a nomogram adjustment, in which the spherical portion (when written in plus cylinder notation) is reduced by 10% to 15% based on the patient age and refractive error. For example, for a 35-year-old patient with a refraction of −8.00 + 2.00 × 90, the treatment would be adjusted so that the sphere would be reduced by 10% to −7.20 + 2.00 × 90.

Initially, an exposure time of 2 minutes was used in prophylactic cases of MMC. Recently our group began evaluating shorter exposure times of MMC in prophylactic cases in an attempt to further minimize potential toxicity. Early results indicate that with 7 months of follow-up, there is no difference in haze formation rates between exposure times of 12 seconds (10% of the original exposure) and 60 seconds. Of course, because corneal haze following surface ablation is a late-onset phenomenon in many cases, no long-term conclusions can be made at this time. However, if a shorter exposure time can minimize scar

formation, it would certainly be preferable because it would further reduce any potential dose-dependent complications of MMC.

There is considerable evidence of the toxicity of MMC in the literature. Corneal edema, glaucoma, corneal perforation, iritis, and photophobia following the use of MMC in pterygium surgery has been described by Rubinfield et al. All of these adverse effects were due to prolonged topical administration of MMC. However, a single-dose of MMC has been reported by Dougherty et al. to have produced a corneoscleral melt in a patient undergoing pterygium surgery.

We feel that our protocol is fundamentally different from previous ophthalmic applications of MMC. In pterygium surgery, the MMC is often used chronically in the postoperative course. Our protocol abandoned this concept because MMC penetrates an intact epithelium poorly, and because we felt that chronic instillation would result in prolonged contact with other ocular surface structures, the most important of which is the limbus. The majority of complications that have been reported occurred following limbal application of MMC for indications such as pterygium surgery. Because the limbus is a highly vascular region, the complications seen are likely to be due to ischemia of the limbal vessels, which may initiate an inflammatory cascade that could potentially lead to release of proteolytic enzymes, and result in a corneoscleral melt. In addition, MMC contact with the stem cell population at the limbus might result in delayed reepithelialization, which is another risk factor for corneal melt. Our protocol involves application to only the central, avascular cornea, and meticulous care to prevent MMC contact with any other ocular structure. MMC is delivered via a corneal light shield, which serves to limit the contact of MMC to only the central 6 mm of the cornea. A Merocel spear is not recommended for MMC application due to its propensity to allow MMC to leak onto the limbus and conjunctiva. Copious irrigation of the ocular surface with 30 mL of balanced salt solution is likely to remove any residual MMC.

Furthermore, it is imperative to utilize the correct concentration of MMC. In our series, a single intraoperative dose of 0.02% MMC was utilized for exactly 2 minutes, followed by copious irrigation. Our experience with patients who have received MMC treatment for post-PRK haze removal have shown no long-term adverse effects over 8 years, and no patients in the prophylactic group experienced any toxic adverse effects related to MMC administration. Reepithelialization was complete in all eyes by the fifth postoperative day, which is similar to our experience with other PRK and LASEK patients who were not treated with MMC. Safety studies conducted by various investigators reveal that over the short term, corneal and endothelial toxicity is absent as evidenced clinically and with confocal microscopic evaluation.

Patients should be advised that the use of MMC to prevent or treat corneal haze is off-label. The long-term effects are not well known. The benefits and risks should be included in the informed consent and the discussion well documented in the chart.

The role of MMC has expanded recently in refractive surgery. Its first major application was in preventing haze recurrence after PRK and RK. Use of MMC in conjunction with transepithelial PTK/PRK has also proven to be effective in treating patients with complicated LASIK flaps. The results of our case series demonstrate that MMC is effective in reducing the incidence of haze in those eyes that are most likely to develop this visually disabling complication. Certainly, longer follow-up and treatment of greater numbers of patients will help support the validity of this technique.

SUGGESTED READINGS

Candal EM, Majmudar PA. Surface ablation with prophylactic MMC for high myopia and high-risk patients. In: Probst L, ed. *LASIK: advances,* *controversies and custom*. Thorofare, NJ, Slack; 2004: 325–332.

Carones F, Vigo L, Scandola E, et al. Evaluation of the prophylactic use of mitomycin-C to inhibit haze formation after photorefractive keratectomy. *J Cataract Refract Surg*. 2002; 28:2088–2095.

Dougherty PJ, Hardten DR, Lindstrom RL. Corneoscleral melt after pterygium surgery using a single intraoperative application of mitomycin-C. *Cornea*. 1996; 15:537–540.

Gambato C, Ghirlando A, Moretto E, Busato F, Midena E. Mitomycin C modulation of corneal wound healing after photorefractive keratectomy in highly myopic eyes. *Ophthalmology*. 2005;112:208–218.

Kapadia MS, Wilson SE. Transepithelial photorefractive keratectomy for treatment of thin flaps or caps after complicated laser *in situ* keratomileusis. *Am J Ophthalmology*. 1998;126:827–829.

Lane H, Swale J, Majmudar P. Prophylactic use of mitomycin-C in the management of a buttonholed LASIK flap. *J Cataract Refract Surg*. 2003;29: 387–389.

Lee D. *Personal communication*, Yonsei Eye Center, Seoul, Republic of South Korea, 2002.

Majmudar PA, Forstot SL, Nirankari VS, et al. Topical mitomycin-C for subepithelial fibrosis after corneal surgery. *Ophthalmology*. 2000;107:89–94.

Muller LT, Candal EM, Epstein RJ, et al. Transepithelial phototherapeutic keratectomy/photorefractive keratectomy with adjunctive mitomycin-C for complicated LASIK flaps. *J Cataract Refract Surg*. 2005; 31:291–295.

Rubinfield RS, Pfister RR, Stein RM, et al. Serious complications of topical mitomycin-C after pterygium surgery. *Ophthalmology*. 1992;99:1647–1654.

Talamo JH, Gollamudi S, Green WR, et al. Modulation of corneal wound healing after excimer laser keratomileusis using topical mitomycin-C and steroids. *Arch Ophthalmol*. 1991;109:1141–1146.

Zolotaryov AV. Prophylactic intraoperative MMC: on the way to haze-free PRK? *Am Acad Ophthalmology*, annual meeting, 2002.

Retreatment of Patients after Primary Refractive Surgery

Michael Rosenberg, M.D.

This chapter will review retreatment of the refractive surgery patient who has symptomatic ametropia following refractive surgery. The management of other LASIK-related complications is covered in detail in the complications chapter (Chapter 5).

The most important factors determining patient satisfaction after refractive surgery are realistic vision expectations before surgery and a thorough understanding of the process. This includes an understanding of the type and frequency of potential complications of retreatment. It is the responsibility of the surgeon to communicate the expected vision goals of the surgery for each specific patient. Accordingly, the philosophy of each surgeon, and his or her comfort with retreatment, is the single most important factor in determining the ultimate outcome for any given patient. Most physicians performing refractive surgery can be generally described as aggressive or conservative with regard to outcomes. Aggressive surgeons will set high expectations—for example, at least a 98% probability of uncorrected vision of 20/25 or better. To achieve these results, a relatively higher probability of retreatment must be expected. More conservative surgeons may set lower goals—for example, the ability to pass a driving test without restrictions or to perform the majority of visual tasks without spectacles or contact lenses. Patients willing to accept the less rigorous goals can expect a lower probability of retreatment. Nevertheless, patients who preoperatively seem willing to accept the possibility of a less than ideal outcome are frequently dissatisfied after surgery. Not only do they see worse than they did with spectacles or contact lenses, but they have night vision symptoms resulting from residual refractive error.

For these reasons, it is imperative that every physician performing refractive surgery be comfortable with the concept of retreatment and be knowledgeable about the various techniques available. Patients who attain the highest level of postoperative visual function will be active ambassadors for the refractive surgeon. This will increase both patient referrals and the success of the practice. Patients who achieve less than expected results after surgery are more likely to lack enthusiasm for the procedure and will communicate that feeling to the detriment of their surgeon and the field of refractive surgery.

It is hoped that the information in this chapter will allow the reader to be enthusiastic about retreatment and receive the gratification that comes from patient outcomes that are "wonderful" rather than just "okay."

INDICATIONS

The basic indications for retreatment of a patient after primary refractive surgery are patient dissatisfaction, a problem that can be fixed with a retreatment technique, and a realistic expectation on the part of the patient and the surgeon that the benefit of the retreatment procedure outweighs the risk. The patient must have decreased vision that, when corrected with appropriate refraction, results in good visual acuity. The residual refractive error must be treatable by an approved laser protocol or by appropriate incisional surgery.

In some cases the result following initial surgery may be consistent with the preoperative discussion of expectations, but the patient is still unhappy. This may occur in patients who are given soft outcome predictions. For instance, they may be told "If you have refractive surgery, you will be able to do virtually everything you need to do without glasses, including driving." A soft end point sounds good during the consultation. However, it may not sound so good after treatment, when a patient with preoperative best-corrected visual acuity of 20/20 has a postoperative uncorrected visual acuity of 20/25– and night vision issues. The patient can drive without glasses, but is not comfortable. In these situations, the physician must choose between several options: Remind the patient of the preoperative discussion, convince the patient that all is fine, or proceed with retreatment. A surgeon who fails to present the option of retreatment either because of an unwillingness to do a retreatment or because of a lack of comfort with the techniques will leave the patient with the perception of a less than satisfactory result. This surgeon misses the opportunity to provide the patient with a result perceived to be excellent.

Refractive surgery is a process rather than an event and this should be communicated to the patient before surgery. The surgeon should present the patient with the option of retreatment rather than waiting for the patient to request the procedure. This will instill confidence and ultimately leave the patient with a very positive experience.

On the other hand, many refractive surgeons do not believe in encouraging retreatment for a patient with less than 20/20 visual acuity or some other surgically induced vision abnormality unless the patient expresses discontent. While this patient may not become an ambassador for LASIK surgery, there will also be no added risk due to retreatment. In the unlikely event that a retreatment problem were to develop, a patient might wonder why he or she was encouraged to have a second surgery in the absence of complaint. As surgeons become more comfortable with flap lifting and limbal relaxing incision (LRI) techniques and with designing a customized retreatment surgery

for their patients, it becomes easier to recommend the additional surgery. The majority of patients do benefit from retreatment when it is properly planned and executed.

Residual refractive errors result from initial overcorrection, undercorrection, or regression. The likelihood of postoperative ametropia in the immediate postoperative period increases with the degree of correction. Regression refers to minimal or no refractive error in the immediate postoperative period, and late, slow drift in the direction of the primary refractive state. The larger the correction the patient has preoperatively, the greater the likelihood of regression.

There are multiple reasons for immediate overcorrection or undercorrection. Inaccurate refraction may result from surgeon or technician error, or inadequate cycloplegia. Failure to calibrate the laser properly may lead to insufficient or excessive laser energy. Overcorrections may result from dehydration of the stromal bed during the procedure, particularly when the ablation time is lengthy. This is potentiated by low humidity in the laser suite or prolonged elevation of a flap during LASIK prior to initiating treatment. Undercorrections may be related to overhydration of the cornea due to high humidity or excessive irrigation prior to initiating treatment. Many myopia treatment nomograms were geared toward a slight undercorrection. They were developed to avoid overcorrection of myopia at a time when treatment of hyperopia was not available.

To optimize postoperative results, it is essential for each surgeon to develop a standardized LASIK technique, and to develop an individual nomogram based on the postoperative results, the equipment being used, and the conditions in the laser suite. This requires tight control and maintenance of both temperature and humidity.

COMMON POSTOPERATIVE VISION PROBLEMS

There are certain common situations in which patients voice dissatisfaction, despite apparently good outcomes. These include the following:

- Asymmetry of visual acuity
- Night vision symptoms

- Oblique astigmatism
- Unrecognized anisometropia
- Asthenopia in overcorrected prepresbyopic patients.

We should emphasize that evaluation of the true residual refractive error should always be on the basis of a cycloplegic refraction. Whether the subsequent retreatment is based on the cycloplegic refraction or manifest refraction requires some surgical judgment.

Asymmetry of Visual Acuity

A patient who has very sharp 20/20 visual acuity or better in one eye but weak 20/25 acuity in the other eye will frequently complain about the weaker eye. This is especially significant when the weak eye is the dominant eye. In the binocular situation, the brain will choose to derive most visual information on the basis of input from the dominant eye and thus the overall satisfaction will be dependent on the acuity in that eye. Generally no amount of reassurance will satisfy a patient, who is able to alternately cover each eye. This comparison will be done in perpetuity until the weaker eye is corrected. Patients may be convinced not to have retreatment of a mildly myopic nondominant eye, especially if they have early presbyopic symptoms.

Night Vision Symptoms

Uncorrected refractive error is the most common cause of persistent nighttime haloes and glare. Night vision issues are one of the more significant concerns of patients contemplating refractive surgery. Persistent complaints about night vision from a patient with good visual acuity, but a residual refractive error, should be addressed with retreatment. As an example, a patient with a visual acuity of 20/20− who has a refraction of −0.50 + 1.25 × 75 degress may have star-bursting related to the residual cylinder. This becomes more evident at night when the pupil is larger. Effective treatment of these patients will reduce the number of patients with night vision problems following laser vision correction.

Oblique Astigmatism

Patients with oblique astigmatism frequently complain of subjective visual disturbance out of proportion to visual acuity. The accurate identification and measurement of residual oblique astigmatism requires cycloplegia and careful refraction by an experienced refractionist. Patients with astigmatism "with-the-rule" or "against-the-rule" will usually have either a vertical or a horizontal border in relative focus, providing sufficient visual clues in a world that is oriented vertically and horizontally. Patients with oblique astigmatism have equal defocus of vertical and horizontal borders, creating a more generalized blur.

Unrecognized Anisometropia

Patients with anisometropia will frequently have subjective complaints despite apparently good visual acuity when tested monocularly without cycloplegia. Overcorrected myopes with hyperopia in one eye may read the Snellen chart quite easily until dilated, and may not show a significant refractive error on manifest refraction. A young patient with a postoperative refractive error may have postoperative hyperopia with or without astigmatism of up to +1.00 to +1.25 D and still have 20/15 visual acuity. It is incumbent on the physician to perform a cycloplegic refraction on any patient with unexplained visual complaints, regardless of the uncorrected visual acuity. It is also important to perform at least one cycloplegic examination on every patient at a time when the refractive error is likely stable, and before the patient is released from postoperative care. Symptomatic patients with unrecognized overcorrection may return several years after discharge, with reduced acuity and dissatisfaction creating a situation in which accurate explanation of the issues is awkward, and correction by retreatment somewhat more difficult.

Asthenopia in Uncorrected Prepresbyopic Patients

Patients with symmetric overcorrection and hyperopia may have good acuity and vague symptoms, especially if there is some degree of persistent astigmatism. Timely cycloplegic refraction will identify these patients and permit prompt retreatment.

In summary the measurement of good uncorrected visual acuity is not the sole factor in identifying patients who are candidates for possible retreatment. Careful consideration of patient symptoms combined with careful refraction, with and without cycloplegia, is necessary to ensure that patients will have optimal refractive outcomes.

EVALUATION

The most important prerequisite for retreatment is refractive stability. The stability of refraction should be determined on the basis of cycloplegic refraction to avoid undercorrection of accommodating hyperopic patients and the overcorrection of accommodating myopic patients. The surgeon should determine whether the retreatment will be based on the cycloplegic or the manifest refraction. Moderately myopic patients (up to -7.00 D) may be retreated as soon as two refractions, 1 month apart, are stable and as soon as 2 to 3 months after an initial uncomplicated LASIK. For patients with greater amounts of myopia, patients treated for hyperopia, patients treated with PRK, and patients with complications from the initial treatment (e.g., corneal abrasion), retreatment should be postponed until refractive, topographic, and anatomic corneal stability are observed. For patients with significant confounding abnormalities such as visually significant striae, keratitis, or epithelial ingrowth, appropriate treatment of the abnormality is required before retreatment with the laser. In some cases

treatment of these problems will correct the residual refractive error.

Prior to potential retreatment, a thorough examination should include the following: monocular visual acuities (UCVA), best spectacle-corrected visual acuities (BCSVA), manifest and cycloplegic refraction, keratometry, corneal topography, slit-lamp examination, central and peripheral pachymetry, corneal topography, and preferably wavefront evaluation. Table 4.1 provides a checklist that summarizes these retreatment examination tasks.

Keratometry should be done to help predict the postoperative contour after retreatment. Caution is advised if the predicted average keratometry value would be greater than 50.00 D in a hyperopic patient or less than 35.00 D in a myopic patient. Remember the conversion factor of 0.7 or 0.8 multiplied by the spherical equivalent of the refraction. Corneal topography must be used to rule out the presence of cornea ectasia.

The slit-lamp examination is important to rule out corneal pathology that could explain reduced visual acuity, such as surface disruption, striae, interface debris or inflammation, or epithelial ingrowth. The presence of cataract could also explain a shift in refractive error, night vision disturbance, or decreased acuity and should be identified before additional cornea surgery is considered.

If available, wavefront evaluation can be helpful as a technique for determining the residual refractive error. It also determines the type and amount of higher order aberrations (HOAs). It can be used to retreat the patient with a custom ablation. The VISX

Table 4.1   Preoperative examination checklist for LASIK retreatment

Monocular uncorrected visual acuity
Best spectacle-corrected visual acuity
Manifest refraction
Cycloplegic refraction
Keratometry to be certain cornea will not
    be too steep ($\geq$50.00 D) or too flat
    ($\leq$35.00 D) after retreatment
Slit-lamp examination to rule out surface
    disruption, striae, interface debris or
    inflammation, ingrowth, or cataract

Corneal topography to rule out ectasia
Ultrasonic pachymetry centrally to determine
    RST; and peripherally, if LRI considered
Wavefront scan to determine refraction,
    HOAs, create PreVue lens, or prepare for
    custom retreatment

WaveScan system can be used to prepare a PreVue lens, which the patient can use preoperatively to help determine the value of a custom retreatment.

Ultrasonic pachymetry is especially important after prior refractive surgery. Orbscan pachymetry should never be relied on to calculate residual stromal thickness (RST) or flap thickness. Corneal thickness must be adequate in the areas in which retreatment will occur, the central cornea (myopia), midperipheral cornea (hyperopia and astigmatism), or peripheral cornea (if incisional correction is indicated). The RST is calculated using the non–nomogram-adjusted refractive error, taking into consideration the diameter of the treatment zones. Ideally the flap thickness in LASIK patients has been determined by subtraction pachymetry during the initial treatment. If it has not, knowledge of the instrument use to create the flap, the specific microkeratome and head, or the IntraLase flap settings may provide enough information to estimate the adequacy of the remaining cornea. Some patients must be counseled that intraoperative pachymetry will be performed at the time of retreatment and if inadequate stromal thickness is present, retreatment will not be performed.

The actual retreatment of the undercorrected myopic patient should not be nomogram adjusted; that is, the manifest or the cycloplegic refraction without adjustment is used.

The complications of retreatment should be carefully explained to the patient. Infection is quite rare; however, the risk of epithelial ingrowth is more likely than after a primary procedure, presumably due to manipulation associated with scoring and lifting of the original flap. Assuming the initial flap of a LASIK procedure was well constructed, the likelihood of a defective flap after relifting is quite low. The character of the flap is slightly less flexible than after the initial surgery. As a result, if handled carefully, the likelihood of postoperative striae is less than after a primary procedure and repositioning is often easier. Ideally, most patients with less than satisfactory results from a primary refractive procedure will require only one retreatment, but if adequate corneal thickness is present, additional retreatment is possible.

SURGICAL TECHNIQUES FOR RETREATMENT

Multiple techniques are available to surgeons for patients requiring retreatment. The range of FDA-approved laser treatments is broad enough on most lasers to allow a standard laser correction for most retreatment patients. Some lasers have narrower approved treatment ranges, and an occasional patient treated on these lasers will require off-label approaches to retreatment. Surgeons should be well acquainted with the approved treatment range on their available laser and the options available for off-label ablation should this be a consideration. Various techniques are listed next and each technique is discussed in detail in the subsections that follow.

The most common techniques used for retreatment are:

- Standard laser retreatment beneath a previously made LASIK flap
- Standard surface retreatment after primary surface ablation
- Limbal relaxing incision.

Less commonly needed techniques used for retreatment are:

- LASIK or surface ablation in patients having undergone previous radial keratotomy
- LASIK in patients having undergone prior surface treatment
- Surface retreatment in patients having undergone prior LASIK
- Custom surface or LASIK retreatment of patients having had prior conventional treatment.

Standard Excimer Laser Retreatment beneath a Previously Made LASIK Flap

The patient is seated at the slit lamp and topical anesthetic is instilled in both eyes. If the patient is to have a custom retreatment or has a significant amount of astigmatism, a sterile marking pen is used to mark the 3 and 9 o' clock positions at the limbus with the aid of a horizontally directed slit beam. The cornea is then illuminated with a broad, obliquely directed beam. The patient is asked to look toward the direction of the hinge, and the edge of the flap is usually easily identified as a faint gray or white curvilinear opacity. Occasionally, this may be difficult to see, especially if the flap edge is located near the limbus within the vascular arcade, or within a corneal arcus. In this instance the flap edge can usually be seen elsewhere on the cornea where the edge of the flap is located further from the limbus. The patient may have to look in different directions to enable the surgeon to identify a distinct flap edge.

Occasionally, the flap is still difficult to discern. Gentle pressure with an instrument on the peripheral cornea near the estimated position of the flap edge will distort the cornea and make the edge evident. The flap edge is marked using the tip of a #25 sterile hypodermic needle bevel up, scoring the flap for at least one clock hour. Some surgeons prefer a Sinsky hook. A Machat LASIK retreatment spatula (Asico AE-2830) (Fig. 4.1) or a Sinsky hook is positioned at an acute angle to the stroma at the scratch mark and moved along the scored edge until an easily identifiable area of separation of at least one clock hour is created. Some physicians do the entire procedure, including the flap lift, under the laser microscope, but the optics of the slit lamp are far superior, and corneal epithelial injury is less likely when this part of the procedure is performed at the slit lamp.

Once the flap is elevated, the patient is positioned under the laser microscope and is prepped and draped. The cornea is marked over the flap edge in the same manner as for a primary treatment. The Machat LASIK retreatment spatula, Sinskey hook, or a Rosenfeld

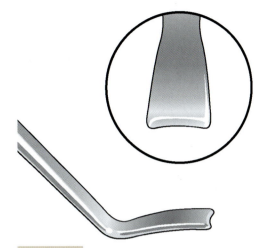

Rosenfeld glide dissector (Storz E9086).

glide dissector (Storz E9086) (Fig. 4.2) is placed in the initial area of separation and passed in circumferential fashion, breaking the epithelium at the flap edge and separating the flap edge from the underlying bed, until the hinge is encountered on each side.

After appropriate positioning of the laser, the flap is either grasped and gently lifted using a forceps 180 degrees from the hinge, or a spatula is passed under the flap from one edge to the other at the hinge, sweeping toward the free edge, lifting and folding the flap back at the hinge. If the initial flap was made with a mechanical microkeratome, the lift is usually easy. Only rarely is it necessary to use a spatula to break adhesions under the flap before the lift is made. Some patients who are retreated within the first 6 months have more resistance than patients lifted after several years. It is therefore wise to lift the flap slowly to avoid inadvertent flap trauma. However, this author has lifted flaps 7 years after primary surgery with little difficulty. Usually the greatest resistance is encountered at the flap edge in patients with large flaps where the edge falls in or near the limbal arcade and there is some degree of vessel associated scarring.

If the flap has been made with a femtosecond laser, the epithelium is more adherent at the flap edge. The cornea is therefore more prone to epithelial disruption. Either scoring the flap edge more extensively before lifting or

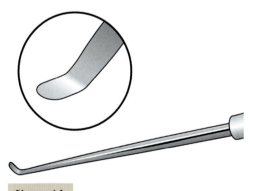

Machat LASIK retreatment spatula (Asico AE-2830).

lifting with greater care is advised. It is also advisable to use a spatulated instrument passed across the bed prior the lift. If there is resistance near the hinge, a dry Merocel sponge can be placed on the undersurface of the flap and it can be "peeled" toward the hinge.

The refractive procedure is performed in the usual manner. Some surgeons prefer to slow the laser for low treatments to reduce the chance of decentration caused by patient eye movement. As previously stated, no nomogram adjustment should be used for myopia correction. For patients being retreated for hyperopia, whether the result of overcorrection of primary myopia or undercorrection of primary hyperopia, a nomogram adjustment is usually advised based on the surgeon's personal outcome experience.

Before the flap is replaced, a dry Merocel sponge is used to push from the periphery of the stromal bed toward the epithelial margin of the flap to remove any epithelial cells inadvertently introduced onto the bed. The flap is replaced. It usually repositions easily and seems to be significantly more resistant to swelling during repositioning. The placement of a bandage contact lens overnight is a good idea to provide increased comfort and promote epithelialization. In addition, maintaining a secure flap that is resistant to movement by blink or inadvertent patient contact may reduce the incidence of epithelial ingrowth. In the absence of a significant corneal abrasion, the soft contact lens is not associated with an increased risk of diffuse lamellar keratitis (DLK). When the epithelium is minimally disrupted, some surgeons prefer not to use a contact lens.

Postoperative care consists of topical prednisolone 1% and a topical fluoroquinolone four times daily just as is done after primary treatment. Topical ketorolac tromethamine 0.5% (Acular) is instilled at the end of procedure and lubricants are used at least four times a day. Patients who have undergone retreatment often have less discomfort than was present with the original procedure. However, significant discomfort may occur when epithelial disruption is moderate or marked, or if the contact lens is too tight. Patients typically recognize the visual improvement immediately or shortly after removal of the contact lens.

Because flaps may be relifted even years after the primary procedure, there is broad consensus within the refractive community that recutting should be avoided unless absolutely necessary. If there is a question about the quality or viability of the flap based on the clinical appearance, surface retreatment with or without mitomycin-C is usually a preferred alternative.

Surface Retreatment after Primary Surface Ablation

Retreatment is performed in a fashion identical to the primary treatment. The patient is given an oral nonsteroid anti-inflammatory agent 1 hour prior to surgery. After instillation of topical anesthesia, a 7- or 9-mm optical zone marker (Asico AE 2713) is placed on the cornea centered on the pupil. The marker may be filled with topical anesthetic to loosen the epithelial attachments. The epithelium is then mechanically debrided with a Beaver blade or alternatively with an Amoils brush. Another approach is to fill the marker with a 20% alcohol solution and allow it to remain for 20 seconds. The toxicity of the solution is significantly greater as contact with the ocular surface increases beyond this time interval. Caution the patient about moving the eyes so the solution will not leak beyond the debridement area. The alcohol is removed from the well with a spear and the cornea irrigated with cold balanced salt solution. After drying with a Merocel sponge, the edge marked with the zone marker is easily visualized, and the reticle of the laser microscope is used to check for adequate centration.

Using the Machat LASIK retreatment spatula, the epithelium is removed with much less force than with simple mechanical removal. It may be preserved as a sheet if the surgeon wishes to replace it after the treatment, such as in laser epithelial keratomileusis (LASEK). The bed is inspected to ensure that no epithelial remnants are present and the treatment is applied. If more than 1 minute of time is required to remove the epithelium, a moist sponge should be gently wiped across the stromal bed to avoid excessive dehydration. No nomogram adjustment on the cycloplegic refraction is used in PRK. Following the application of the laser, the cornea is irrigated for 1 minute with chilled balanced salt solution and a chilled contact lens is placed. Some physicians advocate chilling the cornea with a "Popsicle" of frozen sterile balance salt. Postoperative medications include a topical fluoroquinolone four times daily, ketorolac 0.5% (Acular) four times daily, topical prednisolone 1% twice a day, artificial tears, and dilute anesthetic drops. The anesthetic drops may be prepared by adding topical anesthetic to a bottle of artificial tears to formulate a 10% or 20% concentration or alternatively it can be obtained from a compounding pharmacy. It should be used only if needed, no more than four times per day, and only during the first couple of days.

There is no consensus regarding the use of mitomycin-C for retreatment after primary PRK. If significant haze is present, treatment of the haze with topical steroids or mitomycin-C should precede any laser retreatment. It is most commonly used in patients at risk for scar formation after surface ablation for retreatment or in primary surface treatment requiring an ablation depth greater than 70 to 75 µm. Refer to the chapter on mitomycin (Chapter 3) for a more complete discussion on the use of mitomycin-C in refractive surgery.

Limbal Relaxing Incisions

Limbal relaxing incisions (LRIs) are made just inside the limbus. The incisions are made in the axis of the steepest meridian, that is, the axis of plus cylinder. Pachymetry should be performed at the limbus at each end of the steep meridian. The standard LRI is performed using a knife with a diamond blade that has 600 µm exposed. One of the keys to a successful LRI is achieving the maximum 600-µm depth. Knowing that the thickness of the cornea is greater than 600 µm at the incision site allows the surgeon to use the LRI instrument appropriately.

Topical anesthetic is instilled in both eyes and, with the patient seated at the slit lamp, the 3 and 6 o'clock meridians are marked using the horizontal slit beam and sterile marking pen. The LRI may be done under the microscope of the laser or under an operating microscope in a minor surgery suite. After marking, the patient reclines under the microscope and is prepped with

povidone iodine and draped. A Mendez degree gauge (Asico AE-2765) or equivalent instrument is aligned with the previously made marks at 180 degrees, and a marking pen is used to mark the limbus at each end of the axis of the steep meridian (plus cylinder). An LRI circumferential marker of 30, 45, or 60 degrees is inked and used to mark the cornea so that the center of the marker is bisected by the mark at the end of the steep meridian.

The circumferential size of the marker and number of incisions, one or two, is determined according to the specific astigmatic nomogram used. A number of nomograms exist. Nomograms designed to correct astigmatism in patients undergoing cataract surgery are applicable. The Nichamin nomogram (Table 4.2) is a popular one. Other nomograms are available and others can be found on the Internet by searching for "astigmatic nomograms." The circumferential mark should be in clear cornea, preferably just central to the normal limbal vessels. The LRI knife is inserted to full depth perpendicular to the corneal surface at one end of the LRI mark and moved to the other end of the mark. The incision is gently spread with a forceps to verify depth and absence of a perforation. The patient should be examined at the slit lamp immediately postoperatively to confirm normal anterior chamber depth and globe integrity. Postoperative drops include topical fluoroquinolone and prednisolone 1% four times daily for 1 week. The patient should be examined the next day and 1 week later. The effect is usually noted within 1 to 2 days.

LASIK or Surface Ablation after Prior Radial Keratotomy

Patients having had previous radial keratotomy (RK) may be good candidates for retreatment if their vision is correctable with refraction or a hard contact lens. While acuity may be improved by retreatment, symptoms of glare and night vision problems caused by incisions or scarring within the central corneal cannot be expected to improve. If the BSCVA is good, LASIK can be considered provided the RK incisions are well healed and

Table 4.2	Nichamin intralimbal arcuate astigmatic nomogram

WITH-THE-RULE				AGAINST-THE-RULE				
PREOP-ERATIVE CYL (D)	Paired Incisions in Degrees of Arc				PREOP-ERATIVE CYL (D)	Paired Incisions in Degrees of Arc			
	20–30	31–40	41–50	51–60 yrs.		20–30	31–40	41–50	51–60 yrs.
0.75	40	35	35	30	0.75	45	40	40	35
1.00	45	40	40	35	1.00	50	45	45	40
1.25	55	50	45	40	1.25	55	55	50	45
1.50	60	55	50	45	1.50	60	60	55	50
1.75	65	60	55	50	1.75	65	65	60	55
2.00	70	65	60	55	2.00	70	70	65	60
2.25	75	70	65	60	2.25	75	75	70	65
2.50	80	75	70	65	2.50	80	80	75	70
2.75	85	80	75	70	2.75	85	85	80	75
3.00	90	90	85	80	3.00	90	90	85	80

Source: Printed with permission of Louis D. "Skip" Nichamin, M.D.

narrow. Wider scars, a large number of incisions, and epithelial plugging within the incisions increase the risk of instability of the segments of the corneal flap; that is, the flap may break into segments when lifted. The risk of epithelial ingrowth under a LASIK flap may be increased if a large epithelial plug fills one or more incisions and is then transected when the flap is cut.

In patients having LASIK following RK, a microkeratome should be used rather than a femtosecond laser since the lifting of the flap after the laser treatment requires more forceful manipulation. If corneal thickness permits, a thicker flap will decrease the risk of instability. It is best to use a spatula under the flap to lift in order to maintain alignment of the flap segments. It is not unusual to have some slight segment movement on lifting and replacing the flap. If the segments are carefully repositioned and a bandage contact lens applied, healing is usually uneventful.

Patients with multiple incisions or best-corrected visual acuity with a contact lens are better candidates for surface treatment. Use of a VISX PreVue lens is helpful because it allows the patient to make a subjective decision about the quality of vision after the proposed custom surface retreatment. Mechanical debridement of the epithelium should be avoided. The use of alcohol and gentle debridement is less traumatic. Mitomycin-C may reduce the incidence of haze following a surface ablation. The treatment may need to be reduced to avoid overcorrection (refer to Chapter 3 on the use of mitomycin-C).

LASIK Retreatment after Prior Surface Treatment

This is indicated for PRK patients with adequate corneal thickness. A typical patient may have had myopic PRK because LASIK was unavailable at the time of surgery. Another example would be a patient whose central cornea was judged too thin for LASIK, but now requires hyperopic retreatment for an overcorrection and there is sufficient peripheral corneal thickness. The original central keratometric measurements rather than the values after primary keratorefractive treatment should be the basis for deciding the microkeratome ring size. Although not an accurate measurement of the peripheral cornea, these readings are a better indicator of the peripheral corneal steepness where the blade will engage the cornea. Flaps created with the femtosecond laser are not influenced by keratometric values. The excimer procedure is performed exactly as a primary treatment.

Surface Retreatment after Prior LASIK

This situation occurs in patients with inadequate corneal thickness for treatment under a flap, or in patients with poor quality flaps that may be further compromised by relifting. Access and review of the original preoperative and intraoperative records by the retreating surgeon is important in order to understand the flap quality and thickness and the risk of further flap compromise. While many surgeons use mitomycin-C routinely for surface retreatment after LASIK, the peer-reviewed literature does not support the clear benefit or necessity of mitomycin-C in these patients. Treatment is performed as described previously for primary PRK, except for the need to protect the flap by avoiding mechanical epithelial debridement.

Custom Surface or LASIK Retreatment after Prior Conventional Treatment

Some patients continue to complain of poor-quality daytime or nighttime vision after primary treatment despite good visual acuity and minimal to no refractive error. These patients are candidates for custom retreatment if an acceptable treatment plan can be generated after wavefront analysis. The use of a PreVue lens in this situation can demonstrate to the patient the potential benefit of custom retreatment. This goes a long way toward alleviating physician and patient anxiety about the results of treatment.

4

LASIK Complications and Management

Christopher J. Rapuano, M.D.

INTRODUCTION

The significant advantages of LASIK over PRK are somewhat tempered by the increased complexity of the surgery, which increases the type and severity of complications. While the risk of complications is low, when a complication occurs, it needs to be managed appropriately to achieve the best chance of a satisfactory result. Additionally, surgeons should continue to strive to minimize complications. This chapter will focus on intraoperative and postoperative complications and their causes, prevention, and management. It may be helpful for the reader to refer to the chapter on retreatment (Chapter 4) as needed for a more detailed discussion of indications and technique related to relifting a LASIK flap.

INTRAOPERATIVE COMPLICATIONS

Shredded Flap

A shredded flap is one of the most feared complications of LASIK. It is typically only recognized after the microkeratome has made its pass and is removed from the eye. The surgeon may notice the flap to be somewhat irregular. Otherwise, it becomes obvious when the surgeon attempts to lift the flap and does not find a standard flap attached at a hinge.

Causes

- **Poor suction (pseudosuction).** Most, if not all, modern microkeratome systems alert the surgeon when the machine senses adequate suction on the eye and will not allow the microkeratome to pass unless suction is achieved. However, if the suction port or ports are occluded by conjunctiva, the machine can measure full suction without the intraocular pressure (IOP) being adequately elevated. This situation is termed *pseudosuction*. Patients with redundant or boggy conjunctiva, such as might occur in association with thyroid orbitopathy, are at greater risk for pseudosuction.
- **Poor blade quality.** If a pass is made with an imperfect blade, the result may be a poor-quality flap. The exact condition of the blade will impact both the nature and the degree of flap damage.

Prevention

- **Obtain sufficient exposure.** Poor suction can occur due to difficulty positioning the microkeratome onto the eye. This is more likely to occur when exposure is inadequate. The surgeon may notice a hissing sound, if suction is insufficient.
- **Press the ring firmly against the globe.** Firm posterior pressure on the suction ring presses the redundant conjunctiva against the sclera. This may help reduce the risk of pseudosuction.
- **Triple check the IOP:**
  - First: As the pressure in the eye is increasing, the surgeon should monitor the pupil, which often dilates slightly and then remains enlarged.
  - Second: Once the machine registers full suction, the IOP should be high enough

to obstruct blood flow to the eye and the patient will usually notice the vision dimming or even blacking out.

- Third: Check the IOP. This can be done with a Barraquer tonometer, pneumotonometer, TonoPen, or even with digital palpation. The pressure should be >65 mmHg to obtain a quality flap with a blade microkeratome.
- **Check the blade.** The surgeon or an experienced technician should always check the quality of the blade prior to seating it in the microkeratome.

Management

- **DO NOT LASER.**
- **Replace flap pieces as best as you can.** The goal is to put all of the pieces of the shredded flap back into their original location. This is often quite difficult because there may be multiple small fragments of essentially clear cornea.
- **Place a bandage soft contact lens (BSCL).** The BSCL is usually removed 1 to 7 days later. Topical antibiotic and topical corticosteroid eyedrops are applied in routine fashion with the lens in place and after the lens is removed.

Long-Term Management

Later options include no refractive surgery, transepithelial PRK with or without mitomycin-C, and LASIK with a microkeratome or femtosecond laser.

Buttonhole Flap

Buttonhole flaps (Fig. 5.1) have been described in eyes with normal corneal curvature, but steep corneas appear to be at increased risk. The surgeon must always closely examine the quality of the flap as it is being lifted and reflected. Special attention should be paid to the central and paracentral cornea, looking for a full-thickness (easy to detect) and partial-thickness (harder to detect) buttonhole. Buttonholes are easier to detect on the stromal bed appearing as an area of elevation or a smooth island of tissue, but can also be seen as an irregularity or hole in the underside of the flap as it is lifted (Fig. 5.2). Although rare, buttonholes can occur even with the femtosecond laser.

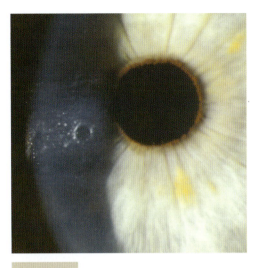

Figure 5.1

Flap buttonhole. (Courtesy of Christopher Rapuano, M.D.)

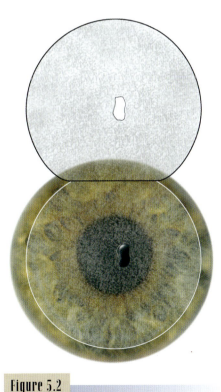

Figure 5.2

Smooth, elevated contour of a full-thickness buttonhole noted in the stromal bed, with a corresponding hole noted in the flap.

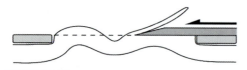

Figure 5.3

Proposed mechanism of the buttonhole. It is presumed that an at-risk cornea will buckle in advance of the microkeratome pass, resulting in an isolated area in which the flap is not cut.

Cause

- **Steep cornea** ($\geq$48.00 D). The proposed mechanism for steep corneas predisposing to buttonholes is that when suction is applied, the steepness allows a large amount of tissue to be "pushed up," above the plane of the suction ring. As this large quantity of cornea is flattened by the microkeratome during the pass, the tissue buckles slightly under the plane of the blade and is thereby uncut, creating a buttonhole (Fig 5.3).

Prevention

- **Use an appropriate suction ring** (e.g., use an 8.5-mm suction ring when $K > 45.00$ D). Most microkeratome systems are designed with a variety of suction rings. Smaller rings do not allow as much corneal tissue to protrude anteriorly. Follow the manufacturer's recommendations regarding which suction ring size to use based on the keratometry readings.
- **Femtosecond laser** (e.g., IntraLase). The risk of a buttonhole is less because the applanating lens flattens the cornea within the suction ring and there is no mechanical pass across the cornea to induce a buckling of tissue. A buttonhole can occur if a corneal facet was present and the flap is thin. The epithelial plug can become dislodged as carbon dioxide is produced in the flap. Also an unusually rough flap dissection could result in a traumatic buttonhole. These are very rare situations. In general, the femtosecond laser is much safer than a blade microkeratome for the patient with a steep cornea.

- **PRK/epithelial-sparing surface ablation.** If steep keratometry readings are noted preoperatively, the surgeon may want to avoid the possibility of a LASIK flap complication and perform a surface ablation.

Management

- **DO NOT LASER.**
- **Replace the flap as best as you can.**
- **Place a BSCL, in the event of a full-thickness buttonhole.** The BSCL is usually removed 1 to 7 days later.

Long-Term Management

Later options include no refractive surgery, transepithelial PRK (with or without mitomycin-C), and LASIK (with a microkeratome with a thicker plate or femtosecond laser).

Short or Decentered Flap with an Edge in Laser Treatment Zone

The LASIK flap needs to be properly centered and large enough to accommodate the entire well-centered laser ablation. A 6-mm-diameter ablation does not require as large a flap as an 8-mm-diameter wavefront custom ablation or a 9-mm hyperopic correction.

Causes

- **Poor centration of the microkeratome.** The microkeratome should be centered on the pupil or slightly decentered toward the hinge. The suction ring may slip slightly as suction is being applied to the eye or the globe might rotate under the ring.
- **Small flap.** The flap may be too small to allow the full laser ablation size. This may be due to inadequate suction before the pass or a flat corneal contour with keratometry readings $\leq$40.00 D.
- **Incomplete flap.** Loss of suction during the microkeratome pass might result in a foreshortened flap. An incomplete flap can occur with the femtosecond laser if the applanation pressure is light, if fluid is present under the applanation lens, or if the meniscus is too close to the flap edge. Refer to the section in Chapter 2 on the femtosecond laser for a more complete discussion.

Management

- **Use the reticle.** Use the reticle to determine if the treatment zone will fit entirely beneath the flap. If the hinge is slightly encroaching within a large (e.g., 8- or 9-mm diameter) ablation zone, then the laser treatment can most likely proceed safely. The hinge should be covered with a hinge protector when the treatment zone is large. Ablation of the hinge should be prevented to avoid a doubly treated area. Laser system software that can design a hinge-sparing ablation may exist on the particular excimer laser being used (see Alcon laser section in Chapter 2). Check with the medical director of the laser center.
- **DO NOT LASER if flap size is inadequate.** If the flap does not cover the vast majority of the treatment zone, it is best to abort the excimer procedure.
- **Do not attempt another blade microkeratome pass during the same surgery session.** The femtosecond laser is an exception in this situation. At the first sign of a significant incomplete laser ablation, stop the femtosecond laser. Using the same applanation cone, the laser can be reset, the surface dried, and, if good applanation can be achieved, another laser pass attempted. Usually an adequate flap can be created with this second pass; however, if the stromal bed appears very irregular it may be best to abort the excimer procedure.
- **Do not try a lamellar dissection to increase flap diameter.** Attempting to increase the flap diameter with a blade is very likely to cause irregular astigmatism and poor vision. In some cases after a femtosecond laser flap has been created, a small area of incomplete ablation can successfully be bluntly dissected.
- **Replace the flap.** If the flap is inadequate, replace it as one would replace a routine LASIK flap.

Late Management

Later options include no refractive surgery. After waiting for 6 months one could attempt to repeat microkeratome LASIK with a larger and thicker flap. Finally, surface ablation with or without mitomycin-C could be considered.

Surface ablation over a previous flap increases the risk of haze.

Free Cap

Automated lamellar keratoplasty, the predecessor to LASIK, and original LASIK techniques were performed with free caps. The current hinged flap technique improved wound alignment and the safety of the LASIK procedure. While there are reports of free caps occurring in eyes with normal corneal curvature, the risk is increased in patients with flat corneas.

The presence of a free cap (see Fig. 1, Case 66, Chapter 7) is not always a disaster, particularly if it is discovered right away and prompt, appropriate action taken. The surgeon must immediately recognize that a free cap was created before the technician removes and disassembles the microkeratome, potentially losing the cap. Noting that part of the corneal ink mark is missing following the microkeratome pass and observing an irregular light reflex as the microkeratome is removed from the eye are key. The free cap must be gently removed from the microkeratome unit and placed epithelial side down on a thin layer of saline. If the ink marks are disappearing, they may need to be augmented to ensure correct cap placement. If the cap looks like a jigsaw puzzle piece, it should fit perfectly on the stromal bed when it is replaced. If it does not, the cap may be upside down.

Causes

- **Flat cornea ($\leq$40 D).**
- **Poor microkeratome suction.**
- **Improper settings for the microkeratome.** If the settings (e.g., ring size on the console does not match the size used, incorrect hinge width) of the microkeratome are incorrect, there is an increased risk of flap complications.
- **Torn hinge**

Prevention

- **Use a large suction ring on a flat cornea** (e.g., 9.5 mm). The proposed mechanism for flat corneas increasing the risk of free caps is that when suction is applied, the flat contour

Poorly Adherent Flap

A poorly adherent flap noted immediately after surgery is more likely to become displaced postoperatively. It is wise to make sure the flap is well aligned and stable in position prior to the patient leaving the laser center.

Causes

- **Overhydration of the flap.** Excessive irrigation of the flap interface and lifting and replacing the flap multiple times increases flap hydration and can lead to poor adherence.
- **Trauma to the flap from the eyelid speculum.** During speculum removal the flap can be displaced, requiring careful repositioning. Care should be taken to lift the eyelid speculum away from the cornea during removal to prevent hitting the flap.
- **Endothelial dysfunction** (e.g., Fuchs' corneal dystrophy). Reduced endothelial pump function may decrease flap adherence. A thick cornea, central pachymetry ≥650 μm, noted preoperatively should prompt a further evaluation with specular microscopy to rule out a low endothelial cell count. A thick cornea due to endothelial dysfunction may result in postoperative flap instability after LASIK surgery.

Prevention

- **Keep the flap irrigation and manipulation to a minimum.**
- **Remove the eyelash drapes and eyelid speculum very carefully, avoiding contact with the flap edge.**
- **Avoid topical brimonidine,** which can increase the risk of flap displacement.
- **Avoid LASIK in patients with endothelial dysfunction.**

Management

- **Let flap "dry" in good position for a few minutes prior to carefully removing the eyelid speculum.**
- **Consider placing a BSCL on the eye if the flap does not appear secure.**
- **Insist that the patient wear protective glasses and nighttime goggles postoperatively and avoid touching or rubbing the eyes.**

POSTOPERATIVE COMPLICATIONS

Complications that usually occur soon after surgery include a displaced flap, infection, DLK, and flap striae. Other complications that occur later include dry eye syndrome/neurotrophic keratopathy, epithelial ingrowth, pressure-induced keratitis, and ectasia. Postoperative vision complaints that may be considered complications by patients include poor unaided visual acuity due to inadequate correction of refractive error or regression of refractive effect; poor night vision due to glare, haloes, or decreased contrast sensitivity; photophobia; and ghosting. Refer to the retreatment chapter (Chapter 4) for a more detailed discussion of the management of patients with these complaints.

Flap Displacement

A displaced flap can occur any time after surgery from the first day to years later. The most common symptoms of a dislodged flap are acute pain and decreased vision, which may be mild to severe depending on the severity of the displacement. It can range from a small area of folding at the flap edge to a completely dislodged flap, only adherent at the hinge. Rarely, the flap can be entirely avulsed.

Causes

- **Trauma is the main cause of a dislodged flap.** The sooner after surgery, the less trauma it takes to move a flap. In fact, in the first few days postoperatively, the patient may not recall any trauma. The injury could be as minor as rubbing the eye. After months or years, it typically requires a distinct and memorable jab to the eye.
- **There are anecdotal reports of a very arid environment, such as a sauna, causing flap dislocation soon after LASIK.**

Prevention

- **Remind patients to be cautious about getting hit or poked in the eye.**
- **Patients should wear eye protection (glasses and nighttime goggles),** especially during activities where there is risk of ocular trauma.

Management

- **A dislodged flap should be repositioned as soon as possible.** A small fold at the flap edge that occurred a few hours prior may be simply repositioned at the slit lamp, for example, with a cellulose sponge or a fine spatula. A more extensive displacement or one that occurred days before most likely requires repositioning under an operating microscope. The displaced flap should be folded back, and the underside of the flap and the stromal bed need to scraped carefully but aggressively (e.g., with a Tooke knife or Beaver No. 15 blade) to remove any epithelial cells that may have grown in. If flap folds are present, they should be stretched out as much as possible. The flap is repositioned and the interface irrigated. Let the flap adhere for at least 5 minutes, because it is often edematous and prone to slippage. Consider placement of a BSCL.

- **The flap can be sutured in place if it is not adhering well.**

Infection

Infection is one of the most dreaded postoperative complications of LASIK. Symptoms include pain, redness, and decreased vision. The symptoms may be acute or gradual in onset and they may begin days or weeks after surgery. Infection can originate on the ocular surface or in the flap interface. It typically begins with an infiltrate that may be single or multiple and can become confluent (Fig. 5.4). There may also be an anterior chamber reaction.

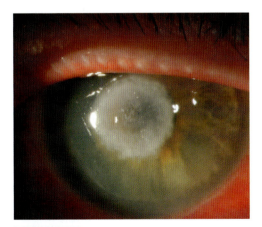

Figure 5.4

Fungal infection of a LASIK flap. (Courtesy of Christopher Rapuano, M.D.)

Causes

- **Bacteria.** Typically early onset, within 3 to 5 days; usually begins as a single superficial infiltrate. Epithelial defects, contact lens use, and blepharitis likely predispose the patient to bacterial infections.
- **Atypical mycobacteria.** Usually later onset, after 2 to 4 weeks; may have multiple discrete infiltrates initially, often in the interface.
- **Fungus.** Typically later onset, after 2 to 4 weeks; may be associated with prolonged steroid use.
- **Recurrent HSV.** May present as an epithelial dendrite or stromal inflammation.

Prevention

- **Treatment of underlying blepharitis** prior to surgery may decrease the risk of infection or sterile inflammation.
- **Preoperative and postoperative topical antibiotics** also may decrease the risk of infection.
- **Povidone iodine prep before surgery.**
- **Preoperative and postoperative treatment of dry eye syndrome** also may decrease the risk of infection.
- **Limiting the duration of topical steroid use** increases the resistance to infection.

Management

- **Small peripheral superficial infiltrates can be treated with frequent broad-spectrum topical antibiotics** (e.g., a fluoroquinolone or fortified antibiotics). Larger, deeper, or more central surface infiltrates should be cultured and treated aggressively.
- **Infiltrates in the flap interface require lifting of the flap, culture of the infiltrate in the interface, irrigation of the interface with antibiotics, and replacement of the flap.** The patient should receive frequent broadspectrum topical antibiotics that are effective against atypical mycobacteria (e.g., amikacin or clarithromycin)
- **Close follow-up is required for all suspected infections.**
- **Remove the flap if the condition is not responding to antibiotics or if the flap becomes necrotic.** The flap may be a barrier to antibiotic treatment of a deeper infection.
- **Infection needs to be differentiated from DLK** (see next section).

5

Diffuse Lamellar Keratitis

Diffuse lamellar keratitis is also known as diffuse interface keratitis, diffuse interstitial keratitis, and "Sands of the Sahara" syndrome. It is a nonspecific sterile inflammatory response to a corneal insult. The insult can vary greatly from apparently uncomplicated LASIK flap creation with a microkeratome or femtosecond laser to foreign material in the interface or an epithelial defect. The onset of DLK is typically within a few days of surgery. Corneal trauma, epithelial erosion, or corneal infection months or years after LASIK can also induce DLK. Symptoms range from none to mild photophobia and/ or mild decreased vision to more severe decreased vision. Signs include diffuse haze at the flap interface that usually begins peripherally or paracentrally, and migrates centrally. It often appears "wave-like." There is minimal to no anterior chamber reaction. As DLK progresses the interface inflammation coalesces into clumps of inflammatory material. The view of iris details can become obscured. Ultimately, melting of the flap overlying the opacity can occur.

Causes

The cause is multifactorial and includes:

- **Bacterial endo/exotoxins from a sterilizer,** which can cause epidemics of DLK.
- **Meibomian secretions.**
- **Cleaner/oils from microkeratome.**
- **Epithelial defect,** either from the surgery or later from trauma or recurrent erosion syndrome.
- **Excessive femtosecond laser energy.**
- **Infectious keratitis, either related to the surgery or months or years later.** Bacterial, adenoviral, and HSV keratitis can cause a secondary sterile interface inflammation (DLK) in addition to the active infection.

Prevention

- **Appropriate sterilization techniques.**
- **Appropriate cleaning of microkeratome equipment.** Disposable microkeratomes may decrease the risk of DLK.
- **Treat and control lid margin inflammation and acne rosacea preoperatively.**

- **Avoid intraoperative epithelial defects** (see earlier section).
- **Avoid postoperative trauma.**
- **Properly adjust the energy level of the femtosecond laser.**

Grading and Treatment

The severity of DLK varies from mild to severe and has been divided into grades. Treatment depends on the severity of the inflammation. Needless to say, if the underlying cause is known it should be addressed. The general principles of treatment are use of corticosteroids (topical and/or oral), coverage with topical antibiotics, lifting the flap in more severe cases to remove inflammatory material, and close follow-up in all cases. DLK generally resolves over several days to a few weeks. Except for the very mild cases, the condition usually progresses before resolving, despite the use of steroids. The surgeon is advised to have a low threshold for lifting the flap, scraping the interface and undersurface of the flap, and irrigating. Lifting the flap sooner rather than later cannot be overemphasized. The goal of treatment is not simply to clear the inflammation, but also to preserve the refractive correction. Delay in treatment can result in stromal thinning with a hyperopic shift and rarely corneal scarring. It is important to explain to the patient the potential seriousness of this condition and the need for aggressive treatment and careful follow-up. The various grades, an illustration of each, and the suggested treatment at each grade follows:

- **Grade 1** (Fig. 5.5): Mild keratitis, typically peripheral, minimal to no symptoms. Tx: Topical prednisolone 1% every 1–2 hours while awake. Follow up within 1 to 2 days.
- **Grade 2** (Figs. 5.6 and 5.7): Moderate infiltration, extending to the central cornea, decreased visual acuity, and/or photophobia. Tx: Topical prednisolone 1% every hour. Consider adding oral prednisone 60 mg/day. Follow up in 1 day.
- **Grade 3** (Figs. 5.8 and 5.9): Significant infiltration, central involvement, clumping of inflammation obscuring iris detail, further decrease in visual function. Tx: Topical prednisolone 1% every hour, oral prednisone

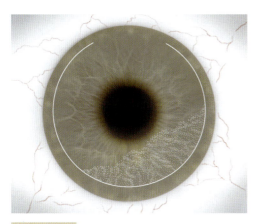

Figure 5.5

DLK grade 1: fine cell in flap interface not involving visual axis.

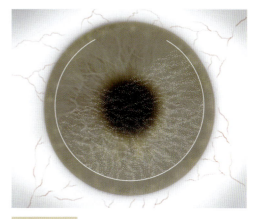

Figure 5.6

DLK grade 2: fine interface cell involving the central cornea.

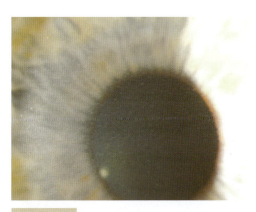

Figure 5.7

Clinical appearance of DLK grade 2. (Courtesy of Christopher Rapuano, M.D.)

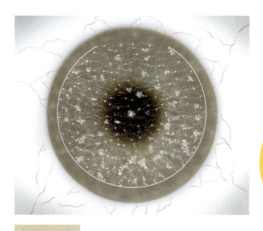

Figure 5.8

DLK grade 3: clumping of cellular material within part or the entire interface.

5

60 mg/day, lift flap and brush stromal bed and undersurface of the flap with a Merocel sponge or gently scrape with a blunt Machat PRK/LASIK spatula (Asico AE-2769), irrigate interface copiously, obtain culture if considering infection. Follow up in 1 day.

- **Grade 4** (Fig. 5.10): Dense white infiltrate centrally with or without melting, marked loss of visual function. Tx: Lift flap, scrape interface debris, culture, and irrigate. Place a drop of steroid on the stromal bed. Topical

prednisolone 1% every hour. Continue oral steroids. Follow up in 1 day.

Pressure-Induced Stromal Keratitis

After LASIK, elevated IOP can cause a sterile pressure-induced stromal keratitis (PISK) that can mimic DLK. The typical history is that the patient was initially placed on topical steroids to treat DLK. The IOP is not routinely measured. A few weeks go by and the stromal keratitis worsens. The IOP is still not measured and the steroids are increased to treat the "DLK."

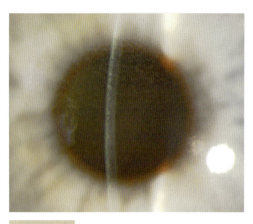

Figure 5.9

Clinical appearance of DLK grade 3. (Courtesy of Christopher Rapuano, M.D.)

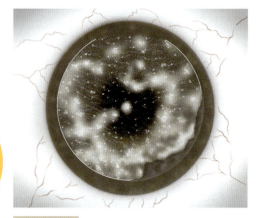

Figure 5.10

DLK grade 4: dense infiltrate prevents view of underlying iris detail. Keratolysis can also be seen as illustrated in this drawing.

Cause

- **Elevated intraocular pressure, often a steroid response.** A fluid cleft may develop in the flap interface. This fluid cleft causes a falsely low IOP measurement with Goldmann applanation tonometry.

Prevention

- **Routinely check the IOP approximately 1 week after LASIK,** especially if the patient is using topical steroids, and definitely if DLK is not responding as expected.

- **Consider checking the IOP with a TonoPen centrally and peripherally.** A Goldmann tonometer placed outside the flap may also reveal elevated IOP.

Management

- **Taper and stop the topical steroids quickly.**
- **Treat the elevated IOP.** The stromal keratitis should resolve soon after the IOP returns to normal.

Microstriae

When a LASIK flap is created, it fits perfectly on the stromal bed beneath it. However, in myopic LASIK the underlying stromal bed is flattened, and in hyperopic LASIK it is steepened. Therefore, the flap and the bed no longer have the exact same curvature. When the flap is replaced on the stromal bed after the laser ablation, it must conform to a new shape. This can result in the formation of tiny folds or microstriae. They are commonly seen after LASIK, especially after treatment of high refractive errors, where the "mismatch" is greatest. They often have a "cracked mud" appearance best seen with indirect or retro-illumination (Fig. 5.11) or after instillation of fluorescein. Occasionally they can also appear

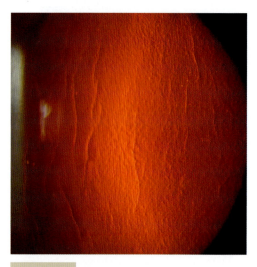

Figure 5.11

Microstriae demonstrated on retroillumination in patient 10 days postoperatively to correct –9.50 + 0.50 × 180. (Courtesy of Robert Feder, M.D.)

5

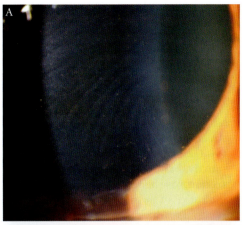

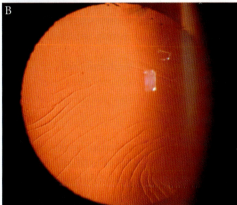

Figure 5.12

Macrostriae. **A:** Macrostriae are seen on direct slit-lamp illumination in a patient with BCVA 20/30–. **B:** The same cornea in retroillumination. (Courtesy of Paul Bryar, M.D.)

as fine parallel lines. Microstriae are thought not to affect visual acuity.

Causes
- **Mild flap-bed mismatch once the flap is replaced after the laser ablation.**
- **Epithelial defects may cause flap swelling,** which can accentuate the mismatch and increase the risk of microstriae.

Prevention
- **Impossible to completely prevent.** Make sure the flap is well seated after it is replaced. Check both the ink mark alignment and the trough width around the entire flap.

- **Prevent epithelial defects as discussed earlier.**

Management
- **None required because microstriae are not felt to affect vision.** However, if central striae are seen at the slit lamp immediately after surgery, refloating the flap is advisable. If vision is affected, see next section on macrostriae.

Macrostriae

In contrast to microstriae, macrostriae [also called folds (Figs. 5.12A and B)] can significantly decrease visual acuity as well as the quality of vision and often require treatment. They result from a grossly misaligned flap and can cause a significant irregularity in the tear film, thereby affecting visual function.

Causes
- **Poor flap alignment at the time of surgery.**
- **Minor trauma after surgery.** May be associated with eyedrop instillation, wiping the eye, or bumping the eye.
- **Idiopathic.** Occasionally striae that appear as microstriae on slit-lamp examination cause some irregular astigmatism to occur for unclear reasons.

Prevention
- At the time of surgery, **make certain that the flap is well positioned, marks are well aligned, and the edge gutters are symmetrical.**
- As the eyelash drapes and eyelid speculum are removed, **encourage the patient to continue looking at the fixation light to avoid contact of the drape or speculum with the flap edge.** Lift the speculum upward during removal to prevent bumping the cornea and displacing the flap.
- **Instruct the patient how to safely instill drops, use eye protection, and avoid eye rubbing and trauma.**

Management
- **Lifting and realigning the flap into proper position** works well when it occurs at the time of surgery or is noted and fixed soon after surgery.

5

- If symptomatic macrostriae are noted on postoperative day 1, **the flap should be lifted and "stretched" under an operating microscope.** Some surgeons will attempt to smooth out striae at the slit lamp. Use of hypertonic and hypotonic solutions to dehydrate or hydrate the flap prior to "ironing it out" have been advocated by some surgeons.
- If the striae are still present, **consideration should be given to removing the central epithelium,** because the epithelium may be "holding" the striae in position. Understand the associated risks of slow healing and DLK.
- **Excimer laser PTK** has been used to treat the gray zone between micro- and macrostriae, where the flap does not appear grossly displaced, but the vision seems to be affected. This procedure does risk a hyperopic shift in refractive error.
- Some surgeons have advocated **heating the flap to really "iron" it.**
- An excellent technique for recalcitrant striae is **suturing the flap.** The flap is lifted, stretched, and then sutured into position with approximately seven interrupted 10-0 nylon sutures. Some surgeons use a running antitorque suture. Sutures should be left in place for 4 to 6 weeks.

Dry Eye Syndrome/Neurotrophic Epitheliopathy

Irritation, dryness, grittiness, and foreign body sensation are common symptoms after LASIK surgery, particularly when the flap is created with the femtosecond laser. The symptoms can last from several days to months, but usually go back to baseline by 6 months. Rarely patients can be very unhappy due to prolonged and/or severe symptoms.

Causes

- **During LASIK, the corneal nerves are transected creating a neurotrophic cornea, which can result in a neurotrophic epitheliopathy.**
- **This neurotrophic effect decreases the feedback loop to the lacrimal glands and can cause a secondary decrease in tear production and a dry eye condition.**

- **The surface of the reshaped cornea may not hold the tear film as well as before, causing secondary wetting problems.**
- **The microkeratome may damage the goblet cells and microvilli, causing a corneal surface problem.**

Predisposing Factors

- **An abnormally low Schirmer's test result, low tear break-up time (TBUT), and conjunctival and corneal staining with fluorescein, rose bengal, or lissamine green** are indicative of possible preoperative dry eye syndrome, which predisposes the patient to such problems postoperatively.
- **Low ambient humidity** such as occurs in desert climates or during winter months in northern climates.
- **Blepharitis** and **meibomianitis** may also predispose to surface problems after LASIK surgery.

Prevention

- **Treat dry eye syndrome preoperatively with a combination of artificial tear supplements, topical cyclosporine (Restasis), and punctal plugs.**
- **Treat blepharitis preoperatively.**
- **Consider performing a nasal hinge LASIK flap,** because theoretically it transects fewer corneal nerves than a superior hinge. The consequence, however, may be an increased incidence of flap displacement.
- **Consider a surface ablation procedure,** because as it induces less neurotrophic effect and consequently is less likely to compromise tear function.
- **Consider avoiding keratorefractive surgery** in a patient with a higher risk of postoperative dry eye problems, when the surface problems cannot be satisfactorily improved prior to surgery.

Management

- **To control the commonly encountered superficial punctate keratopathy (SPK) and dry eye symptoms during the first few months after LASIK, patients should all receive frequent preservative-free tears to use during the first postoperative month.** The tears can be changed to minimally preserved tears and their frequency decreased as the SPK and dry eye symptoms improve.

- **Artificial tear gels and ointments may be required,** if the tear supplements are not enough.
- **Cyclosporine 0.05% (Restasis) drops twice daily can be very effective in improving tear production and symptoms in patients with dry eyes after LASIK.** While the effect of the cyclosporine can take up to 1 month to observe, the onset of beneficial effects from the vehicle (marketed as Endura) is much quicker.
- **Punctal plugs, either long-acting collagen plugs or permanent plugs, can be inserted to improve SPK and symptoms.**
- **A personal humidifier at the workstation can be helpful for patients who spend hours in front of the computer.**
- **Encourage good hydration in patients who exercise heavily.**
- **Avoid dehydration in patients on oral diuretic agents and, if possible, reduce the dose of oral allergy medications or other drugs that have anticholinergic side effects.**
- Fortunately, the symptoms improve with time in most patients.

Glare/Haloes

Glare, haloes, or starbursts around lights, especially in dim illumination, are common for 2 to 6 weeks after LASIK. These symptoms are most frequently noted during nighttime driving. The symptoms generally improve after 6 weeks and then return to "baseline." Patients often have similar symptoms prior to LASIK, but may not notice them until after surgery.

Predisposing Factors

- **High degrees of myopia** are often treated with smaller effective optical zones that increase the likelihood of symptoms.
- **High degrees of astigmatism** may also shrink the optical zone and increase glare and halo symptoms.
- **Large pupils in dim illumination,** generally thought to be greater than 6.5 mm, may also increase the chance of glare and haloes. The scientific data on this issue are conflicting.
- **Older age** may increase the risk of these symptoms.

- **Residual refractive error** causes defocus that may mimic or worsen glare and halo symptoms. This is a major cause of night vision problems.
- Other factors are certainly involved but have yet to be identified.

Prevention

- **Prior to surgery, inquire about glare and haloes, especially when driving at night.** If symptoms are denied, encourage the patient to pay attention to the quality of vision at night. Awareness of night vision preoperatively can help form a basis for comparison after surgery. If they do have symptoms, have them draw a representation of the visual symptoms and put this drawing in the chart.
- **In patients at higher risk for these symptoms or with significant concerns, consider performing unilateral surgery on the nondominant eye.** If the patient is happy with the result the fellow eye can be treated.
- **When treating astigmatism, mark the 3 and 9 o'clock axes on the eye preoperatively to help compensate for intraoperative cyclotorsion.** This will help to properly align the astigmatic treatment. New laser software with iris registration should improve the alignment of astigmatism correction.
- **Use a larger optical zone (e.g., 6.5 mm) and blend zone (e.g., 8.0 mm) when possible.**
- **Custom LASIK may reduce the preexisting higher order aberrations (HOAs) thought to be associated with night vision symptoms.** Custom LASIK also may induce fewer HOAs than conventional LASIK.

Management

- **Treat ametropia.** Whether due to initial undercorrection or overcorrection, or due to regression, defocus is a common source of vision problems at night. Treatment can be as simple as a pair of glasses worn only for night driving. An enhancement procedure once the cornea has stabilized will have a beneficial effect at night to the extent that defocus is improved or eliminated. (See Chapter 4.)
- **Preventing excessive pupil enlargement in dim light with topical brimonidine drops**

5

or shrinking the pupil size with dilute pilocarpine (1/2% to 1/32%) can significantly improve symptoms in some patients.

- A wavefront- or topography-guided peripheral blend or optical zone enlargement may improve glare and halo symptoms, particularly if HOAs are high. If a custom PreVue lens (VISX) is available, the patient can use this at night to determine the potential value of a custom treatment.
- The symptoms often improve with time. Whether this is due to cornea remodeling, brain adaptation, or a gradual decrease in pupil size over time is unclear.

Epithelial Ingrowth

Epithelial ingrowth occurs when epithelial cells grow under the LASIK flap (see Cases 68 and 69 in Chapter 7). It is commonly noted at the flap edge, advancing less than 0.5 mm inward. It typically grows centrally and/or circumferentially from a fistulous epithelial tract at the flap edge. It can also be seen as an island of epithelium, presumably implanted at the time of surgery. When it is extends beyond 1 to 2 mm from the flap edge, it can cause problems. If it reaches the paracentral cornea, it can cause elevation of the flap and irregular astigmatism. If the epithelium reaches the central cornea, it can actually block the vision. The sheet of epithelium in the interface can also impede nutrients from reaching the flap. This lack of nutrients can cause SPK or even flap necrosis. This is not usually serious at the flap edge, but centrally it can significantly affect vision. It is rather uncommon after primary procedures, but occurs with increased frequency after enhancement surgery.

Cause

- Epithelium under the flap from a fistulous tract at the flap edge or implantation of epithelial cells at the time of primary or enhancement surgery.

Predisposing Factors

- An undetected underturned flap edge that is not remedied immediately following surgery.
- An intraoperative epithelial defect, especially at the flap edge, increases the risk that

epithelium will grow under the flap and not over it.

- Anterior basement membrane dystrophy increases the risk of loose epithelium and epithelial defects during surgery.
- A flap buttonhole can allow epithelium to grow under the flap.
- Flap dehiscence patients are at high risk of epithelial ingrowth because epithelium grows over the stromal bed during the time the flap is out of position. If it is not thoroughly removed prior to replacement of the flap, it will continue to grow beneath the flap.
- Free cap.
- Enhancement surgery increases the risk of epithelial ingrowth because when the flap is lifted, the epithelial edges are ragged. These ragged edges tend to heal somewhat more slowly, increasing the risk that some cells will grow under the flap.
- Hyperopic ablations tend to be wider than myopic ablations, and occasionally the laser treatment spills out onto the epithelium outside the stromal bed. This epithelial damage may cause difficulty with healing, thereby increasing the risk of ingrowth.
- Older patients have been shown to have a higher tendency toward epithelial ingrowth, perhaps because the epithelium may in general be somewhat less adherent.

Prevention

- Use a bandage contact lens to facilitate rapid healing if epithelial irregularities occur during surgery.
- Take steps to avoid epithelial defects and buttonholes. See earlier sections.
- Meticulous epithelial tag replacement at the time of enhancement surgery.
- Educate the patient regarding avoiding trauma to the flap.
- Create large flaps for hyperopic treatment to avoid ablating the epithelium.

Management

- Treatment is required when the epithelial ingrowth is causing problems either with flap health (SPK, epithelial defect, flap necrosis) or vision (irregular astigmatism or central opacity). Serious consideration should be given to treating ingrowth greater than 2 mm from flap edge.

- **Surgical treatment of primary epithelial ingrowth:**
  - At the slit lamp, mark the involved area with a small amount of dye and lift the edge of the flap with a Sinskey hook or Machat LASIK enhancement spatula (Asico AE-2830).
  - Under the laser microscope, mark the flap edge for later realignment, gently open the edge of the flap with a Rosenfeld Glide Dissector (Storz E9086) or other blunt instrument designed for this purpose and lift the flap with a cyclodialysis spatula.
  - Aggressively, but carefully, remove all epithelial cells from the stroma and underside of the flap. A Tooke knife or sharp blade is very helpful, but special care must be taken when scraping the underside of the flap to avoid damaging it. A Machat PRK/LASIK spatula (Asico AE 2769) also works well.
  - Replace the flap, irrigate the interface, and line up all the epithelial tags. Consider placing a bandage soft contact lens, especially if the epithelial edges are ragged.
- **Surgical treatment of recurrent epithelial ingrowth:**
  - Consider repeating the lift and scrape procedure described in the preceding item.
  - Consider suturing the flap. The technique is identical to the one just described with the addition of interrupted or a running suture to secure the flap edge.
  - Some surgeons use absolute alcohol or PTK to eliminate residual epithelial cells; however, these can damage the cornea.
  - Some surgeons use fibrin glue at the flap edge to prevent recurrent epithelial ingrowth.

Corneal Ectasia

Corneal ectasia is a thinning and protrusion of the cornea, similar to what is seen in keratoconus, which can occur after LASIK. It leads to irregular astigmatism and may be progressive.

Cause
- **LASIK surgery weakens the corneal stroma,** leading to progressive corneal thinning and protrusion.

Predisposing Factors
- **Forme fruste keratoconus, also called subclinical keratoconus, and pellucid marginal degeneration greatly increase the risk of progressive ectasia following LASIK.** (Refer to the section on preoperative evaluation in Chapter 1 as well as the corneal topography section in Chapter 2.)
- **A residual stromal bed thickness less than 250 μm likely weakens the cornea excessively and increases the risk of ectasia.** The stromal bed thickness is related to the thickness of the flap and the amount of tissue removed with the excimer laser. The safety of this 250 μm barrier has not been proven. Some patients may require a thicker barrier. Some surgeons prefer a residual stromal thickness of 300 μm.
- **Treatment of high myopia and use of thick flaps decrease the residual stromal bed thickness.**
- **A residual stromal bed thickness of less than 50% of the original corneal thickness may also excessively weaken the cornea and predispose to ectasia.**

Prevention
- **Review the preoperative corneal topography,** carefully looking for signs of mild keratoconus and pellucid marginal degeneration.
- **Measure the corneal thickness preoperatively and confirm it intraoperatively.** Calculate the expected residual bed thickness for each patient and make sure it is >250 μm and >50% of the original corneal thickness.
- **Always use the refraction prior to nomogram adjustment to calculate ablation depth and do not use the ablation depth calculated by the laser.** This is the nomogram-adjusted ablation depth.
- **Consider measuring the flap thickness intraoperatively using the subtraction technique (Chapter 1) to be sure there is adequate residual stromal bed thickness for the planned ablation.**

5

Alternatives to LASIK Refractive Surgery

Lawrence Gans, M.D.

INTRODUCTION

Excimer laser refractive surgery, and LASIK in particular, is the most popular refractive procedure worldwide. However, alternate procedures are available for favorably modifying the refractive properties of the eye, and when laser vision correction is not appropriate, these procedures become valuable tools for the refractive surgeon. This chapter is an introduction to help the reader understand the role that these alternatives can play to help the patient achieve better uncorrected vision.

SURFACE ABLATION: PRK/LASEK/ EPI-LASIK

The various names for keratorefractive surface ablation with the excimer laser are derived from the technique used to handle the epithelial layer. The first U.S. FDA approval for refractive surgery with the excimer laser was for photorefractive keratectomy (PRK). This procedure involves the mechanical removal of the epithelium followed by excimer ablation of the underlying surface stroma. Although the mechanical removal was initially done with a blade, a battery-operated rotating brush was developed to facilitate epithelial removal. Later, the use of dilute ethanol (20%), applied to the surface for 20 to 30 seconds, was introduced to facilitate mechanical epithelial removal. Limiting the duration of contact with the epithelium, removing the alcohol, and copiously irrigating the corneal surface minimize corneal toxicity. The alcohol

pretreatment effectively loosens the adhesion of the basal epithelial cells so the layer can be gently swept aside. An alternate technique uses the excimer laser to partially remove the epithelium prior to the refractive ablation. This requires the mechanical removal of the remaining epithelium from the ablation zone and was, therefore, termed Laser-Scrape.

With any technique that involves the removal of the epithelium, there is associated postoperative pain and delay of vision recovery until the epithelial layer is healed and optically smooth. In the hopes that preserving the epithelium and returning it to the surface following the laser ablation would minimize the soreness and hasten the visual recovery, techniques were developed that allowed the epithelial surface to be lifted as a sheet and then replaced over the treated surface. When this is performed with chemical loosening of the epithelium and mechanical lifting of the flap, it is called LASEK (laser epithelial keratomileusis). When it is performed using an epithelial keratome, it is known as Epi-LASIK. The epithelial keratome uses an oscillating blunt dissector to separate the sheet of epithelium from Bowman's layer. A water-jet device can also be used to create an epithelial flap.

Several advantages make surface ablation an important alternative to LASIK. The long-term postoperative results of surface ablation surgery are comparable to those of LASIK particularly for myopic corrections of ≤ -5.00 D. Because no stromal flap is created, risks such as striae, flap displacement, diffuse lamellar keratitis (DLK), and epithelial ingrowth are eliminated. This is also true of the risk of flap segmentation problems, which can occur after LASIK in post-RK patients.

An important advantage of PRK is that more stromal tissue is available for safe laser ablation. If a typical LASIK flap measures 100 to 180 μm in thickness including the 50- to 60-μm epithelial layer, a surface procedure can be performed with an additional 40 to 130 μm of stromal tissue available for ablation. This is particularly helpful in treating patients with relatively thin corneas or patients with higher refractive errors. Because customized wavefront-based LASIK surgery requires the ablation of more stromal tissue, surface ablation may be the preferred option in order to accommodate the treatment. The surgeon should be advised that custom PRK has not been as carefully evaluated as custom LASIK.

Less severe and less prolonged dry eye problems are encountered after surface treatment, which is advantageous in patients who have preexisting tear film problems. When there is no suction ring to raise the intraocular pressure, there is less concern for ischemic complications to the optic nerve, and this may be more suitable for patients with risk factors for glaucoma or other optic nerve disease. A suction ring should not be used on a patient with a filtering bleb; therefore PRK would be preferred over LASIK in this rare circumstance.

The cost for equipment needed to prepare the corneal surface for surgery can be much less than that for LASIK. However, epithelial keratomes for Epi-LASIK can approach the cost of a microkeratome for LASIK. The per-case cost is generally less with epithelial keratomes.

The three major disadvantages of surface ablation are postoperative discomfort, slow visual rehabilitation, and the risk of stromal scarring. The removal of surface epithelium by any technique is associated with postoperative pain. This can range from mild to severe and may last for several days until the epithelium has healed. Pain can be minimized with bandage contact lenses, oral analgesics, cold compresses, oral and topical nonsteroidal anti-inflammatory medications, and even dilute topical anesthetics. Immediately following surface ablation, the vision can be quite good with uncorrected visual acuity (UCVA) in the range of 20/40 to

20/60. As the epithelium heals during the next few days, the vision becomes hazier as the central optical zone becomes rough and irregular. The initial epithelial layer is somewhat thickened but gradually smooths out to achieve better optical quality in the subsequent weeks after surgery. The UCVA after the first week is typically 20/40 and may take 2 or more weeks to achieve 20/20 or better vision. Retreatment should not be considered for 6 months after PRK, because of the time necessary for complete healing to occur.

Stromal scarring in the form of reticular haze occurs with increasing frequency and severity with myopic corrections above −5.00 D (≥75-μm ablation depth) and is more common with broad-beam laser procedures. It is less frequent with spot lasers but still occurs with higher corrections. Several measures can minimize the incidence and severity of this scarring even at higher corrections. These include irrigating the cornea with chilled BSS after the ablation, the use of oral ascorbic acid (1,000 mg daily), and the use of a topical steroid for at least a month following surgery. Prolonged topical steroid use increases the risk of IOP elevation that can become quite severe. Mitomycin-C can be applied to the bare stroma after the ablation is completed to provide potent protection from stromal scarring, but nomogram adjustments may be needed to prevent overcorrections (see Chapter 3). Enhancements after surface surgery require the patient to go through the same process with discomfort and slow return of useful vision. During the enhancement procedure the surgeon should be prepared for the rougher appearance of the bared stroma within the previous ablation zone.

The technique for PRK or LASEK involves centering a well or blunt trephine, slightly larger than the planned ablation diameter, on the corneal surface. This is filled with 20% ethanol and held in place for 20 seconds. The solution is then removed and the surface washed with chilled BSS. If an epithelial flap is to be prepared, the edges are bluntly dissected centrally to create an intact epithelial layer that is reflected away from the treatment zone. Alternately, the epithelium is just wiped from the surface. The laser ablation is performed. For procedures with ablation depths

6

over 75 μm, mitomycin-C 0.02% on a cellulose sponge can then applied to the stromal surface for 12 to 45 seconds. The surface is irrigated again with chilled BSS. A bandage contact lens is placed on the cornea and the procedure is complete.

Oral celecoxib 200 mg/day beginning the day prior to surgery and continuing for 1 to 2 days after surgery will help with discomfort. Cold compresses can be used as well. Oral ascorbic acid 1,000 mg/day beginning the day of surgery is continued for 1 month. Topical antibiotic and steroid eyedrops are used four times daily. The antibiotic can be discontinued once the epithelium is healed but the steroid is continued for at least a 1 month. The bandage contact lens is removed when the epithelium is intact, usually on the fourth postoperative day.

Bilateral surgery can be done, but the patient must be thoroughly prepared preoperatively for the visual disability that will likely occur during the first week after surgery. Sequential surgery and LASIK in the fellow eye are two approaches that may be preferable.

INCISIONAL PROCEDURES

Astigmatic Keratotomy and Limbal Relaxing Keratotomy

Astigmatic keratotomy (AK) is an extension of the relaxing incision procedure long used by corneal transplant surgeons to correct post-keratoplasty astigmatism. Straight or arcuate tangential incisions are made in the steep meridian to cause an axial change in the astigmatism. The number and pattern of these incisions, along with their distance from the visual axis, determine the amount of correction obtained. In addition to flattening the steep meridian, these incisions also produce a steepening in the orthogonal meridian (90 degrees away) resulting in what is termed *coupling*. The ratio of the amount of flattening in the steep meridian where the incision is placed to the amount of steepening in the orthogonal meridian is termed the *coupling ratio*. The coupling ratio varies with the type of incision produced and is an important predictor of the spherical equivalent change that will result from the astigmatic surgery. A coupling ratio of 1:1 will have no change in the spherical

equivalent. For example, an eye that begins at $-4.00 + 4.00 \times 90°$ (spherical equivalent of -2.00 D) and undergoes successful AK should end up at approximately -2.00 D. Short and straight tangential incisions tend to produce less orthogonal steepening than do longer or arcuate incisions.

The procedure is performed with a thin diamond blade that has a rectangular or trapezoidal tip with cutting edges at the base and the sides to allow the knife to slide predictably at the same depth along the curved circumference of the cornea. The guarded edge is set with a micrometer or is set at a fixed length to produce an incision 90% to 95% of the corneal pachymetry for midperipheral incisions (AK), and arbitrarily at 600 μm for limbal relaxing incisions (LRIs). The 3 and 9 o' clock limbus is marked at the slit lamp so that adjustment for intraoperative cyclotorsion movements can be made. The steep meridian is confirmed with intraoperative keratoscopy or a Mendez gauge, and the incision track is marked on the corneal surface. Incisions are commonly performed in pairs with one on either side of the visual axis and both centered on the steep meridian. The incisions are generally made at the edge of a 7-mm optical zone to minimize visual symptoms, but can be made at a smaller optical zone for greater amounts of correction.

Astigmatic keratotomy can correct mild to moderate cylinder reliably with few objectionable symptoms. When performed at the time of cataract surgery with a standard lens implant, the LRI procedure helps produce an emmetropic result for patients with corneal astigmatism. When the attempted correction exceeds 2 D, the number of incisions and the need to be closer to the optical zone result in objectionable visual symptoms. LRI is an effective way to treat low degrees of post-LASIK mixed astigmatism. Because of the coupling effect, both the sphere and the cylinder are corrected. This can be done without incurring the risk of flap relift or the expense of excimer laser retreatment (see Chapter 4).

Radial Keratotomy

Radial keratotomy (RK) was the first surgical procedure widely performed in the United States for the correction of myopia. The early popularity of this procedure led to the evolution of refractive surgery as a means to reduce or eliminate the need for corrective lenses. The procedure has fallen into disfavor due to the short- and long-term corneal instability encountered, particularly when larger degrees of correction are attempted. This is discussed in greater detail later.

Radial incisions in the peripheral cornea correct myopia by producing a peripheral bulge and central flattening of the anterior refractive surface. This central corneal flattening can correct mild to moderate degrees of myopia. By altering the length and number of incisions created, the surgeon controls the amount of refractive correction produced.

A wide range of factors influence the effectiveness of the surgery. These include the age of the patient (older patients experience greater effects for the same amount of surgery), gender (some have said women experience greater effects), the depth, and the incision profile at the central end of the incision. The surgeon needs to select the number of incisions and the optical zone, which is the clear, unincised area of central cornea, based on the characteristics of the particular eye. RK surgeons developed personal nomograms to help produce consistent results with their individual technique. Radial keratotomy can correct myopia from -0.50 to as high as -8.00 D or more, but in practice it is only useful up to about -4.00 D before disturbing visual symptoms interfere with the refractive correction.

The surgery is performed with the patient recumbent. Topical anesthesia is applied and the patient is instructed to fixate on a target. An ink mark is made with an optical zone marker to delineate the optical zone centered on the entrance pupil of the eye. The surgeon stabilizes the globe with a forceps or fixation ring and creates the incisions using a guarded diamond knife blade. The exposed portion of the blade is set with a micrometer to ideally create an incision that is 85% to 95% of the corneal thickness as determined by pachymetry. Modern RK knives have a thin diamond blade with a sharp front vertical edge for incisions made from the limbus to the optical zone (Russian technique) or a sharp angled edge for incisions made from the optical zone to the periphery (American technique). The former produces a more vertical incision profile centrally and thus gives greater refractive effect. The latter minimizes the risk of the incision entering the optical zone with any unintended eye movement. Bidirectional blades (with a shortened sharp edge on the vertical side) allow the incision to be created first with the American technique moving away from the optical zone and then back with the Russian technique to give the vertical incision profile centrally. The shortened sharp edge of the vertical side stops the blade when the original entry point is reached at the optical zone mark. Commonly four to eight radial incisions are created.

RK has several inherent side effects that make photoablative surgery much more desirable. The incisions weaken the peripheral cornea to cause the bending that flattens the central curvature to correct myopia. From morning to evening that bending may vary to produce the diurnal fluctuation mentioned earlier. It is not uncommon for RK patients to be relatively hyperopic in the morning and more myopic by evening. The fluctuations increase with higher attempted corrections using more numerous and longer incisions. The incisions can heal with epithelial plugs growing into the depths of the incisions. Some incisions may not be created perpendicular to the corneal surface. In each of these situations, the incisions can become opaque, resulting in glare. In the avascular cornea these incisions are never completely healed and can split open with ocular trauma or during penetrating keratoplasty. Infections, if they occur, can rapidly progress toward the posterior stroma.

One of the most disturbing after effects of RK is the long-term instability, with some eyes becoming significantly hyperopic in future years. Former RK patients are presenting to refractive surgeons for correction of progressive hyperopia. LASIK can be done if the incisions are fine, that is, without large epithelial plugs. PRK is another option, but it can result in haze. Mitomycin-C 0.02% solution applied to the treatment zone after the PRK ablation can reduce this risk (see Chapter 3). Conductive keratoplasty is not recommended for consecutive hyperopia after RK. Intraocular lens (IOL) procedures such as phakic IOL insertion or refractive lens exchange are additional alternatives. Despite the hyperopic correction, the risk of retinal detachment in these previously myopic patients must be considered if clear lens exchange is planned. Irregular astigmatism and continued progressive effect make some of these patients difficult to treat.

As an alternative to LASIK, RK does have a few advantages. The cost of the equipment is minimal and there are no royalties to pay when performing the procedure. In RK the visual axis is spared and there is no loss of tissue or significant loss of keratocytes.

Hexagonal keratotomy was an incisional technique once used to correct hyperopia in which a series of six tangential incisions in a hexagonal pattern around the visual axis was made to induce central steepening. This procedure, however, produced significant vision problems such as polyopia, glare, irregular astigmatism, and inaccurate results and was subsequently abandoned.

THERMAL PROCEDURES

The use of heat to change the shape of the cornea is more than 100 years old, but only recent advances in technology have allowed the controlled application of heat to predictably change the corneal shape without causing necrosis and scarring. The goal is to apply heat to the midperipheral cornea to induce shrinking, which secondarily steepens the central cornea, correcting hyperopia.

Conductive Keratoplasty

Conductive keratoplasty (CK) is a nonlaser procedure that uses radiofrequency (RF) energy to create the thermal shrinking of collagen that alters the corneal contour. RF energy can be controlled very precisely to produce a safe, predictable effect in the tissue. The ViewPoint CK System (Refractec, Inc., Irvine, CA) is relatively inexpensive and includes the RF generator with an eyelid speculum and probe tip to perform the surgery. The probe, or Keratoplast, has a metal tip that is 90 μm wide and has a guard that allows exposure of 450 μm

to penetrate the corneal stroma. The RF energy pulse moves from the exposed portion of the metal tip inserted into the corneal stroma and passes through the tissue back into the eyelid speculum that acts as the return path for the current to the generator box. The resistance of the tissue to the passage of the RF energy produces the heat that causes a column of contraction around the Keratoplast posteriorly to the 450-μm depth.

CK is performed in the office with topical anesthesia. A corneal marker defines a pattern of eight spots in a series of rings centered on the entrance pupil. Originally the rings were at 6.0-, 7.0-, and 8.0-mm optical zones. The number of rings used for treatment defines the intended correction. More recently a modified technique termed *Light Touch* CK uses rings of spots only at 7.00 and 8.00 mm. The surgeon inserts the Keratoplast at each spot on the cornea and depresses a foot pedal to get the CK unit to deliver the energy. It typically takes about 2 minutes to perform each ring.

CK is able to induce up to 3 D of myopia. This procedure can be used for the correction of a corresponding amount of hyperopia, or to induce myopia for the correction of presbyopia. The latter is termed NearVision CK (NVCK) and is typically performed on the nondominant eye in a plano-presbyope to provide "blended vision" where both eyes are used together for distance and near. With the Light Touch CK technique, a single 8-mm ring will produce 1 D of steepening and two rings at 7 and 8 mm gives slightly more than 2 D. These rings are farther from the visual axis and are less likely to induce astigmatism or produce glare than the original CK performed at 6 and 7 mm.

The advantage of CK over hyperopic LASIK is that it is less expensive to perform and does not involve surgery on the central cornea. In the FDA trials of CK, the efficacy data were similar to that of LASIK, and the safety variables were superior. As an off-label use, the surgeon can vary the pattern of spots to correct astigmatism by applying more spots, or moving them closer to the visual axis, in the flatter meridian.

The correction of corneal astigmatism cannot be predicted accurately using CK, but intraoperative keratoscopy can confirm the astigmatic effect at the time of the surgery. The FDA limits the ViewPoint CK System RF generator to a fixed energy level in the United States, but the generators available outside of the United States allow manipulation of the energy for treatment spots.

CK can also correct postkeratoplasty astigmatism when combined with traditional relaxing incisions. The CK spots are applied just central to the graft wound on both sides of the flat meridian after creation of the relaxing incisions. The CK spots act like compression sutures to enhance the effect of the relaxing incisions. The number of spots applied is directed by intraoperative keratoscopy.

CK can be performed after myopic LASIK or PRK to treat overcorrections. The effect of CK spots is dramatically increased in eyes that have had laser vision correction and thus the diameter of the CK treatment ring can be increased to 9 mm or more and still produce steepening of a diopter or more. Because the peripheral cornea is not thinned significantly by myopic laser correction, there should generally be sufficient thickness (>450 μm), but peripheral pachymetry should confirm this.

NVCK is more commonly used in patients who became plano-presbyopes because of laser vision correction. The patient who had LASIK years ago to eliminate the need for glasses at age 38 was happy until age 44 and now needs reading glasses. NVCK is an alternative to LASIK enhancement to induce myopia in the eye preferred for reading to produce monovision. There is a significant difference in the result of NVCK performed after LASIK surgery from the results in eyes that have not had prior refractive surgery. In the FDA studies for NearVision CK in patients with no prior surgery, two thirds of patients retained 20/30 uncorrected distance acuity in the treated eye while achieving J3 or better near vision. This does not occur with NVCK in eyes that have had prior LASIK. After laser refractive surgery, the effect of CK is more like monovision contact lenses where the reading-corrected eye loses significant distance acuity.

The data in the FDA studies of CK showed similar refractive efficacy to that of LASIK for previously untreated eyes, and the safety variables were superior. Attempts to use CK in eyes that have had a hyperopic shift from previous RK surgery have produced very poor results. Eyes with peripheral thinning from marginal degenerations or keratoconus should not be treated with CK.

Holmium LTK

The holmium−yttrium-aluminum-garnet (Ho-YAG) laser produces light in the infrared spectrum (2,100 nm) and was developed with a contact (Summit Technology, Inc., Waltham, MA) and a noncontact (Sunrise Technologies International, Inc., Fremont, CA) delivery system. Only the Sunrise Hyperion LTK system received FDA approval for refractive surgery. The laser delivers eight simultaneous spots in a ring centered on the entrance pupil. One or two rings at 6.0 and 7.0 mm were used to flatten the peripheral cornea and thus steepen the central optical zone for the correction of spherical hyperopia up to +2.50 D. Unfortunately, the thermal effect of the laser was mostly superficial and the resulting correction was often disappointing and short lived. The procedure took a few seconds but could not be varied from the programmed patterns approved by the FDA. The laser is expensive and now is rarely used.

AUGMENTATION PROCEDURES

Intrastromal Ring Segments

Intrastromal ring segments, Intacs (Addition Technology, Des Plaines, IL) and Ferrara rings (Ferrara Ophthalmics/Ltda., BeloHorizonte, Brazil) are used to treat low amounts of spherical myopia, to delay the need for keratoplasty in keratoconus, and to treat laser-induced corneal ectasia. These semicircular (Intacs = 150-degree arc; Ferrara rings = 160-degree arc) ring segments made of PMMA are placed within a stromal pocket or channel created in the midperiphery of the cornea (Fig. 6.1). The amount of correction produced is determined by the thickness of the segments, which steepen the peripheral cornea to flatten the optical zone.

Intacs were first FDA approved for the correction of spherical myopia up to −3.00 D. The stromal pockets are prepared

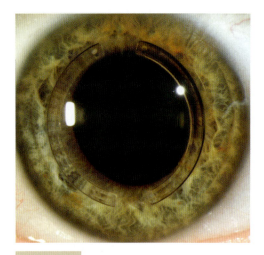

Figure 6.1

Intrastromal ring segments (Intacs). (Courtesy of Addition Technology, Inc.)

that the ring segments can be easily removed or exchanged to reverse or modify the refractive result and the central cornea is untouched by the procedure.

The disadvantages of Intacs have kept it from becoming popular. They can only correct low levels of myopia without astigmatism. It requires expensive equipment and special training to create the lamellar channels. There is a small risk of the ring dissecting out of the channel anteriorly or posteriorly during insertion. It can be associated with complaints of chronic postoperative discomfort and/or glare. The ring segments are visible with close observation, which is a cosmetic objection to some. Finally, white channel deposits adjacent to the Intacs can occur that may also be cosmetically significant.

Ring segments have some specialized uses beyond the correction of low myopia. They can be used to correct small amounts of residual myopia following LASIK, where the remaining central stromal bed is too thin for further laser ablation. Ring segments are FDA approved under a human device exemption for patients with keratoconus to improve uncorrected acuity and to facilitate contact lens correction. This can delay the need for corneal transplantation in some patients but does not arrest the progression of the disease. Intacs have also been used to help manage cases of corneal ectasia following LASIK. Radial inserts for the correction of hyperopia are currently being evaluated.

with a special set of instruments to create a lamellar channel at about two-thirds stromal depth having a 7.5-mm diameter around the geometric center of the cornea. Ferrara rings can be placed at a 5-mm diameter for greater myopic correction. The procedure is performed with topical anesthesia. A 1.0-mm radial incision is made at 68% of the pachymetry reading where the insertion is to be started. A suction ring is applied to stabilize the globe at the appropriate pressure and to guide the tip of the dissector as it creates the channels in each direction away from the starting incision. The ring segment will then slide into place through the lamellar channel, and the radial incision may be secured with a single nylon suture.

Alternatively the lamellar channels can be created with a femtosecond Nd-YAG laser (IntraLase) using a programmed photodisruption of the collagen layers. This simplifies the preparation of the channels. The amount of correction can also be increased by using a femtosecond laser to create narrower intrastromal channels.

Visual outcomes with Intacs for low levels of myopia are similar to those achieved with conventional LASIK. Above −2.25 D of correction, patients are more likely to complain of glare, photophobia, and polyopia. The advantage of Intacs over LASIK is

Keratophakia

Keratophakia is a procedure in which a lens is placed within the corneal stroma to favorably alter the anterior refracting surface. The intrastromal lens can be created from homoplastic donor corneal tissue or alloplastic, synthetic material. The donor corneal tissue is prepared on a cryolathe where it is ground into the shape of a plus power lens. Alternatively, synthetic material (e.g., hydrogel) is produced with the desired refractive power in a 5.0- to 5.5-mm-diameter lenticule. A corneal flap or pocket is created and the lenticule is centered over the pupil. The flap or pocket is closed to secure the lenticule in place.

Homoplastic keratophakia is rarely performed because of the cost and technical difficulty associated with the use of the cryo-lathe. Alloplastic keratophakia with a PermaVision hydrogel lens (Anamed, Inc., Lake Forest, CA) is still undergoing clinical trials in the United States for the correction of hyperopia up to +6.00 D. As an alternative to hyperopic LASIK, this procedure offers the potential to reverse or modify the correction with removal or exchange of the lenticule.

Epikeratoplasty

This procedure was developed to avoid the need for lamellar corneal dissection. It was dubbed "the living contact lens" because it was prepared from human donor corneal stroma and permanently attached to the patient's corneal surface to act as a contact lens for the correction of various refractive conditions. The donor tissue was cryolathed in a commercial process and lyophilized for later use in surgery. The patient's cornea was prepared by removing the central epithelium and creating a peripheral corneal groove. The rehydrated lenticule would then fit onto the cornea surface and the edges would be sutured into the peripheral groove or pocket. The patient's epithelium would then grow over the surface of the epikeratoplasty to provide a new anterior refractive surface for the cornea.

The results of surgery were most promising for aphakic patients for whom lens implantation was not appropriate. The procedure was plagued with healing problems, unpredictable refractive results, and poor postoperative vision. The manufacturer of the commercially prepared lenticules abandoned production and now the procedure is only performed in centers that still have a cryolathe to create their own lenticules.

Orthokeratology

Orthokeratology is a nonsurgical alternative to correct low levels of spherical myopia. A rigid gas permeable contact lens (Paragon CRT) with a flatter base curve than the corneal curvature is worn during sleep to produce a temporary correction of myopia when the lens is removed on awakening. It is most appropriate for individuals adverse to surgery with spherical myopia up to −2.50 D. Orthokeratology effect is temporary and vision will blur with

regression, but the lenses can be reinserted to restore the correction. Most patients complain of discomfort with these lenses. Its effective range is similar to that of Intacs and shares the advantage over LASIK of potential reversibility. These lenses have also been reported to improve vision in eyes with undercorrected LASIK surgery. There have been reports of bacterial keratitis with the use of these lenses.

Lens Implantation: Clear Lens Exchange

With the evolution of cataract surgery to include astigmatism-neutral incisions and highly accurate biometry came the expectation that surgeons could reduce the patient's dependence on glasses after surgery. Thus cataract surgery is becoming a refractive procedure as well as one for visual rehabilitation. Safety issues associated with peribulbar and retrobulbar anesthesia are avoided with topical, clear corneal surgery. Foldable IOLs can be implanted through small, self-sealing incisions so that the recovery of useful vision occurs soon after the completion of the procedure. There are, however, recent reports of an increased incidence of endophthalmitis occurring with these incisions. Nevertheless, the relatively high degree of safety and the relative simplicity of the process for the patient have led to the use of clear lens extraction and prosthetic implantation for purely refractive purposes.

Clear lens exchange may be an option when contraindications to corneal refractive surgery exist, such as when the cornea is too thin, flat, or steep; or if the degree of refractive error is beyond the limit of safety and predictability for excimer laser ablation. The exchange of the patient's clear lens with an IOL of appropriate power can correct a wider range of refractive conditions than the laser and it is not dependent on the corneal contour except for predicting the proper lens power. It requires equipment and skills that most refractive surgeons already possess and the start-up costs are significantly less than those for excimer laser surgery.

Refractive astigmatism will be adequately corrected if its source is lenticular in nature. Astigmatism may potentially increase postoperatively if corneal astigmatism is unmasked by extraction of the lens. Because the purpose of the surgery is refractive in nature, the surgeon must have a plan for dealing with astigmatism. Astigmatism ≤1 D may be corrected by placing the wound in the axis of plus cylinder. LRI or toric IOL implantation may be required for astigmatic corrections up to 2.50 D. Toric IOLs are discussed in a later section. For correction of greater degrees of astigmatism, a keratorefractive procedure may be considered (see later section on bioptics). Patients with large spherical corrections preoperatively may not be as bothered by small amounts of residual correction after surgery.

A plan for near vision correction must be developed preoperatively. Prepresbyopic patients must understand that extraction of the crystalline lens will be associated with loss of accommodation and near acuity. The preservation of accommodation is an advantage of phakic IOL surgery. The clear lens exchange patient has several options available including the use of reading glasses, monovision using monofocal IOLs to create low myopia in the nondominant eye, multifocal IOL insertion, and use of the accommodating IOL. These more sophisticated IOLs are discussed in the next section.

The patient must understand that usually this surgery is performed as a bilateral procedure that is done sequentially and not simultaneously. The risks associated with intraocular surgery must be explained and the patient should understand the more invasive nature of this surgery. The risk of IOL power miscalculation should be addressed. Patients with a history of iritis, glaucoma, or risk factors for retinal detachment may be poor candidates for this surgery.

The surgery is essentially the same as for cataract removal, though the accuracy of the biometry and lens power calculation is most critical to produce the ideal refractive result. Noncontact techniques such as emersion A-scan ultrasonography and optical biometry with the IOL Master (Carl Zeiss Meditec Inc., Dublin, CA) can be more accurate than traditional contact ultrasonography. The IOL Master is of particular value in eyes that have had previous refractive surgery.

Hyperopic patients may have a crowded anterior chamber and may get the added benefit of deepening their chamber angle after surgery. Particular caution is advised when treating myopic patients, because of the risk of retinal detachment. This risk increases with the degree of myopia, the number of years after surgery, and after postoperative capsulotomy. Some surgeons advise clear lens exchange only for hyperopic patients, for which the risk of retinal detachment is reduced.

Selection of lens implant material may be important for highly myopic eyes at risk for future retinal problems. Silicone IOLs can fog during pars plana vitrectomy when gas is placed in the vitreous for pneumatic retinopexy. These lenses will also lose their refractive interface if the eye is filled with silicone oil. Recent improvements in lens implant optics can also reduce glare and troublesome night vision symptoms associated with some earlier lens implant designs. The Bausch & Lomb SofPort AO and the AMO Advanced Medical Optics Tecnis Z9000 are examples of lenses designed to reduce spherical aberration.

Clear lens extraction in the moderate to markedly myopic patient with long axial lengths can be technically more challenging than in patients with nuclear cataracts. The anterior chambers can become quite deep, particularly if the chamber is overfilled with viscoelastic and the irrigation bottle is set high. A small anterior capsulotomy may make subincisional cortex or epinucleus difficult to aspirate. Finally, wide swings in anterior chamber depth may make capsular rupture more likely. Attention to fluidics is essential in order to reduce this risk. If the phaco machine cannot be sufficiently adjusted to maintain the anterior chamber depth, CruiseControl (STAAR Surgical Co., Monrovia, CA) a specially designed aspiration filter can be interposed between the aspiration port on the phacoemulsification handpiece and the aspiration tubing.

ADVANCED TECHNOLOGY INTRAOCULAR LENSES

Toric Intraocular Lenses

The STAAR Toric IOL is currently the only FDA-approved IOL designed for the correction of astigmatism following lens extraction. The lens is a foldable, plate-haptic, silicone IOL inserted into the eye with an injector. After insertion the lens is rotated to the axis of plus corneal astigmatism. Two linear marks near the optic on both sides indicate the axis of the cylindrical IOL power. The axis and power of the cylindrical correction required are based on keratometry and topography, and not on refraction. The precision of the alignment along the steep corneal meridian may be within 10 degree of ideal and still provide excellent refractive results. The lens has a 6.0-mm optic and is available in a 10.8-mm (TF) or 11.2-mm (TL) length. The lenses are available in powers from +10.00 D to +28.00 D with cylindrical power of +2.0 D and +3.5 D. The IOL can correct about 1.4 D of astigmatism at the corneal plane with the lower cylindrical power lens and about 2.3 D with the higher power IOL. The lens is intended for implantation in the capsular bag.

The major drawback of this lens had been IOL rotation that caused either a reduction of effect or increased astigmatism if the rotation was extensive. This problem has been greatly reduced since the addition of a large fenestration in each end of the IOL within the haptic, which encourages capsular fixation. The larger lens length also reduces the incidence of rotation. Removing all of the viscoelastic at the conclusion of the case, making certain the wound is watertight, is also essential. Finally many surgeons insert this lens upside down. The anterior surface of the IOL is better able to resist lens rotation. Inserting the lens in this way may result in a slight reduction in the correction achieved.

Another possible problem with the plate-haptic, posterior chamber IOL (PCIOL) is extrusion into the posterior segment if a large posterior capsulotomy is created postoperatively. Caution is advised when performing a laser capsulotomy in order to avoid this complication.

Multifocal Intraocular Lenses

The Array lens (AMO, Inc., Santa Ana, CA) was the first FDA-approved multifocal IOL in the United States. This distant-dominant, 6.0-mm silicone posterior chamber has a +3.50 D add power and focuses 50% of the incoming light for distance, 30% for near, and 20% for intermediate. To obtain adequate near function, the pupil should be ≥4.0 mm.

Remember that pupil diameter tends to decrease with increasing age. Bilateral surgery usually results in the greatest patient satisfaction. The quality of vision diminishes in low-contrast situations and the overall quality of vision may not be as good as with a monofocal IOL. Patients have more glare and haloes with these lenses, but over several months the symptoms tend to diminish. With all multifocal lenses good centration is essential to achieve the best possible postoperative vision. Accurate biometry is also required for the patient to achieve the ideal focal range. These lenses are not dependent on ciliary muscle contraction for the near vision correction.

The ReZoom lens (AMO, Inc.) is a recently FDA-approved, second-generation, zonal refractive multifocal acrylic IOL (Fig. 6.2). It is also distance dominant, but has five expanded optical zones. Zones 1, 3, and 5 are for distance correction and 2 and 4 are for near correction, while transition areas between

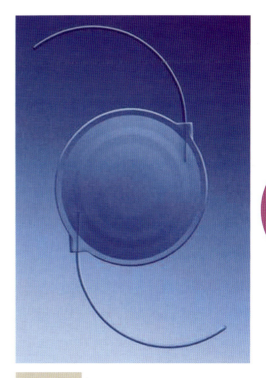

Figure 6.2

The ReZoom zonal refractive multifocal acrylic IOL. (Courtesy of AMO, Inc.)

6

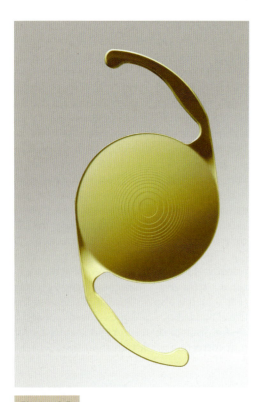

Figure 6.3

The AcrySof ReSTOR is an apodized, diffractive, acrylic multifocal IOL. (Courtesy of Alcon.)

peripheral part of the 6.0-mm optic is a refractive distance lens. The lens is distance dominant at night when the pupil is enlarged; however, adequate near correction is maintained. When the pupil is smaller the light focus is split between distance and near. Therefore, the lens function is less dependent on pupil size than a zonal refractive IOL. The lens has an add power of 3.2 D at the spectacle plane. Intermediate correction with the ReSTOR is not as robust as distance and near correction.

Accommodative Intraocular Lenses

Unlike the multifocal lenses, an accommodative IOL depends on movement of the lens optic within the eye to achieve a change in refractive power. The FDA-approved Crystalens (Eyeonics, Inc., Aliso Viejo, CA) is the first accommodative IOL available in the United States (Fig. 6.4). Others are being investigated. The Crystalens has a biconvex silicone optic

zones correct vision at the intermediate distance. This 13.00-mm modified C style PCIOL has a 6.0-mm optic and produces about 2.8 D of accommodative effect. This newer multifocal is an improvement over the Array lens because patients supposedly have a broad range of quality vision correction and they experience less glare and fewer haloes and starbursts.

The AcrySof ReSTOR (Alcon, Fort Worth, TX) is also a foldable, acrylic multifocal IOL that has also received FDA approval (Fig. 6.3). In contrast to the ReZoom, the central 3.6 mm of the ReSTOR is an apodized diffractive lens. Apodization technology is used to smooth the step heights of this diffractive IOL to improve image quality through enhanced light utilization, thereby reducing visual disturbances. The postoperative incidence of bothersome glare and haloes is reportedly 5%. It is recommended that this lens be used in both eyes to obtain the optimal effect. The

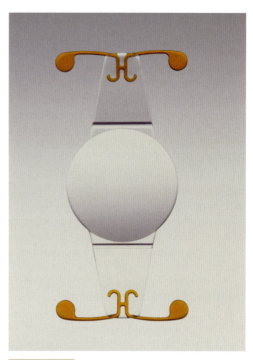

Figure 6.4

The Crystalens accommodating IOL. (Courtesy of Eyeonics, Inc.)

measuring only 4.5 mm. The lens powers range from +10.00 to +30.00 D in +0.50-D steps. Because of its posterior location within the eye, there does not appear to be more glare than would occur with a standard 6.0-mm optic. It has a modified plate-haptic IOL with a grooved hinge on either side of the optic that allows the lens to flex and the optic to move anteriorly when the ciliary muscle contracts. This movement increases the effective lens power thereby achieving its accommodative effect. It is estimated that 1 mm of anterior displacement results in 2 D of accommodative power. The lens has a small T-shaped polyamide portion at each end of the 11.5-mm lens to ensure adequate capsular bag fixation.

The lens is placed in the eye without an inserter. The capsulorrhexis must be ≤5.5 mm for the lens to function properly. The pupil must be dilated for at least 10 days postoperatively to ensure that there is no premature anterior vaulting of the lens, allowing the lens to fixate in a position to maximize distance correction. If, soon after surgery, the lens flexes anteriorly due to wound leak, large capsulorrhexis, or inadequate cycloplegia, the lens will not function properly. Patients generally should experience good distance acuity soon after surgery, but reading glasses will be needed initially, and the patient may be weaned off of these after 2 to 4 weeks. The accommodative effect of the lens increases over time during the first postoperative year.

Phakic Intraocular Lenses

The phakic IOL (PIOL) is capable of correcting a much larger range of refractive error than LASIK and the quality of corrected vision does not drop off at the extremes of the myopic or hyperopic treatment range. Table 6.1 summarizes the various PIOLs and their treatment ranges. The PIOL does, however, require intraocular surgery for insertion, and the PIOL procedure lacks the fine-tuning capability of LASIK. Keratorefractive procedures can be used to fine-tune the results after PIOL insertion surgery once they have stabilized.

Patients may not be suitable candidates for LASIK surgery because the cornea is too

Table 6.1	Phakic IOL Treatment Ranges			
Position of PIOL	Style	Available Power	Optic Size (mm)	Length (mm)
Angle-supported	NuVita MA20	7−20 D myopia	5.0 (4.5)	12−13.5 (0.5)
	Vivarte	7−20 D myopia	5.5	12.0−13.0 (0.5)
	93A or ZSAL-4	6−22 D myopia	5.5 (5.0)	13.0
	MCR 200 "phakic 6"	2−25 D myopia	6.0	12.0−14.0 (0.5)
	MCR 200 "phakic 6"	2−10 D hyperopia	6.0	12.0−14.0 (0.5)
Iris-supported (Verisyse AMO)	Artisan model 204	3−15.5 D myopia	5.0 or 6.0	8.5
	Artisan model 206	3−23.5 D myopia	5.0 or 6.0	8.5
	Artisan model 203	3−12 D hyperopia	5.0 or 6.0	8.5
	Artisan toric IOL	Custom combinations ≤+7.0	5.0 or 6.0	8.5
Sulcus-supported	Visian ICL	3−23 D myopia	4.65−5.5	12.1, 12.6, 13.2, 13.7
	Visian ICL	3−20 D hyperopia	5.5	12.1, 12.6, 13.2, 13.7
	Visian ICL	3− 20 D myopia with 1− 4 D astigmatism	4.65−5.5	12.1, 12.6, 13.2, 13.7
	PRL	3−20 D myopia	4.75−5.5	10.8 and 11.3
	PRL	4−15 D hyperopia	4.5	10.6

Source: Adapted with permission from the American Academy of Ophthalmology.

thin to accommodate the desired refractive correction. The refractive correction may exceed the approved treatment range on the available laser. Tear deficiency or corneal neovascularization may also disqualify the patient for LASIK. Keratorefractive surgery may be ill advised if the resultant keratometry measurements would be <35.00 or >50.00 D. The patient may be a candidate for a PIOL in each of these situations. Therefore, the PIOL has the potential to extend the limits of refractive surgery beyond what LASIK can safely treat.

Unlike a clear lens exchange procedure with a monofocal IOL, the patient retains accommodation. This is particularly important for the younger prepresbyopic patient. The PIOL is removable if IOL exchange or cataract surgery becomes necessary. The surgical skills required are similar to those used in small incision cataract surgery and the start-up costs involved are far less than those required for the purchase of an excimer laser.

Patients should be informed that, in contrast to LASIK surgery, this is intraocular surgery with all of its associated risks. Informed consent written specifically for this procedure should be reviewed and completed by the patient at least several days prior to surgery. Bilateral sequential surgery will be required unless the patient has marked anisometropia and is either a candidate for LASIK in the fellow eye or does not require refractive correction in the fellow eye. Patients with iritis, rubeosis iridis, glaucoma, cataract, or endothelial dystrophy are poor candidates for this procedure. The more accurate the preoperative biometry and other measurements, the better the refractive outcome. Most lens manufacturers have their own proprietary methods of determining the proper IOL power based on preoperative measurements.

PIOLs have been available outside the United States for years. They are positioned in three basic locations: the anterior chamber angle vaulting over the iris and crystalline lens, fixation on the iris surface, and in the ciliary sulcus between the iris and the crystalline lens. To date in the United States only two PIOLS, Verisyse and Visian Implantable Collamer Lens have received FDA approval. The Verisyse lens (distributed by AMO, Inc.) also known as the Artisan lens (Ophtec BV, Groningen, The Netherlands) has received approval. This is an

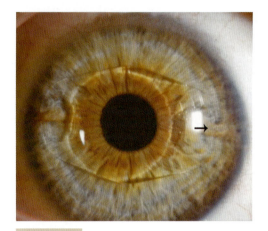

Figure 6.5

The Verisyse (also known as Artisan) iris-supported phakic IOL. The arrow indicates a knuckle of iris enclavated within lens haptics. (Courtesy of AMO, Inc.)

iris-supported lens that has the advantage of being a one-size-fits-all IOL (Fig. 6.5). A foldable version and a toric version are currently under investigation. The main disadvantage of the currently approved PMMA lens is that it requires a large incision for insertion, which could induce astigmatism. It also requires an anterior chamber depth of ≥3.2 mm for safe insertion. The technique of enclavation, in which a small knuckle of iris is incorporated into the clawlike haptics on either side of the lens, is a specialized surgical skill that must be mastered. Fixation in this way allows the pupil to move freely.

This lens design has a long track record of safety and has been used internationally for many years as a popular lens for secondary implantation to correct surgical aphakia. Because the iris supports the lens, and the pupil is constricted pharmacologically during implantation, there is little risk of trauma to the crystalline lens leading to cataract. But the enclavation technique is challenging, and it is critical to achieve a stable, secure, and accurate position for the lens.

The anterior chamber PIOLs (ACPIOLs) are foldable and can be inserted through a small clear cornea wound. They are dependent on accurate sizing to achieve a proper fit. The white-to-white distance has been shown to be inaccurate. Scheimpflug photography (see

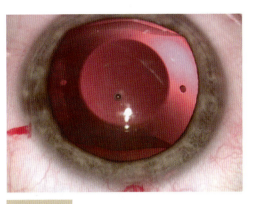

Figure 6.6

The Visian ICL in position in the ciliary sulcus anterior to the crystalline lens. (Courtesy of STAAR Surgical.)

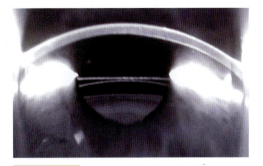

Figure 6.7

Scheimpflug photography shows PIOL optic (Visian ICL) in the posterior chamber vaulting over the crystalline lens. (Courtesy of STAAR Surgical.)

topography section in Chapter 2) and ultrasound biomicroscopy are currently being used for more accurate sizing of PIOLs. New, more accurate ways of measuring the anterior segment structures are being developed. An adequate anterior chamber depth is necessary to implant this lens. The risks associated with implantation include endothelial cell loss, pupil ovalization, and pupillary block.

The posterior chamber PIOLs (PCPIOLs), for example, the FDA-approved Visian ICL (STAAR; Fig. 6.6) and the PRL (CIBA), are flexible and can also be inserted through a small clear cornea incision. The Visian ICL is available outside the United States in a toric version capable of correcting up to 6 D of astigmatism. The lens fits in the posterior chamber with the haptics in the ciliary sulcus and the optic vaulting the crystalline lens (Fig. 6.7). Modifications in the Visian ICL have resulted in a lens design with a low incidence of cataract. However, this remains a risk along with pupillary block.

Preoperative prophylactic laser peripheral iridotomies are recommended for all the PIOL types to reduce the risk of pupillary block. A summary of the risks associated with each of the PIOLs is presented in Table 6.2.

Bioptics

Zaldivar described the combined use of lens implantation followed at a later time by laser refractive surgery and used the term *bioptics*. Originally, bioptics referred to insertion of a PCPIOL followed by LASIK. Güell used the term *adjustable refractive surgery* (ARS) to describe his technique of creating a LASIK flap and then inserting an iris-fixated PIOL. He would later perform the exclmer procedure as an enhancement, if needed. This flap-first technique was designed to reduce the risk of corneal endothelial trauma caused by using a microkeratome in the presence of an iris-fixated PIOL. Over time *bioptics* has come to mean the combination of any two refractive procedures. Bioptics is particularly useful for expanding the range of lens surgery, adding additional myopic, hyperopic, and astigmatism correction beyond the available lens implant powers. It also adds the fine-tuning capability of a keratorefractive procedure. Keratorefractive surgery can be done with less risk of ectasia in patients with high myopia or thin corneas. Interestingly, the highly myopic patients can increase lines of BCVA presumably due to image magnification. The results of bioptics and ARS are presented in Table 6.3.

6

Table 6.2   Incidence of complications with PIOLs

Lens Model	Eyes	Glare/Haloes	Pupil Ovalization	Mean Endothelial Cell Loss	Cataract	Pigment Dispersion	IOP Elevation
ACPIOL							
Alió et al., 1999[1] ZB5M/MF/ZSAL-4	263	20% at 1 y 10% at 7 y	5.9%	8.4% at 7 y			
Baikoff et al., 1998[2] ZB5M	134 35	18.8% at 1 y 12.5% at 3 y	9.9% at 1 y 27.5% at 3 y	4.6% at 3 y			
Pérez-Santonja et al., 2000[3] ZSAL-4	23	26.1% at 2 y	17.4% at 2 y	4.2 % at 2 y	3%	18.7%	15.6%
Iris-Fixated IOL							
Menezo et al., 1998[4] Iris-claw lens	111	1.8%		13.4% at 4 y		12.8%	5.3%
Manche, 2002[5] Artisan IOL	228	3.5% 5.0-mm optic 4.1% 6.0-mm optic		2.6% at 2 y			
Budo et al., 2000[6] Artisan IOL	518	13.7% at 3 y (249 eyes)		2.4% at 1 y; 0.7% at 3 y	2.4% (249 eyes)		
PCPIOL							
Vukich, 2003[7] Visian ICL	257			No corneal edema from 1–24 mo	6.7% ASC at 2 y		
Arne, 2000[8] Visian ICL	58	54.3%		<3.9% at 1 y	3.4% ASC	15.5%	3.4%
Zaldivar et al., 1998[9] Visian ICL	124	2.4%	Not available	2.4%		Not available	11.3%

Source: Adapted with permission from the American Academy of Ophthalmology.

[1] Alió IL, De La Hoz F, Pérez-Santonja JJ, et al. Phakic anterior chamber lenses for the correction of myopia: a 7-year cumulative analysis of complications in 263 cases. *Ophthalmology*. 1999;106:458–466.

[2] Baikoff G, Arne IL, Bokobza Y, et al. Angle-fixated anterior chamber phakic intraocular lens for myopia of −7 to −19 diopters. *J Cataract Refract Surg*. 1998;14:282–293.

[3] Pérez-Santonja JJ, Alió JL, Jimenez-Alfaro I, et al. Surgical correction of severe myopia with an angle-supported phakic intraocular lens. *J Cataract Refract Surg*. 2000;26:1288–1302.

[4] Menezo JL, Cisneros AL, Rodriguez-Salvador, V. Endothelial study of iris-claw phakic lens: 4 year follow-up. *J Cataract Refract Surg*. 1998;24:1039–1049.

[5] Manche EE. The Artisan anterior chamber lens. Presented at Subspecialty Day: Refractive Surgery, Back to the Future, Orlando, FL, 2002. San Francisco: American Academy of Ophthalmology.

[6] Budo C, Hessloehl JC, Izak M, et al. Multicenter study of the Artisan phakic intraocular lens. *J Cataract Refract Surg*. 2000;26:1163–1171.

[7] Vukich JA, Ticlittom ISG. U.S. Food and Drug Administration clinical trial of the implantable contact lens for moderate to high myopia. *Ophthalmology*. 2003;110:255–266.

[8] Arne JL, Lesueur LC. Phakic posterior chamber lenses for high myopia: functional and anatomical outcomes. *J Cataract Refract Surg*. 2000;26:369–374.

[9] Zaldivar R, Davidorf JM, Oscherow S. Posterior chamber phakic intraocular lens for myopia of −8 to −19 diopters. *J Refract Surg*. 1998;14:294.

Table 6.5   Bioptics results

	Number of Eyes	Mean Preoperative Sph Eq (Range)	UCVA $\geq$ 20/40	Gain $\geq$ 2 Lines of BCVA	Loss $\geq$ 2 Lines of BCVA
Bioptics (Zaldivar et al.,1999[1])	67	−23.00 D (−18.75 to −35.00 D)	69% (46)	76% (51)	0%
ARS (Güell et al., 2001[2])	26	−18.42 D (−16.00 to −23.00 D)	77% (20)	42% (11)	0%
ICL with LASIK or PRK (Chayet, 2001[3])	37	−17.74 D (−9.75 to −28.00 D)	89.1% (33)	64.8% (24)	3% (1)

Source: Adapted with permission from the American Academy of Ophthalmology.
[1] Zaldivar R, Davidorf JM, Oscherow S, et al. Combined posterior chamber phakic intraocular lens and laser *in situ* keratomileusis: bioptics for extreme myopia. *J Refract Surg.* 1999;15:299–308.
[2] Güell JI, Vázquez M, Gris O. Adjustable refractive surgery: 6-mm Artisan lens plus laser *in situ* keratomileusis for the correction of high myopia. *Ophthalmology.* 2001;108:945–952.
[3] Chayet, A. Presented at Refractive Surgery Subspecialty Day. 2001.

6

Case Section

Anthony Cirino, M.D., Robert S. Feder, M.D., Lawrence Gans, M.D., Colman Kraff, M.D., Marian Macsai, M.D.,
Parag Majmudar, M.D., Christopher J. Rapuano, M.D., Michael Rosenberg, M.D., Steven Rosenfeld, M.D.,
Jonathan Rubenstein, M.D., and Michael Vrabec, M.D., F.A.C.S.

In this section cases are presented for study. The cases have been prepared by the editors and the contributors and at times will reflect the opinions and preferences of the individual author. The reader is presented with one way—but not the only way—to work the case. Each patient is unique and surgery should always be designed with the specific patient in mind.

The cases are arranged in order of complexity from easiest to more difficult. Preoperative decision making is emphasized in the first half of the case section. The later cases emphasize intraoperative and postoperative management. It can be assumed in each case that the risks of surgery have been presented to the patient, that they were understood, and that the patient wishes to proceed with surgery. Unless otherwise indicated, the patient has been out of contact lenses long enough for the given refractions to be stable. However, not every patient presented is a candidate for LASIK surgery. The reader will need to make that determination. The most accurate way of determining flap thickness and residual stromal thickness is by performing intraoperative pachymetry. For the sake of discussion, a preoperative estimate of residual stromal thickness is shown as preoperative pachymetry minus plate thickness and estimated ablation depth. The reader should be aware that this is only an estimate and is not a substitute for intraoperative pachymetry.

The best learning experience will occur if the reader, with paper and pencil in hand, actively studies each case history and examination and develops a surgical strategy before reading the discussion and treatment plan. The reader should work the case as if the patient had presented in the office. The variables or challenges that must be considered in developing a surgical plan should be identified. The key questions to be answered in each case are as follows: Is this patient a good candidate for LASIK surgery? How should the flap be created? What treatment zone is most appropriate? What is the approximate ablation depth? What is the overall plan for surgery in the language the scrub technician and laser engineer can use? For example, specify the microkeratome ring and plate sizes as well as the ablation zone. Are there any special considerations in the case?

Each case is followed by a narrative discussion and most cases provide a tabular summary of the surgical plan. The equipment used to carry out the plan is specified. Readers should refer to the various sections pertaining to the equipment available in their own laser center. At the conclusion of each case, a series of take-home points is listed.

An alternative way to use the case section is to use the various case indexes. Three charts are provided: one for preoperative patient characteristics (pages 129–131), one for intraoperative and postoperative conditions (pages 214–216), and one for equipment (page 132). Both the case number and the page number indicate the cases containing specific variables. Readers can match the variables from a patient they will treat with the specific relevant cases in the book. For example, a reader concerned about the management of a patient with corneal neovascularization can locate this variable in the chart and be directed to all of the cases in which corneal neovascularization is discussed. These indices will hopefully allow the reader to easily access those specific cases and discussions that will be most relevant. It is our hope that studying these cases will be a satisfying experience, both challenging and rewarding.

Preoperative Planning Index			
Patient Characteristic	Case Number	Page Number	Contributor
Amblyopia	21	166	Colman Kraff
	34	190	Robert S. Feder
Anemia	28	180	Robert S. Feder and Anthony Cirino
Anisometropia	37	195	Robert S. Feder and Anthony Cirino
Astigmatism	15	154	Marian Macsai
	18	159	Anthony Cirino and Robert S. Feder
Astigmatism disparity (M vs. C)	14	152	Robert S. Feder
	30	183	Robert S. Feder
Astigmatism, lenticular	14	152	Robert S. Feder
Astigmatism, mixed	34	190	Robert S. Feder
	35	191	Marian Macsai
	36	193	Robert S. Feder
Bioptics	38	196	Lawrence Gans
Blepharitis	3	136	Jonathan Rubenstein
	11	148	Robert S. Feder and Anthony Cirino
	14	152	Robert S. Feder
Blepharospasm	22	168	Steven Rosenfeld
	24	171	Robert S. Feder
Clear lens exchange	39	198	Lawrence Gans
	40	200	Lawrence Gans
Corneal ectasia	25	173	Parag Majmudar
	26	174	Robert S. Feder and Anthony Cirino
Deep set eyes	9	145	Robert S. Feder
	30	183	Robert S. Feder
Diabetes	41	202	Robert S. Feder
Disc drusen	18	159	Anthony Cirino and Robert S. Feder
Dry eye	3	136	Jonathan Rubenstein
	16	155	Robert S. Feder and Anthony Cirino
	17	157	Robert S. Feder
	33	188	Marian Macsai
Epithelial defect	32	186	Robert S. Feder
	33	188	Marian Macsai
Esophoria	11	148	Robert S. Feder and Anthony Cirino
	30	183	Robert S. Feder
Exotropia	24	171	Robert S. Feder
Flat cornea	6	140	Parag Majmudar
	7	142	Robert S. Feder and Anthony Cirino
	9	145	Robert S. Feder
	29	181	Colman Kraff
	25	173	Parag Majmudar
Forme fruste KCN	26	174	Robert S. Feder and Anthony Cirino
	38	196	Lawrence Gans

continued

Equipment Index					
	Microkeratome				
	Becton Dickinson	**Hansatome**	**Moria**	**Nidek Amadeus**	**IntraLase**	**None**
Laser						
VISX		Cases 1, 2, 4, 7, 9, 11, 14, 16, 26, 28, 30, 34, 36, 41, 43, 48, 53	Case 42	Cases 45, 46	Cases 11, 13, 17, 19, 30, 44	Cases 18, 24, 26, 27, 30, 32
VISX Custom		Cases 21, 29	Case 22		Cases 12, 72	Cases 55, 49, 49, 50
B&L		Case 6				Cases 52, 67
Alcon	Case 3					Cases 23, 51
NIDEK		Case 33		Cases 5, 15, 35		
LRI						Cases 38, 54, 65
PIOL						Cases 37, 38
CLE						Cases 27, 40
CK						Case 56

PREOPERATIVE DECISION MAKING

CASE 1

A 35-year-old woman with a history of myopia and a 20-year history of soft contact lens wear expresses interest in LASIK surgery. Assume she has been out of her contacts long enough for the refractions to have stabilized.

W	OD–6.25 20/20+ OS –6.25 20/20–	**Uncorrected Va** 20/400 OU
M	OD–5.50 + 0.50 x 40° 20/15 OS –5.25 20/15–	
C	OD–5.25 20/15 OS –4.75 20/15–	
K	OD 44.50 x 180°/44.87 x 90° OS 44.50 x 180°/44.75 x 90°	

Pachymetry	**Topography**	**Scotopic Pupils**
OD 541 µm OS 531 µm	No cone OU	OD 5.0 mm OS 5.0 mm

Additional Examination
Excellent exposure with a normal slit-lamp examination, intraocular pressure (IOP), and fundus examination.

Discussion

This is a fairly straightforward patient with myopia. While astigmatism appears in the manifest refraction, the cycloplegic refraction will be used in determining the laser treatment. Many surgeons prefer not to change the cylinder from the manifest refraction. Alternatively the patient could have a postcycloplegic refraction prior to surgery to check the astigmatism.

The small scotopic pupil allows the surgeon to choose a small treatment zone. This will help preserve corneal tissue. Because there is no peripheral pathology and the corneal diameter is presumably of normal size, a larger ring can be used. This will create a larger flap that may be desirable in the event future retreatment is necessary. Notice that this patient appears to be moderately overcorrected in her present spectacles. Relaxing accommodation may take some time. It is helpful to warn the patient preoperatively that the full vision correction will not occur instantaneously but may occur over several days to a couple of weeks.

Surgical Plan

	Right Eye	Left Eye	Comments
Ring size	8.5 or 9.5 mm	8.5 or 9.5 mm	If perilimbal neovascularization or a small corneal diameter, choose 8.5-mm ring
Plate size	160 or 180 μm	160 or 180 μm	Hansatome flap may be thinner than plate size
Ablation zone	6.0 mm	6.0 mm	Ablation zone > scotopic pupil
Cycloplegic RX	−5.25 D	−4.75 D	
Calculations: Sphere in cycloplegic refraction is reduced by the VISX nomogram	−5.25 × 6% = −0.315 −5.25 + 0.32 = −4.93	−4.75 × 6% = −0.285 −4.75 + 0.29 = −4.46	Refer to VISX laser discussion in Chapter 2 and the nomogram (Table 2.11, page 35) for the amount of reduction
Adjusted correction is entered into VISX laser	−4.93 D	−4.46 D	
Ablation depth Use non–nomogram-adjusted spherical equivalent	From Table 2.13: 66 μm Using calculation: −5.25 D × 12 μm/D = 63 μm	From Table 2.13: 60 μm Calculation: −4.75 D × 12 μm/D = 57 μm	Most cases will use the calculation method for ablation depth
Residual stromal thickness (RST)	541 μm − 160 μm − 66 μm = 315 μm >250 μm	531 μm − 160 μm − 60 μm = 311 μm >250 μm	Intraoperative pachymetry best for RST calculation

Take-Home Points

1. Always use the cycloplegic refraction before making the nomogram adjustment in calculating the ablation depth.
2. Using an ablation zone slightly larger than the scotopic pupil minimizes tissue removal.
3. A larger flap is desirable in case a retreatment requires a larger treatment zone. However, when the flap edge is near the limbus, the flap may be more difficult to relift.
4. Warn the patient overcorrected in spectacles or glasses about the possibility of a slower postoperative visual recovery.

7

A 38-year-old woman has worn rigid gas-permeable hard contact lenses for 15 years and presents for LASIK evaluation. The patient is highly myopic and feels vulnerable and disabled without her contact lenses. The past ocular history has been completely uneventful. There has specifically been no history of corneal ulceration, abrasion, or keratitis. Her general health is excellent. After consultation and detailed explanation of the risks of surgery, the patient is anxious to proceed with LASIK. She was kept out of contact lenses until the corneal contour and refraction stabilized.

		Uncorrected Va
W	OD−10.25 + 1.25 x 4° 20/25 − OS −10.25 + 0.75 x 150° 20/30 −	CF 3′ CF 3′
M	OD−9.50 + 0.50 x 180° 20/15 − OS −9.75 + 0.75 x 1 35° 20/15	
C	OD− 9.75 + 0.50 x 160° 20/15 − Vertex distance 12 mm OS − 9.50 + 0.50 x 120° 20/20 Vertex distance 12 mm	
K	OD 44.87 x 90°/44.50 x 180° OS 43.87 x 40°/44.50 x 130°	

Pachymetry	Topography	Scotopic Pupils
OD 564 μm OS 555 μm	Against-the-rule astigmatism OU; no cone OU	OD 5.0 mm OS 5.0 mm

Additional Examination

The external eye appears healthy. The lids are lax and the palpebral fissure is wide. The exposure is excellent. The slit-lamp examination shows subepithelial haze OD with minimal thinning near the limbus superiorly extending for 1 clock hour. There is no active keratitis and no corneal neovascularization. The anterior segment is otherwise normal in both eyes. The lids and lashes are normal with no evidence of blepharitis or meibomian gland disease. The IOP and dilated fundus examinations are normal.

Discussion

The treatment of high myopia requires an adequate corneal thickness and corneal steepness in order to ensure that the cornea will not be too thin or flat postoperatively. If the corneal thickness is inadequate, the cornea is too flat, or the degree of myopia is too great, consider an alternative to LASIK such as insertion of a phakic IOL (see Chapter 6 on alternatives to LASIK). Clear lens exchange in an extreme myope may have an unacceptably high risk of retinal detachment over the long term.

The highly myopic patient may have excessive myopic correction in spectacles or contact lenses, which can only be uncovered with a full cycloplegic refraction. It is also important to measure the vertex distance. Most excimer lasers have a default vertex distance at the spectacle plane. If the measured vertex distance is different than the default, an adjustment is required. For greatest accuracy central pachymetry should be measured at the time of surgery. Do not rely on the pachymetry performed on a different day to calculate flap thickness. Many

7

factors including contact lens wear, time of day, and ambient humidity can impact corneal thickness.

To estimate the postoperative corneal contour, multiply the spherical equivalent by 0.7 or, to be even more conservative, 0.8. Subtract this product from the average of the preoperative keratometry values. If the result is <35.00 D, the cornea may be too flat after surgery. Highly myopic patients are more likely to regress postoperatively; therefore, in anticipation of possible regression, it is useful to make certain that there is sufficient corneal steepness and thickness to support retreatment. If there is not much room for retreatment, the patient must be warned of the limitation on enhancement and the consequence of untreated regression. Because the pupil is rather small in this case, a smaller ablation zone can be used. This will mean the ablation will not be as deep and will leave more residual stroma.

This patient has an old scar in the right cornea. She denies inflammation, infection, or erosion. Because the scarring is superficial and well out of the ablation zone, it is not a contraindication to surgery. The surgeon should always attempt to determine the cause of such a scar by obtaining a complete history and performing a thorough examination.

Surgical Plan

	Right Eye	Left Eye	Comments
Ring size	9.5 mm	9.5 mm	Hansatome
Plate size	160 μm	160 μm	Hansatome flap is usually thinner than the plate thickness.
Ablation zone	6.0 mm	6.0 mm	VISX STAR S4
Calculations with nomogram correction (enter into VISX)	-9.50 D × 11% = 1.05 $-9.75 + 1.05 = 8.70$ $-8.70 + 0.50 × 180$	$-9.25 × 11\% = 1.02$ $-9.50 + 1.02 = 8.48$ $-8.48 + 0.50 × 135$	Use cylinder axis of the manifest or split the difference between M and C
Ablation depth	9.50 D × 12 μm/D = 114 μm	9.25D × 12 μm/D = 111 μm	Always use non–nomogram-adjusted spherical equivalent to calculate ablation depth
Residual stromal thickness	564 μm − 128 μm −114 μm = 322 μm >250 μm	555 μm − 123 μm − 111 μm = 321 μm >250 μm	RST calculated using the central flap thickness measured in surgery

Take-Home Points

1. Make certain the patient will have enough residual stromal thickness for retreatment and will have adequate corneal curvature to support good visual function.
2. Always use the non–nomogram-adjusted spherical equivalent to calculate the ablation depth. Do not rely on the ablation depth calculated by the laser for conventional LASIK.
3. Measure pachymetry intraoperatively. Do not rely on a central pachymetry measurement made on a different day.
4. Do not compromise on patient safety. Consider alternatives to LASIK when necessary. Straight talk with the patient is always the best approach.

Proceed to Case 74 to find out what happened to this patient.

A 40-year-old woman comes desiring refractive surgery. She has worn rigid gas-permeable contact lenses (RGPCL) for more than 15 years and is becoming increasingly intolerant to her contact lenses. She stopped wearing her RGPCLs 4 weeks ago in preparation for her refractive evaluation. She has been treated in the past for Graves disease. She currently takes levothyroxine (Synthroid) and occasional artificial tears.

W	OD−4.25 + 1.00 x 78° OS −2.50 + 0.50 x 125°	**Uncorrected Va** 20/400 20/200
M	OD−4.75 + 1.25 x 70°20/20 OS −3.25 + 0.75 x 135° 20/20	
C	OD−5.00 + 1.50 x 75° 20/20 OS −3.00 + 0.50 x 125° 20/20	
K	OD 41.00 x 170°/43.00 x 80° OS 42.12 x 35°/43.75 x 125°	

Pachymetry	**Topography**	**Scotopic Pupils**
OD 548 µm OS 552 µm	Regular astigmatism OU	OD 6.9 mm OS 6.8 mm

Additional Examination

Her corneas are clear without staining. Her eyelids show 2+ to 3+ blepharitis with meibomianitis. Changes are seen on her eyelids and face consistent with acne rosacea. There is mild upper lid retraction OU without proptosis. The remainder of her ocular examination is normal.

Discussion

This patient's case illustrates a number of important clinical points. This patient has been a long-time RGPCL wearer. These rigid contact lenses may alter the shape of the cornea and mask astigmatism and myopia. Therefore, the surgeon must be sure that the refraction is stable and accurate. The magnitude and axis of the astigmatism must be consistent between the manifest refraction, cycloplegic refraction, and the corneal maps. The corneal maps should show regular astigmatism and no signs of corneal warping. If there is any doubt as to whether the contact lenses have altered the refraction and corneal shape, the patient should stay out of the contacts for a longer period of time and return for repeat refraction and maps until they are all stable and consistent.

This patient is also at risk for postoperative dry eyes. A 40-year-old woman is undergoing early hormonal changes that decrease tear production. She also has increased corneal exposure due to lid retraction resulting from thyroid disease. Lastly, she has posterior blepharitis and abnormal meibomian glands that produce an abnormal lipid component to her tear film and therefore tear film instability. The decreased tear production that normally accompanies a denervated post-LASIK cornea may further contribute to this patient's postoperative dry eye. The patient should be treated aggressively after surgery if signs of dry eye and corneal staining occur. This treatment could include frequent nonpreserved artificial tears and/or topical cyclosporine. Punctal occlusion should be avoided until the posterior blepharitis is treated.

7

Lastly, this patient has posterior blepharitis as a result of the acne rosacea. This increases the chance for diffuse lamellar keratitis (DLK). The rosacea should be treated with eyelid hygiene twice a day combined with oral doxycycline or minocycline. LASIK should be delayed until the lids show clinical improvement.

This patient is a good candidate for custom ablation. Her refractive error falls well within the range for custom ablation and her refraction from the wavefront aberrometer is consistent with her manifest and cycloplegic refraction. She shows enough spherical aberration and coma to benefit from the wavefront-guided treatment. Her corneas are mildly flat and therefore a 9.0-mm suction ring is chosen on the Becton Dickinson K-3000 microkeratome. A 160-μm plate is used to create a slightly thinner flap to avoid any possible masking effects that a thicker flap would have on a custom ablation.

Surgical Plan

	Right Eye	Left Eye	Comments
Considerations	Evaluate for dry eye, treat for rosacea. Proceed only if surface is healthy		
Ring size	9.0 mm	9.0 mm	BD K-3000
Plate size	160 μm	160 μm	Actual flap thickness is usually thinner
Ablation zone	6.5 mm with blend zone	6.5 mm with blend zone	Alcon laser pupils >6.5 mm
Spherical equivalent	−4.25 D	−2.75 D	
CustomCornea treatment based on Alcon wavefront measurements	−4.39 D sphere 1.30 D × 66°	−2.95 D sphere 0.69 D × 132°	The Alcon CustomCornea suggests a 6% reduction of sphere and cylinder; treatment is based on the wavefront data
Nomogram adjustment (6%) at corneal plane in minus cylinder	−2.76 − 1.19 × 156°	−2.04 − 0.65 × 42°	
Ablation depth	80 μm	56 μm	The Alcon software calculates the ablation depth
Residual stromal thickness	548 μm − 160 μm − 80 μm = 308 μm	552 μm − 160 μm − 56 μm = 336 μm	>250 μm

Take-Home Points

1. Be sure that the patient has been out of rigid gas-permeable contact lens long enough to allow the cornea to assume its normal shape.
2. Look for factors that could predispose a patient to postoperative dry eyes and pretreat the patient appropriately.
3. Treat a patient with rosacea with preoperative oral tetracycline and lid hygiene.
4. Consider wavefront-guided ablation if the wavefront-derived refraction is consistent with the manifest refraction and the patient demonstrates higher order aberrations.

A 38-year-old police detective had worn rigid gas-permeable contact lenses for 15 years. He was eager to become less dependent on his contact lenses and glasses prompting a LASIK consultation. He understood the future need for reading glasses and the other associated risks of surgery. After 1 month his refractive error had stabilized and surgery was planned.

		Uncorrected Va
W	OD−2.50 20/20− OS −2.50 20/20−	20/200 20/200
M	OD−3.75 + 1.25 x 87° 20/15 OS −3.25 + 0.75 x 85° 20/15−	
C	OD−3.50 + 1.00 x 85° 20/15− OS −3.25 + 0.75 x 90° 20/15	
K	OD 42.75 x 177°/43.75 x 87° OS 43.00 x 180°/44.00 x 90°	

Pachymetry	Topography	Scotopic Pupils
OD 513 μm OS 509 μm	Regular with-the-rule astigmatism OU	OD 7.0 mm OS 7.0 mm

Discussion

While the pupils are somewhat large and the cornea somewhat thin, the correction is low enough that there is room for a large zone with a blend to extend the treatment to 8.0 mm. This patient, due to his profession, should be specifically warned about the possibility of night vision problems and the effect of a traumatic injury to the flap. He should also be considered for a custom procedure, which may reduce the likelihood of postoperative glare and haloes.

Surgical Plan

	Right Eye	Left Eye	Comments
Ring size	9.5 mm	9.5 mm	
Plate size	160 μm	160 μm	Hansatome flap usually thinner than 160 μm
Ablation zone	6.5 mm with blend	6.5 mm with blend	VISX laser 7.0-mm pupil
Calculations with nomogram correction (enter into VISX laser)	$3.00 D \times 7\% = 0.21 D$ $3.50 D - 0.21 D = 3.29 D$ $-3.29 + 1.00 \times 85$	$2.88 D \times 7\% = 0.20 D$ $3.25 D - 0.20 D = 3.05 D$ $-3.05 + 0.75 \times 90$	
Ablation depth	$45 \mu m + 8 \mu m = 53 \mu m$	$43 \mu m + 8 \mu m = 51 \mu m$	
Residual stromal thickness	$513 \mu m - 160 \mu m$ $- 53 \mu m = 300 \mu m$ $>250 \mu m$	$509 \mu m - 160 \mu m$ $- 51 \mu m = 298 \mu m$ $>250 \mu m$	If flap thinner than 160 μm, RST will be even greater

7

Take-Home Points

1. Emphasize those risks that are relevant to a given patient based on the patient's work and leisure activities.
2. Design the surgery to minimize those risks. In this case use a treatment zone larger than the scotopic pupil and/or consider a custom treatment.

Proceed to Cases 61 and 62 to find out what happened to this patient.

Proceed to Cases 61 and 62 to find out what happened to this patient.

CASE 5

A 30-year-old man, non–contact lens wearer presents with myopic astigmatism. He is anxious to reduce dependency on his glasses as he has two young children that he cannot see in the swimming pool. He is an avid runner and bicycle rider. He is healthy, uses no ocular medications, and is on no systemic medications. The patient was told during a previous LASIK consultation that due to his pupil size he was at great risk for glare and haloes. The patient understands there is a significant risk of nighttime vision disturbances.

		Uncorrected Va
W	OD–4.00 + 0.50 x 90° 20/20	CF
	OS –3.50 + 1.00 x 80° 20/20	20/400
M	OD–3.75 + 0.50 x 90° 20/20	
	OS –3.50 + 0.50 x 90° 20/15	
C	OD–3.50 + 0.50 x 90° 20/20	
	OS –3.50 + 0.50 x 90° 20/15	
K	OD 43.50 x 180°/44.00 x 90°	
	OS 44.00 x 180°/44.50 x 90°	

Pachymetry	Topography	Scotopic Pupils
OD 525 μm	Regular with-the-rule	OD 8.0 mm
OS 539 μm	astigmatism OU	OS 8.0 mm

Additional Examination

The patient has excellent exposure. The external, pupil, motility, slit-lamp, and fundus examinations are normal. The IOP was 16 mmHg OU.

Discussion

This patient is a good candidate for LASIK surgery. His cornea is thick enough and a 160-μm plate with the Nidek MK-2000 microkeratome can be used with no invasion of the posterior 250 μm of the corneal stroma. The large scotopic pupils indicate a need to expand the transition zone of the Nidek EC 5000 laser. Doing so reduces the risk of visual disturbances in the dark. To calculate what should be entered into the laser, the nomogram for myopic astigmatism (Table 2.18, page 76) is followed (see discussion on Nidek laser in Chapter 2). Begin with the cycloplegic refraction of the right eye −3.50 + 0.50 axis 90°. This is converted into negative cylinder and becomes −3.00 − 0.50 axis 180°. This is identified in the Nidek look-up table (available from Nidek) to equate to −2.408 − 0.280 axis 180°. The full cylinder is treated at +0.50 because this is less than 1.25. Because the scotopic pupil is 8.0 mm, the transition zone is expanded to 9.0 mm. A 27% reduction in the spherical component, −2.408 D, is needed because of this expanded transition zone. The spherical component after reduction becomes 1.7578 D, which is rounded up to

1.76 sphere. Therefore, the data entered into the laser are sphere −1.76 D, cylinder −0.50 D, axis 180°, optical zone 6.5 mm, transition zone 9.0 mm. Because the cycloplegic refraction for the left eye is identical, the same data are entered into the laser for the left eye. The only difference between the two eyes is the average keratometry reading, 43.75 D OD and 44.25 D OS.

Surgical Plan

	Right Eye	Left Eye	Comments
Cycloplegic refraction in negative cylinder	−3.00 − 0.50 × 180	−3.00 − 0.50 × 180	
Ring size	9.5 mm	9.5 mm	A larger flap allows for adequate exposure if a hyperopic enhancement is required
Plate size	160 μm	160 μm	
Optical zone	6.5 mm	6.5 mm	Larger treatment zone decreases risk of visual aberrations
Transitional zone	9.0 mm	9.0 mm	1 mm larger than the scotopic pupil measurement
Calculations with Nidek nomogram	2.408 (27%) = 1.76 sphere	2.408 (27%) = 1.76 sphere	Treat full cylinder because it is <1.25 D
Spherical treatment	−1.76 D	−1.76 D	
Cylinder treatment	−0.50 D × 180	−0.50 D × 180	
Approximate ablation depth	50 μm	50 μm	
Residual stromal thickness (RST)	525 μm − 160 μm − 50 μm = 315 μm >250 μm	539 μm − 160 μm − 50 μm = 329 μm >250 μm	
Considerations	MK-2000 130 μm plate remains an option		

Take-Home Points

1. Expansion of the optical and transition zone requires use of a customized nomogram, an example of which can be found in Table 2.18, page 76.
2. Calculation of RST should be performed prior to the LASIK procedure to ensure preservation of 250 μm of residual stroma thickness. Remember that the most accurate determination is made at the time of surgery.

7

CASE 6

A 28-year-old woman presents for laser vision correction. Her past medical history is negative, and her past ocular history is significant for 15 years of soft toric disposable contact lens wear. There is no history of prior ocular trauma, infection, or prior surgery. She is not currently pregnant or nursing. She takes no systemic or ocular medications and has no known drug allergies. She last wore her contact lenses 3 weeks ago.

W	OD −4.50 + 0.50 x 90° 20/25 OS − 4.75 + 0.75 x 90° 20/30	**Uncorrected Va** 20/400 20/400
M	OD −4.75 + 0.50 x 90° 20/20 OS −5.25 + 0.75 x 85° 20/20	
C	OD −4.75 + 0.50 x 90° 20/20 OS −5.25 + 0.75 x 90° 20/20	
K	OD 40.50 x 90°/40.00 x 180° OS 41.50 x 90°/40.50 x 180°	

Pachymetry	**Topography**	**Scotopic Pupils**
OD 535 μm OS 540 μm	Regular bow-tie OU	7.0 mm OU

Additional Examination

The patient does not have deep-set eyes. The palpebral fissure is wide OU. The slit-lamp examination reveals a normal cornea OU with no evidence of guttata or keratoconus. The lenses are clear, and the intraocular pressure is 16 mmHg OU by applanation tonometry. The dilated funduscopic examination is unremarkable. Orbscan evaluation reveals posterior elevation of 22 μm in the right eye, and 26 μm in the left eye.

Discussion

This patient is a very good candidate for laser vision correction, especially LASIK, provided that several points are considered. From a historical perspective, the patient has no other complicating medical or ophthalmic conditions. The length of time that she has been out of her toric contact lenses is adequate with the minimum being 2 weeks. The refractive error is within the range for LASIK, and more importantly has been stable over the past year. Stability is defined as a less than 0.5 D change over the previous 12 months. The corneal thickness is adequate for LASIK at this level of myopia. The topographical analysis is normal in each eye. Orbscan measurements of the posterior elevation may help identify corneas that have forme fruste keratoconus. Remember that posterior elevation in an untreated cornea of 50 μm (0.050 mm) or greater above a "best-fit sphere" are strongly suggestive of FFKC (see discussion of topography in Chapter 2). Values between 40 and 50 μm are suspicious and other criteria should be used to determine whether or not a patient is a candidate for LASIK. A posterior elevation of 22 and 26 μm as in this case is not a reason for concern.

Several issues regarding this patient need to be addressed. The patient's keratometry values are fairly flat. In general, 1 D of excimer ablation will result in flattening of the keratometry by 0.7 to 0.8 D. Although controversial, it is wise to keep the corneal curvature above 35.00 D following LASIK surgery. In this case, the expected postoperative keratometry values should be approximately 36.50 D. Another problem with flat corneal contour relates to the creation of the corneal flap. With a very flat cornea, there is a higher incidence of a small flap or possibly a free cap. To minimize this possibility, a larger diameter suction ring should be used, such as a 9.5-mm ring. The femtosecond laser is a useful alternative, because its use is not dependent on corneal contour.

Another issue is the large pupil size. The Bausch & Lomb (B&L) laser has the capability of treating a wide ablation zone, larger than the scotopic pupil size, and this may help reduce the incidence of glare, haloes, and starbursts. The optical zone determines the depth of ablation, according to Munnerlyn's formula and, therefore, caution is urged in selecting the appropriate zone. The optical zone can be set from 4.5 to 8.0 mm plus a blend zone of 3 additional mm. Therefore, a 6-mm optical zone provides an ablation of 9 × 9 mm, larger than almost all scotopic pupil size. It is the most commonly used optical zone size. In this patient, with 7-mm scotopic pupils, We would select a 6-mm optical zone because the total ablation area is larger than the scotopic pupil size. The selection of a larger optical zone would probably not provide additional benefit and only consume more corneal tissue.

The B&L laser is very accurate. We do not adjust the desired refraction with any nomogram, but each surgeon should make this determination after a careful analysis of their data. We often adjust the target refraction in patients <30 years of age to +0.50 D.

Surgical Plan

	Right Eye	Left Eye	Comments
Ring size	9.5 mm	9.5 mm	Flat contour; use 9.5 to prevent free cap
Plate size	160 µm	160 µm	Hansatome usually cuts 100−120 µm flap
Optical zone	6.0 mm	6.0 mm	B&L laser
Transitional zone	9.0 mm	9.0 mm	Total ablation larger than scotopic pupil
Enter into B&L laser, no nomogram adjustment needed	−5.25 + 0.50 × 90°	−5.75 + 0.75 × 85°	Target + 0.50 D postoperatively
Ablation depth	95 µm	103 µm	
Residual stromal thickness	535 µm − 160 µm − 95 µm = 280 µm >250 µm	540 µm − 160 µm − 103 µm = 277 µm >250 µm	

Take-Home Points

1. Use a 9.5-mm ring for flat corneas in order to prevent free flaps.
2. Select the appropriate optical zone size in order to provide adequate coverage of the scotopic pupil.
3. Always measure intraoperative pachymetry.

CASE 7

A 38-year-old man is interested in refractive surgery. He occasionally wears soft contact lenses. His refraction has been stable for over a year. He has no health problems.

		Uncorrected Va
W	OD −3.75 + 1.75 x 89° 20/20+ OS −4.75 + 2.00 x 81° 20/15	CF 5′ CF 5′
M	OD −3.75 + 1.75 x 100° 20/15 OS −4.50 + 2.00 x 90° 20/15	
C	OD −3.75 + 2.00 x 100° 20/15 OS −4.50 + 2.00 x 85° 20/15−	
K	OD 39.50/41.00 x 94° OS 39.12/41.37 x 94°	

Pachymetry	Topography	Scotopic Pupils
OD 550 µm OS 550 µm	No cone OU	OD 6.0 mm OS 6.0 mm

7

Additional Examination

The patient has slightly deep-set eyes, with lax lids and a wide palpebral fissure. The remainder of the examination was normal.

Discussion

Based on the information given, this patient appears to be a good candidate for LASIK. The presence of astigmatism reduces the laser ablation depth by decreasing the spherical equivalent. In future cases the ablation depth will be determined by the calculation method.

Remember that the width of the astigmatic treatment zone in a conventional treatment with the VISX laser is 4.5 to 5.0 mm, depending on whether the overall treatment zone is 6.0 or 6.5 mm. If the pupil is large and the degree of astigmatism is large, for example, >2 D, nighttime vision issues are possible. The cornea is somewhat flat so a larger ring is necessary to make an ample size flap. The risk of an inadequately small or free cap is greater when the corneal contour is quite flat. If the cornea is very flat, for example, keratometry values <39.00 D, and the degree of correction is low, a surface ablation procedure is a consideration. In this case there is ample tissue, which allows the surgeon the flexibility to choose a 160- or 180-μm plate on the Hansatome. The size of the treatment zone is selected to be slightly larger than the diameter of the scotopic pupil. A slightly deep-set eye would not pose a serious problem particularly if the lids are lax and the palpebral fissure is wide. However, patients with deep-set eyes will be more challenging for beginning LASIK surgeons.

Surgical Plan

	Right Eye	Left Eye	Comments
Ring size	9.5 mm	9.5 mm	Flat contour
Plate size	160 or 180 μm	160 or 180 μm	Actual Hansatome flap likely thinner than the plate
Ablation zone	6.5 mm	6.5 mm	6.0-mm pupils
Spherical equivalent	−2.75 D	−3.50 D	Treat cycloplegic refraction
Calculations: sphere in cycloplegic refraction reduced by nomogram adjustment then enter into VISX laser	$-2.75 \times 7\% = -0.19$ $-3.75 - (-0.19)$ $= -3.56$ $-3.56 + 2.00 \times 100°$	$-3.50 \times 7\% = 0.25$ $-4.50 + 0.25 = -4.25$ $-4.25 + 2.00 \times 90°$ (Use axis from manifest refraction or choose an axis in the middle)	Make sure to reduce the sphere from the cycloplegic refraction by the nomogram adjustment (see discussion on VISX laser in Chapter 2)
Ablation depth Use non−nomogram- adjusted cycloplegic refraction	Using Table 2.14, page 60 = 34 μm Calculation method: 2.75 D × 15 μm/D = 41 μm	Using Table 2.14, page 60 = 42 μm Calculation method: 3.50 D × 15 μm/D = 53 μm	To be conservative, choose the larger of the two values for ablation depth
Residual stromal thickness (RST)	550 μm − 160 μm − 41 μm = 349 μm >250 μm	550 μm − 160 μm − 53 = 337 μm >250 μm	RST >250 μm; intraoperative measurement is recommended

7

Discussion

There are several points worth considering in this case. First, at age 51 this patient is highly likely to experience presbyopic symptoms following bilateral treatment for distance. This patient might do very well if only the dominant left eye is treated for distance. The untreated right eye might serve his intermediate and near vision reasonably well. As a rule patients in this setting are better served with sequential surgery rather than bilateral simultaneous surgery. This allows the patient an opportunity to experience monovision, leaving open the option to subsequently treat the nondominant eye. A preoperative trial of monovision using a contact lens in the dominant eye is often helpful. Second, the corneal contour is relatively flat. Remember that there is an increased risk of a small flap or free cap when the corneal contour is flat. A larger ring is needed to ensure that the flap will be large enough to accommodate a larger treatment zone. Finally, the periorbital anatomy may pose a problem. Remember to check prominence of the brow, relative height of the palpebral fissure, lid laxity, and degree of enophthalmos in determining whether exposure will be adequate. If exposure is an issue, consider going with a more sturdy speculum such as the Murdock (Asico); going without a speculum and the standard ring; using a micro-ring, which has a smaller outer diameter; using a single-piece microkeratome such as the Amadeus (AMO) or the Nidek, which creates a nasal hinge; or consider a surface ablation procedure. Adequate preoperative sedation can help achieve adequate exposure by relaxing periorbital muscles and reducing blepharospasm.

Surgical Plan

	Right Eye	**Left Eye**	**Comments**
Ring size	9.5 mm	9.5 mm	K <45.50 D
Plate size	160 μm	160 μm	
Ablation zone	6.5 mm	6.5 mm	Pupils <6.5 mm
Spherical equivalent	−1.13 D	−2.75 D	
Calculations using nomogram correction	−1.13 D × 7% = −0.08 D −1.25 D + 0.08 D = −1.17 D −1.17 + 0.25 × 175°	−2.75 D × 8% = −0.22 D −2.75 D + 0.22 D = −2.53 D −2.53	Reduce the nomogram adjustment from the sphere in the cycloplegic refraction
Ablation depth	1.13 D × 15 μm/D = 17 μm	2.75 D × 15 μm/D = 41 μm	Use non–nomogram-adjusted cycloplegic refraction to calculate ablation depth
Residual stromal thickness (RST)	OD: 573 μm − 160 μm − 17 μm = 396 μm OS: 572 μm − 160 μm − 41 μm = 371 μm RST >250 μm OU		
Special consideration	Because this patient is of presbyopic age, give strong consideration to treating only the dominant left eye. Right eye can always be treated later.		

Take-Home Points

1. Consider sequential rather than simultaneous treatment if the patient is of presbyopic age and the refractive error of the nondominant eye is suitable for near vision correction.
2. Consider the risk of inadequate flap diameter or free cap if the cornea is flat.
3. Flaps are more difficult to make if the eye is deep set. Remember the various treatment options available in this setting. Discuss the surface ablation option preoperatively.

CASE 10

A 63-year-old man is highly motivated to have refractive surgery to improve his vision. He currently does not wear glasses or contact lenses and functions well. He works full time as an architect. He enjoys fishing and hunting. He drives occasionally and without difficulty during the day but does notice some glare while driving at night.

W None	Uncorrected Va 20/25+ dist; 14 pt near 20/200 dist; 4 pt near
M OD–0.25 + 0.50 x 180° 20/20 OS –2.00 20/20	
C OD pl + 0.50 x 180° 20/20 OS –1.75 20/20–	
K OD 42.62 x 179°/42.00 x 89° OS 43.00 x 180°/43.00 x 90°	

Pachymetry	Topography	Scotopic Pupils
OD 520 μm OS 520 μm	No evidence of keratoconus	OD 5 mm OS 5 mm

Additional Examination
The patient has excellent exposure. The slit-lamp examination, fundus, and IOP are normal.

Discussion
Occasionally a presbyopic-age patient will present with naturally occurring monovision who is highly motivated to have refractive surgery. Although his motivation is high, this man currently functions well during work and leisure activities without correction. Although the patient would be willing to have refractive surgery to correct the left eye, surgery would be ill advised. Because of the loss of near vision postoperatively, this patient would perceive a significant loss of visual function even if the postoperative result were 20/15 OS. While his night driving might improve, he only drives occasionally. His work as an architect would require full-time spectacle use. He would also need reading glasses for fishing. The slight correction in the right eye is too low to treat. This presbyopic patient is not a good candidate for refractive surgery, but might benefit from glasses for night driving.

Take-Home Points
1. Avoid refractive surgery in presbyopic patients who function well without glasses or contact lenses during work and leisure activities.
2. Motivation for refractive surgery does not make a patient a candidate for refractive surgery.
3. The preoperative evaluation is an opportunity to understand the patient's motivations for surgery, determine if the patient will achieve a net gain from the surgery, and educate the patient.
4. A patient properly advised against surgery can be a potential referral source, while a patient made unhappy with surgery will usually speak negatively about the surgeon and the office.

7

A 27-year-old woman presented with a history of myopic astigmatism. She states she wants to be able to drive, water-ski, and work at a computer without contact lenses. She has a history of "lazy eye" OD as a child with no history of strabismus surgery or patching. She also has a history of corneal neovascularization OU. She wears SCL, 2-week disposables, but has tolerated rigid gas-permeable lenses in the past. The patient denies diplopia while wearing contact lenses. Currently she uses no ocular medications.

W	OD −6.25 + 1.00 x 96° 20/20 OS −6.25 + 0.25 x 179° 20/30	**Uncorrected Va** OD CF OS CF
M	OD −6.00 + 1.25 x 90° 20/20+ OS −7.25 20/15−	
C	OD −5.75 + 1.00 x 85° 20/15 OS −6.75 20/15	
K	OD 44.75 x 7°/44.75 x 97° OS 44.50 x 3°/45.00 x 93°	

Pachymetry	**Topography**	**Scotopic Pupils**
OD 549 μm	OD regular astigmatism	OD 7.5 mm
OS 547 μm	OS no cone	OS 7.5 mm

Additional Examination

There appears to be good exposure. There is a 4Δ esophoria in primary position only. There is also superior and inferior pannus <2.0 mm OU and anterior stromal scarring OD without significant thinning extending <1.5 mm from the superior limbus. The refraction is stable out of contact lenses. Mild blepharitis is present in all four lids.

Discussion

This patient is an acceptable candidate for LASIK surgery. The cornea is thick enough to allow the surgeon to use a 180-μm plate; however, a 160-μm plate would leave more room for retreatment if it became necessary. The esophoria is small; however, if the patient developed a large anisometropia postoperatively, fusion may become more challenging for the patient. The large pupil will require a larger treatment zone. With the VISX laser, conventional LASIK would require a 6.5-mm zone with a blend zone extending to 8.0 mm. The myopia OS is within the acceptable range for VISX custom OS for high myopia.

The corneal pannus raises an important concern—namely, the risk of intraoperative bleeding. A flap that is large may cut into the vessels resulting in hemorrhage. (See Chapter 1, page 23, on ring placement for management of intraoperative hemorrhage.) A smaller flap would help avoid the vessels, but may not accommodate the full treatment zone. Because the keratometry indicates that the cornea is not flat, an 8.5-mm ring would probably be adequate to create the necessary flap size reducing the risk of bleeding. Ring decentration to avoid isolated vessels risks a significant flap decentration. The femtosecond laser is advantageous in a case like this, because the flap diameter is more predictable. Also the laser process is less likely to induce problematic bleeding into the interface.

The scarring noted in this patient would likely be in the hinge of a superior-hinged flap and not cause a problem. Whenever scarring is present, even if it is peripheral, the surgeon should attempt to rule out previous herpes simplex disease or other source of chronic keratitis. The blepharitis in this case should be treated and controlled preoperatively and the lids reexamined prior to surgery.

Surgical Plan

	Right Eye	Left Eye	Comments
Ring size	8.5 mm	8.5 mm	Smaller ring to avoid bleeding
Plate size	160 μm	160 μm	More room for retreatment
Ablation zone (VISX laser)	6.5 mm with blend or custom	6.5 mm with blend or custom	Pupils >6.5 mm
Spherical equivalent	−5.25	−6.75	
Calculations with nomogram correction (enter into VISX)	−5.25 × 6% = −0.32 −5.75 + 0.32 = −5.43 −5.43 + 1.00 × 85	−6.75 × 7% = −0.47 −6.75 + 0.47 = −6.28 −6.28	Reduce the sphere of the non–nomogram-adjusted cycloplegic refraction
Ablation depth	5.25 D × 15 μm/D = 79 μm + 8 μm for blend zone = 87 μm	6.75 D × 15 μm/D = 101 μm + 8 μm for blend zone = 109 μm	Remember to add 8 μm additional for blend zone in patient with <10 D; depth with custom may be more
Residual stromal thickness (RST)	549 μm − 160 μm − 87 μm = 302 μm	547 μm − 160 μm − 109 μm = 278 μm	RST >250 μm OU

Take-Home Points

1. Perform a motility examination routinely. Abnormalities should be explained to the patient. Patients who are asymptomatic in contact lenses should do well unless significant anisometropia or distortion has developed that interferes with fusion. Any potential risks should be explained and documented in the chart.
2. When pannus or neovascularization is present, consider flap diameter and its implications. Balance the need to protect the peripheral cornea with the need to accommodate a large treatment zone. IntraLase, if available, can be helpful.
3. Treat blepharitis preoperatively and examine patient before surgery to be certain that the condition is controlled.

CASE 12

A 23-year-old woman presented for LASIK consultation complaining that her contact lenses had become increasingly uncomfortable and as a result her wear times had been declining. She is an accomplished skier and diver and is unable to wear glasses during these activities. She is in good health. She recently saw her eye doctor and was told her eyes were healthy.

W	OD −6.50 + 2.25 x 115° OS −5.50 + 2.00 x 85°	**Uncorrected Va** CF 5' CF 5'
M	OD −6.25 + 2.00 x 115° 20/20 OS −5.75 + 2.50 x 80° 20/20	
WR	OD −6.75 + 2.30 x 120° OS −5.71 + 2.45 x 84°	
C	OD −6.50 + 2.25 x 120° 20/20 OS −5.75 + 2.50 x 85° 20/20	
K	OD 43.00 x 35°/45.75 x 125° OS 42.75 x 175°/45.50 x 85°	

Pachymetry	**Topography**	**Scotopic Pupils**
OD 546 μm OS 548 μm	Regular astigmatism OU	OD 8.7 mm OS 8.8 mm

Additional Examination

The external examination was normal, revealing excellent exposure. The tear function was normal. The slit-lamp examination was unremarkable. The IOP was 12 mm Hg OU and the fundus was normal OU. WaveScan measurement showed 9.2% HOA and RMS 7.64 OD; and 3.4% HOA and RMS 5.29 OS.

Discussion

Review of old records revealed refractive stability for at least 2 years. She had a relatively high RMS (see discussion of custom VISX in Chapter 2) and had pupils that put her into a high-risk category for night vision complaints when combined with her refractive error. After consultation regarding the options, the patient elected to undergo CustomVue LASIK with IntraLase.

The manifest and WaveScan refractions were well matched so no physician adjustment was used. The high RMS value does not influence the treatment plan in this patient. Clinically, any adjustments are based on comparisons of manifest, cycloplegic, and WaveScan refractions.

The flaps and ablations were well centered, and surgery was uncomplicated. The surgeon needs to remember that the clinical situation may vary depending on the method of flap creation. In this case, the IntraLase femtosecond laser was used to create the flap. Often when using the IntraLase a period of waiting is required until the intrastromal gas dissipates enough to allow the tracker to recognize the pupil. If a significant amount of opaque bubble layer is obscuring the view of the pupil, then it is best not to lift the flap immediately, but to instead wait until the gas dissipates. At the 3-month postoperative visit the patient had a UCVA of 20/15 with a plano refraction OU. That patient had no complaints of nighttime glare or haloes.

Surgical Plan

With planned ablation depths of 101 and 83 μm, IntraLase flaps of 120 μm and 9.0 mm in diameter were selected. The CustomVue treatment was set for a 7.0-mm × 6.0-mm optical zone and 9.0-mm ablation zone OU. The 9.0-mm ablation zone was selected to cover the relatively large mesopic pupils.

Take-Home Points

1. The CustomVue platform allows for adjustment of the treatment zone for patients with large pupils.

2. The CustomVue treatment reduces the risk of night vision problems for patients at risk for such problems or in patients who would be bothered by these symptoms.

CASE 13

A 32-year-old woman presents for LASIK consultation with the hopes of being less dependent on her glasses. She does not wear contact lenses.

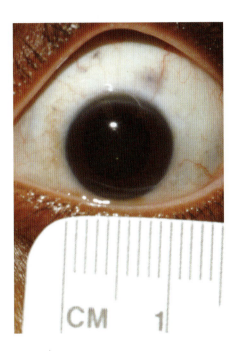

		Uncorrected Va
W	OD –4.50 20/20–	CF 5′
	OS –4.50 20/20–	CF 5′
M	OD –4.75 + 0.75 x 87° 20/15	
	OS –4.50 + 0.50 x 85° 20/15–	
C	OD –4.50 + 0.75 x 85° 20/15–	
	OS –4.25 + 0.50 x 85° 20/15	
K	OD 46.75 x 177°/47.25 x 87°	
	OS 46.50 x 180°/47.00 x 90°	

Pachymetry	Topography	Scotopic Pupils
OD 504 μm	Regular with-the-	OD 7.5 mm
OS 507 μm	rule astigmatism OU	OS 7.5 mm

Case 13, Figure 1

Small corneal diameter. (Courtesy Robert S. Feder, M.D.)

Additional Examination

The external examination reveals excellent exposure with a corneal diameter of 10 mm (Case 13, Fig. 1). The slit-lamp examination shows a clear cornea and the anterior chamber is deep and quiet. The lens appears normal and there is no cataract. The intraocular pressure and fundus examinations are normal.

Discussion

The important findings in this case are the small cornea with relatively steep curvature. The corneas are rather thin and the pupil is large. The key decision is the recognition that use of a mechanical microkeratome might be problematic. The flap must be large enough to accommodate a large treatment zone yet not so large that it extends into the limbus. One could consider using a small ring diameter for the microkeratome to keep the flap from being too large. However, with only slight flap decentration, there is a significant risk of limbal invasion and hemorrhage, because the cornea is small and steep. Other options are probably safer. The most conservative refractive procedure would be PRK in which there is no flap-related risk. A large zone with an added blend could be used and excellent centration should not be difficult to achieve. The patient would need to understand the advantages and disadvantages of sequential and simultaneous surgery.

Another option to consider would be to use the femtosecond laser to make the flap. Remember that the flap diameter with this laser is not dependent on corneal curvature and the diameter can be preset. In addition, with this patient's thin cornea the laser would provide more control over the actual flap thickness. Centration is a concern, however. If the applanation lens was not well centered and the cursor was used to center the ablation, the resultant flap might be too small to accommodate the entire ablation. If the flap edge were too close to the limbus, limbal bleeding might occur or air bubbles might extend into the anterior chamber. Despite these possible risks, the femtosecond laser if available would be a much better choice than a microkeratome for flap creation.

Surgical Plan

	Right Eye	Left Eye	Comments
The patient opts for PRK OU			
Ablation zone	6.5 mm with blend	6.5 mm with blend	VISX STAR S4 laser
No nomogram correction for PRK (enter into VISX)	$-4.50 + 0.75 \times 85°$	$-4.25 + 0.50 \times 85°$	
Ablation depth	$4.13 \, D \times 15 \, \mu m/D$ $= 62 \, \mu m + 8 \, \mu m = 70 \, \mu m$	$60 \, \mu m + 8 \, \mu m$ $= 68 \, \mu m$	Discuss the risk of haze and the need for topical steroids postoperatively
Residual stromal thickness	$504 \, \mu m - 70 \, \mu m$ $= 434 \, \mu m$ $434 \, \mu m$	$507 \, \mu m - 68 \, \mu m$ $= 439 \, \mu m$ $439 \, \mu m$	

Take-Home Points

1. Recognize the special challenge posed by the patient with microcornea.
2. PRK remains an important keratorefractive option in selected cases.
3. The femtosecond laser is safer than the microkeratome in the patient with a small, steep cornea because it offers more control over the flap diameter.

CASE 14

A healthy 31-year-old woman with no significant past medical history had previously worn soft contact lenses for 2 years. She has not worn lenses for 1 month and presents for LASIK consultation.

		Uncorrected Va
W	OD −5.50 + 1.00 x 93° 20/15−	20/400
	OS −4.50 + 0.50 x 75° 20/15	20/400
M	OD −5.00 + 1.00 x 90° 20/15	
	OS −4.50 + 0.50 x 75° 20/15	
C	OD −5.00 + 1.00 x 90° 20/15	
	OS −4.25 + 0.75 x 65° 20/15	
K	OD 42.00 x 180°/45.50 x 90°	
	OS 42.25 x 180°/45.50 x 90°	

Pachymetry	Topography	Scotopic Pupils
OD 528 μm	OD +3.5 D	OD 7.5 mm
OS 537 μm	at 94° regular	OS 7.0 mm
	OS +3.0 D	
	at 89° regular	

7

Additional Examination

There is excellent exposure and the examination is normal except for mild blepharitis and moderate acne rosacea.

Discussion

There are several items of note on the examination. First is the pupil diameter. While some believe pupil size and night vision are not related, many surgeons believe that the treatment diameter should be larger than the pupil size measured in the dark. In this case the VISX laser would treat out to 8.0 mm if a blend zone were used. With CustomVue LASIK the treatment zone could be expanded further if desired. Second, notice that there is substantially more with-the-rule astigmatism on topography and with keratometry than is seen in the cycloplegic refraction. How is this possible? More than likely there is lenticular astigmatism that cancels out some of the corneal astigmatism. If this patient requires cataract surgery in the future, untreated corneal astigmatism may be unmasked. Never treat the astigmatism from keratometry or topography. Some surgeons will choose to use the axis of astigmatism in the manifest refraction, while some will choose an axis midway between the cycloplegic and manifest refractions. Finally, the acne rosacea should be treated with a course of doxycycline provided the patient is not allergic. She should be warned about sun sensitivity, yeast vaginitis, reduction in the effectiveness of oral contraceptives, and risk to the baby if she becomes pregnant. Also it is important to treat significant blepharitis prior to laser surgery.

Surgical Plan

	Right Eye	Left Eye	Comments
Ring size	9.5 mm	9.5 mm	
Plate size	160 μm	160 μm	Actual Hansatome flap often thinner than the plate
Ablation zone	6.5 mm with blend or custom	6.5 mm with blend or custom	Pupils >6.5 mm
Spherical equivalent (SE)	−4.50 D	−3.87 D	
Calculations with nomogram correction (enter into VISX)	−4.50 D × 6% = 0.27 D −5.00 + 0.27 = −4.73 −4.73 + 1.00 × 090	−3.87 D × 6% = 0.23 D −4.25 + 0.23 = −4.02 −4.02 + 0.75 × 065	Reduce sphere of cycloplegic refraction by the calculated nomogram adjustment
Ablation depth	4.50 D × 15 μm/D = 68 μm + 8 μm blend = 76 μm	3.87 D × 15 μm/D = 58 μm + 8 μm blend = 66 μm	Calculate ablation depth using the non–nomogram-adjusted SE
Residual stromal thickness (RST)	528 μm − 160 μm − 76 μm = 292 μm >250 μm	537 μm − 160 μm − 66 μm = 311 μm >250 μm	Intraoperative pachymetry is the most accurate way to determine RST

Take-Home Points

1. A large treatment zone is preferable when the pupil diameter is large.
2. It is worthwhile to note disparities between refractive astigmatism and corneal astigmatism measured with topography and keratometry, but base the treatment on the refractive astigmatism.
3. Treat blepharitis and rosacea prior to surgery.

A 33-year-old mother of three requests laser vision correction to reduce her dependence on her spectacles. She wants to function without glasses, see her children in the swimming pool, and wear makeup without spectacles. She was not successfully fit in either soft contact lenses or rigid gas-permeable contact lenses in the past. She has been told that she has a lot of astigmatism and large pupils. She currently uses no systemic or ocular medications.

		Uncorrected Va
W	OD –6.50 + 2.50 x 135° 20/20 OS –7.00 + 3.25 x 45° 20/20	OD CF OS CF
M	OD –6.25 + 2.25 x 135° 20/20 OS –7.50 + 3.00 x 45° 20/20	
C	OD –6.25 + 2.50 x 135° 20/15 OS –7.25 + 3.25 x 45° 20/15	
K	OD 44.50 x 45°/46.50 x 135° OS 43.50 x 135°/46.50 x 45°	

Pachymetry	Topography	Scotopic Pupils
OD 557 μm OS 568 μm	Regular astigmatism OU	OD 7.5 mm OS 7.5 mm

Additional Examination

The patient has an adequate tear film and normal corneas without neovascularization. She appears to understand that in the future she will need glasses for near activities.

Discussion

This patient is a good candidate for LASIK but her case presents two significant points of discussion. The first is the large amount of oblique astigmatism and the second is her large pupil size in the dark. Her scotopic pupil measures 7.5 mm. To decrease her risk of glare and haloes, the ideal treatment would be 6.5-mm optical zones with an 8.5-mm transition zone, according to the nomogram in Table 2.18, page 76. To determine what the ideal treatment for this patient is, the refraction is converted to negative cylinder for the right eye. The suggested treatment plan would be as follows: The refraction is in negative cylinder: $-3.75 - 2.50 \times 135°$. According to the Nidek LASIK look-up table (see Nidek laser discussion in Chapter 2), this equates to -1.334 sphere -2.806 cylinder. The cylinder is treated as directed by the look-up table due to the fact that there is more than 1.25 D of cylinder in the negative refraction. The spherical component is decreased by 22% according to the nomogram in Table 2.18, page 76, since the transition zone is being expanded to 8.5 mm and a 6.5-mm optical zone is selected. Consequently, the following parameters are entered into the laser for the right eye: spherical treatment: 1.04 D, cylinder treatment: -2.806 D axis 135°, optical zone 6.5 mm, transitional zone 8.5 mm. Following this same protocol for the treatment of the left eye, the refraction is converted to negative cylinder: $-4.00 - 3.25 \times 45°$. The optical zone is set for 6.5 mm, the transitional zone is 8.5 mm, a 22% reduction of sphere found in the Nidek LASIK look-up table is utilized, and the full cylindrical treatment recommended in the Nidek LASIK look-up table is followed. Therefore, the spherical treatment is -0.707 D, cylinder treatment: $-3.753 \times 45°$. This overcorrection of the cylinder is paramount to ideal outcomes.

7

The second area of concern is her high degree of astigmatism. Frequently, astigmatism this high is not well treated by the Nidek excimer laser and may present the need for an enhancement. This requires adequate discussion with the patient preoperatively. In addition, on the day of surgery it is critical that the eye be marked with the patient in the upright position at the slit lamp prior to surgery. These astigmatism markings are then aligned with the curvilinear and horizontal illumination sources on the laser microscope such that the two arcs and the horizontal line intersect in the middle of the pupil and the horizontal line is in alignment with the previously placed limbal marks.

Surgical Plan

	Right Eye	Left Eye	Comments
Cycloplegic refraction in negative cylinder	$-3.75 - 2.50 \times 135°$	$-4.00 - 3.25 \times 45°$	
Ring size	9.5 mm	9.5 mm	
Plate size	160 μm	160 μm	Nidek microkeratome
Optical zone	6.5 mm	6.5 mm	Nidek laser
Transitional zone	8.5 mm	8.5 mm	
Calculations with nomogram	Decrease sphere by 22% treat full cylinder on look-up table $-1.334 - 2.806 \times 135°$	Decrease sphere by 22% treat full cylinder on look-up table $-0.906 - 3.753 \times 45°$	
Spherical treatment	-1.040 D	-0.707 D	
Cylinder treatment	$-2.806 \times 135°$	$-3.753 \times 45°$	Treat full cylinder after marking the cornea and aligning the laser and the patient's head
Approximate ablation depth	75 μm	85 μm	
Residual stromal thickness (RST)	557 μm $-$ 160 μm $-$ 75 mm $=$ 322 μm >250 μm	568 μm $-$ 160 μm $-$ 85 μm $=$ 323 μm >250 μm	

Take-Home Points

1. Expansion of the optical and transition zone requires use of a customized nomogram, an example of which can be found in Table 2.18, page 76.
2. High degrees of astigmatic correction with the Nidek laser are associated with an increased risk of night vision complications. This risk can be reduced by following the full cylindrical correction, recommended in the Nidek LASIK look-up table intended for cylindrical correction >1.25 D. If the cylinder is <1.25 D, treat the full cylinder.

CASE 16

A 43-year-old woman, with an 8-year history of biopsy-proven sarcoidosis, presents with interest in refractive surgery. She was treated for iritis 3 years ago, but there have been no recent episodes of ocular inflammation since that time. She wore soft contact lenses steadily until 2 years ago, when the lenses became increasingly irritating. She now uses them only for sports and social occasions. Last month the patient contracted the flu that was going around her office, but now feels fully recovered. She occasionally uses an oral decongestant for sinus congestion.

		Uncorrected Va
W	OD−5.75 20/30− OS −5.50 + 1.25 x 86° 20/20−	OD CF 5' OS CF 5'
M	OD−5.50 + 0.50 x 65° 20/20+ OS −5.25 + 1.00 x 92° 20/15−	
C	OD−5.25 + 0.75 x 75° 20/20+ OS −5.25 + 1.25 x 92° 20/15−	
K	OD 43.12x 175°/44.00 x 85° OS 42.62 x 180°/43.75 x 90°	

Pachymetry	Topography	Scotopic Pupils
OD 550 μm OS 550 μm	No cone OU	OD 6.5 mm OS 7.0 mm

Additional Examination

There is excellent exposure with a wide palpebral fissure, prominent globes, and lax lids. There is punctate fluorescein staining inferiorly in each eye. The anterior segment, IOP, and fundus examinations are normal.

Discussion

The refractive surgery evaluation should always include the patient's past medical and ophthalmologic history. Both may impact the decision to perform LASIK. In this case the patient has sarcoidosis. There have been no recent episodes of iritis and the fundus examination is normal, however the patient has become contact lens intolerant. Patients often do not offer a history of dry eye even when specifically asked. The clinician must discern whether tear deficiency is present and whether it might affect the surgical outcome. Several of the factors in this case should signal a potential problem with tear function postoperatively. First, sarcoidosis can cause reduction in lacrimal gland tear production. This may have been a factor causing her contact lens intolerance. Second, tear deficiency is more common in middle-aged and older women. Third, she is using oral decongestants, which can dry the mucous membranes. The history of the flu might suggest the consultation is taking place during the winter when the ambient humidity is decreased. Next, the wide fissure and prominent globes will undoubtedly increase the likelihood of evaporation from the ocular surface. Finally, the patient works as a copy editor, requiring her to read all day, further drying the eyes due to exposure.

In short, this patient has many risk factors for dry eye and potential for problems postoperatively. Add to these factors the neurotrophic corneal changes that can result from severing the corneal nerves during flap creation, and the potential for protracted surface irregularity becomes clear. Further evaluation is important in this case. The risk of a postoperative surface abnormality must be explained to the patient. It is prudent to document this in the chart.

The Schirmer test is part of the dry eye evaluation, but it is not the only determinant that should be used. The presence of symptoms particularly at the end of the day, injection of the bulbar conjunctiva within the palpebral fissure, mucous discharge, debris in the tear film, a decreased tear meniscus, and punctate fluorescein staining on the cornea and the conjunctiva are all important factors. Clinical judgment is necessary to determine whether a tear deficiency state can be adequately controlled preoperatively. If various treatment regimens such as tear supplements, topical cyclosporine, punctal plugs, humidifiers, and adequate oral hydration successfully reverse the signs symptoms of dry eye, it may then be safe to proceed with surgery. Remember that a patient with evaporative dry eye due to exposure or poor blink may not respond to tear supplements or plugs as well as the patient with reduced tear production.

7

Given this patient's presbyopic age and profession, it is important to discuss the need for reading glasses or monovision correction. If monovision is considered, remember to try this option in contact lenses preoperatively. The nondominant eye is usually the near eye.

Surgical Plan

	Right Eye	Left Eye	Comments
Considerations	Evaluate for dry eye, consider punctal plugs or other measures, and reevaluate. Proceed only if surface is healthy.		
Ring size	9.5 mm	9.5 mm	Hansatome
Plate size	160 μm or 180 μm	160 μm or 180 μm	Actual flap thickness may be thinner or thicker
Ablation zone	6.5 mm with blend or custom	6.5 mm with blend or custom	VISX STAR S4 Pupils >6.5 mm
Spherical equivalent	−4.88 D	−4.63 D	
Calculations using nomogram adjustment (enter into VISX laser)	$4.88 \times 8\% = 0.39$ $-5.25 + 0.39 = -4.86$ $-4.86 + 0.75 \times 75°$	$4.63 \times 8\% = 0.37$ $-5.25 + 0.36 = -4.89$ $-4.89 + 1.25 \times 92°$	*Some surgeons use cylinder axis from cycloplegic (C) refraction, some use an axis midway between C and M, some use the axis of the M
Ablation depth	$4.88\ D \times 15\ μm/D$ $= 73\ μm$ $+ 8\ μm$ (for blend) $= 81\ μm$	$4.63\ D \times 15\ μm/D$ $= 70\ μm$ $+ 8\ μm$ (for blend) $= 78\ μm$	Use non–nomogram-adjusted SE to calculate ablation depth
Residual stromal thickness (RST) Intraoperative pachymetry is recommended for RST calculation	$550\ μm − 160\ μm$ $− 81\ μm = 309\ μm$ $>250\ μm$	$550\ μm − 160\ μm$ $− 78\ μm = 302\ μm$ $>250\ μm$	If Hansatome flap is thinner than 160 μm, the RST will be greater

Take-Home Points

1. Complete past medical and ocular history is an important part of the preoperative evaluation.
2. Be suspicious for a tear deficiency condition and evaluate properly. Treat the dry eye and reevaluate. Operate only if the surface condition can be normalized. Remember that even if it can, the patient may still experience dry eye symptoms for months or years after surgery.
3. Discuss this condition with the patient and document the discussion in the chart.

7

CASE 17

A 58-year-old woman presents for LASIK consultation, expressing a goal of reducing her dependence on glasses and contact lenses. She wore monovision in contact lenses with the left eye being the near eye. She cannot remember what the monovision correction in the left eye was or where she got the lens. She has not had a problem with dry eye and wears contact lenses

		Uncorrected Va
W	OD –5.25 + 2.00 x 98° 20/25 OS –5.25 + 2.25 x 67° 20/30–	OD CF OS CF
M	OD –5.50 + 2.00 x 100° 20/20– OS –5.25 + 2.00 x 75° 20/20–	
C	OD –5.25 + 2.25 x 90° 20/15– OS –5.25 + 2.25 x 70° 20/20+	
K	OD 45.62 x 175°/48.25 x 85° OS 46.00 x 170°/47.00 x 80°	

Pachymetry	Topography	Scotopic Pupils
OD 489 μm OS 495 μm	No cone OU	OD 5.0 mm OS 5.0 mm

Additional Examination

The intraocular pressure by applanation is 16 mmHg in both eyes. On fundus examination the patient was found to have prominent bilateral optic disc drusen. Visual fields are shown in Case 18, Figures 1A and B.

Discussion

Optic disc drusen may be associated with optic nerve dysfunction. When there is a question of optic nerve dysfunction, always get a baseline visual field to document a possible preoperative field defect. The preoperative fields in each eye appear in Case 18, Figures 1A and 1B. This patient did have an inferior arcuate defect in the left eye and a subtle inferonasal defect in the right. It is not known with certainty the effect IOP elevation during flap creation might have on the optic nerve. Therefore, it is prudent to discuss this with the patient and consider alternative refractive procedures including a surface ablation procedure.

This patient has thinner than average corneas. Some surgeons choose not to perform keratorefractive surgery when the central corneal thickness is less than 500 μm and some choose to avoid keratorefractive surgery when the residual stromal bed will be less than 50% of the preoperative thickness. Some surgeons will not do LASIK surgery if the residual stromal bed is less than 300 μm, while others will use a 250-μm residual stromal bed as their RST reference point. When the cornea is thin relative to the degree of treatment required, it is important to carefully explain the risk of ectasia. It is also important to explain the limitations on retreatment should this become necessary. In this case the moderate astigmatism will reduce the amount of tissue ablation required. The small pupil will allow a smaller treatment zone, which will also reduce the amount of ablation. Choosing a thinner plate will likely ensure a thinner flap, although thin flaps often occur in thin corneas. Using very thin plates in thin corneas may result in unacceptably thin flaps. The variance of flap thickness is less with the femtosecond laser, which can help the surgeon make a flap that is neither too thick nor too thin. However, the suction ring is generally applied for a longer time with the laser than with a mechanical microkeratome. Finally, when LASIK is performed on a patient with a thin cornea, measuring the stromal bed with ultrasonic pachymetry and subtracting this value from the central corneal thickness measured at the time of surgery is necessary to determine the actual flap thickness.

A surface ablation procedure is a viable option here because the cornea is thin, there is optic nerve dysfunction, which potentially could be affected by the increased IOP during LASIK, and the ablation depth is only 50 μm, which would limit the risk of haze. If LASIK was to be considered in this case, it would be wise to get a neuroophthalmology consultation to assess the potential effect of the procedure on the nerve function, discuss the added risk with the patient, and make certain this is documented in the chart. Some surgeons avoid refractive surgery on patients with significant visual field deficits.

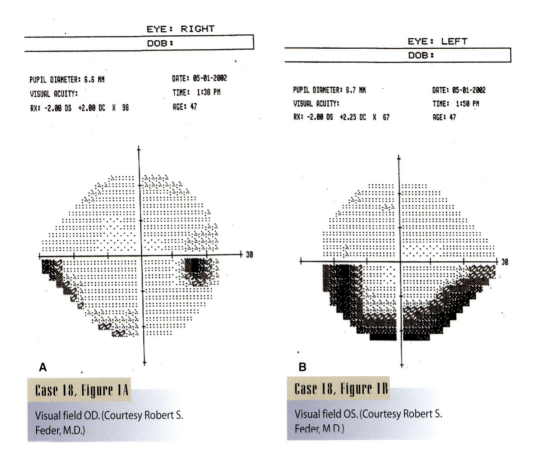

EYE: RIGHT
DOB:

PUPIL DIAMETER: 6.6 MM
VISUAL ACUITY:
RX: -2.00 DS +2.00 DC X 98

DATE: 05-01-2002
TIME: 1:38 PM
AGE: 47

EYE: LEFT
DOB:

PUPIL DIAMETER: 6.7 MM
VISUAL ACUITY:
RX: -2.00 DS +2.25 DC X 67

DATE: 05-01-2002
TIME: 1:50 PM
AGE: 47

A

B

Case 18, Figure 1A

Visual field OD. (Courtesy Robert S. Feder, M.D.)

Case 18, Figure 1B

Visual field OS. (Courtesy Robert S. Feder, M.D.)

Finally, when performing surface ablation or LASIK remember to mark the patient at the slit lamp, when astigmatism is present, in order to identify and compensate for cyclotorsion.

This patient had bilateral PRK OU and the 3-year postoperative visual acuity was 20/20 OU with no progression of visual field defects.

Surgical Plan: LASIK and PRK

	Right Eye	Left Eye	Comments
Ring size	N/A for PRK 8.5 mm for LASIK	N/A for PRK 8.5 mm for LASIK	PRK requires 7.0-mm epithelial debridement
Ablation zone	6.0 mm	6.0 mm	Pupils <6.5 mm
Spherical equivalent	−4.125	−4.125	
Calculations for LASIK with nomogram correction (enter into VISX)	$4.125 \times 8\% = 0.33$ $-5.25 - 0.33 = -4.92$ $-4.92 + 2.25 \times 90°$	$4.125 \times 8\% = 0.33$ $-5.25 - 0.33 = -4.92$ $-4.92 + 2.25 \times 70°$	Make sure to subtract corrected values from sphere of cycloplegic refraction
For PRK (enter cycloplegic refraction into VISX)	$-5.25 + 2.25 \times 90°$	$-5.25 + 2.25 \times 70°$	No need for nomogram correction if doing PRK

7

continued

	Right Eye	Left Eye	Comments
Ablation depth	4.125 D × 12 μm/D = 50 μm	4.125 D × 12 μm/D = 50 μm	No nomogram adjustment for PRK. Always use non–nomogram-adjusted cycloplegic refraction to calculate ablation depth for LASIK
Plate size for LASIK	160 μm	160 μm	If flap too thin on first eye, increase plate thickness or change blade for second eye
Residual stromal thickness (LASIK)	489 μm − 50 μm − 160 μm = 279 μm	495 μm − 50 μm − 160 μm = 285 μm	>250 μm

Take-Home Points

1. Patients with abnormal optic discs, including cupping or disc drusen, require preoperative evaluation, including baseline visual fields.
2. High IOP, which occurs during flap creation, may be undesirable in a patient with optic nerve dysfunction.
3. Thinner flaps result when creating microkeratome flaps on thin corneas.
4. PRK may be a viable option when the cornea is thin or increased IOP is undesirable.
5. In addition to the general risks of refractive surgery, always discuss those specific risks that are unique to the individual patient and document the discussion in the record.

CASE 19

A 35-year-old neurologist presents for LASIK consultation. He enjoys all water sports and is a self-proclaimed "surfer in exile." He wishes to be less dependent on glasses and contact lenses and has worn soft lenses for 15 years. He is in good health and is on no medications. His family history is noncontributory. He mentioned that 6 years previously an eye doctor noted disc asymmetry. Since that time he has received eye care from an optometrist who supplies his contact lenses.

W	OD −5.50 20/25+ OS −6.50 20/25−	**Uncorrected Va** OD CF 5′ OS CF 5′
M	OD −5.00 20/20 OS −6.00 20/20−	
C	OD −5.25 + 0.50 x 90° 20/15 OS −6.00 20/15−	
K	OD 43.25 x 180°/44.00 x 90° OS 43.12 x 30°/44.00 x 120°	

Pachymetry	**Topography**	**Scotopic Pupils**
OD 513 μm OS 512 μm	Regular astigmatism OU	OD 7.5 mm OS 7.0 mm

7

Additional Examination

The external examination was normal with lax lids and a wide palpebral fissure. There was early escape of the pupil response to light OS. Color vision on Ishihara plates was normal in each eye. The slit-lamp examination was entirely normal OU. The IOP was 15 mmHg OD and 14 mmHg OS. The disc photos are shown in Case 19, Figures 1A and B, and the visual fields in Case 19, Figures 2A and B.

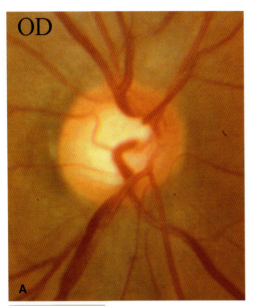
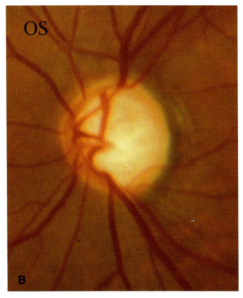

Case 19, Figure 1

Optic disc photos: (A) right disc and (B) left disc. (Courtesy Robert S. Feder, M.D.)

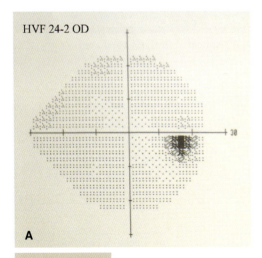
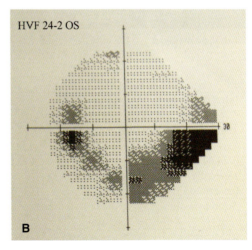

Case 19, Figure 2

Humphrey 24–2 visual field: (A) Visual field OD and (B) Visual field OS. (Courtesy Robert S. Feder, M.D.)

7

Discussion

Extensive glaucomatous cupping OS was seen on the disc photos. There is an inferior arcuate defect OS. The pupillary escape noted OS is another indication of optic nerve dysfunction OS. This patient has normal tension glaucoma. Diurnal pressures were obtained and the maximum measured pressure was 19 mmHg OS. Should refractive surgery be offered to this patient? Several important issues must be carefully considered before answering this question. If LASIK were performed, a significant elevation in IOP would be required in order to create a flap. It is possible for further nerve damage to occur during this period. While the pressure elevation associated with the femtosecond laser is somewhat less than with a microkeratome, it is not uncommon for the Intralase ring to cause a transient loss of vision during flap creation. Further, the suction ring must remain in place on the eye for a longer duration with IntraLase than with the microkeratome. If one were to reject LASIK for this reason, would there be additional risks associated with PRK? Measurement of IOP is not reliable after PRK or LASIK. The actual IOP can be significantly higher than the measured reading. Some advocate measuring the pressure from the peripheral cornea using the TonoPen.

This patient's large pupil and −6.00 D correction necessitate a large ablation zone with a blend resulting in an ablation significantly greater than 75 μm. This carries an increased risk of postoperative haze. Unless mitomycin-C was applied during surgery, the patient would require several months of topical prednisolone 1%. Glaucoma patients are more likely to experience a steroid-induced IOP rise, which might be more difficult to detect postoperatively. If haze were to develop after surgery, visual fields might be less reliable. In short this patient's glaucoma may worsen and be more difficult to follow after keratorefractive surgery. As a neurologist this patient has more insight than the average patient concerning his glaucoma and optic atrophy. Nevertheless, after the risks had been explained he preferred to have LASIK OD and continue to wear his contact lens OS. He understood that he would no longer have binocular vision in spectacles following surgery. He also understood that if glaucoma developed OD, IOP measurement would be less reliable after LASIK.

Surgical Plan

	Right Eye	Left Eye	Comments
IntraLase diameter	9.5 mm	No treatment	IntraLase preferred to create a reliably thinner flap with less IOP elevation
IntraLase depth	110 μm	None	Usually creates a 120-μm flap
Ablation zone	6.5 mm + blend zone	None	VISX STAR S4
Calculations with nomogram correction (enter into VISX)	-5.00 D × 6% = -0.30 D $-5.25 + 0.30$ D= -4.95 D $-4.95 + 0.50$ × 90°		
Ablation depth	-5.00 D ×15 μm/D = 75 μm		
Residual stromal thickness	75 μm + 8 μm = 83 μm 513 μm − 120 μm − 83 μm = 310 μm >250 μm		Intraoperative pachymetry is recommended to determine RST

Take-Home Points

1. A complete eye examination is an important part of the LASIK evaluation.
2. Keratorefractive surgery may make glaucoma more difficult to manage because IOP measurement is unreliable and PRK haze may make fields unreliable; also, steroid-induced IOP elevation may be difficult to detect.
3. It is possible for IOP rise during flap creation to cause further damage to a nerve with extensive glaucomatous damage.

CASE 20

A 32-year-old man presents for LASIK evaluation. His past medical history is negative, but the past ocular history is significant for a 10-year history of disposable soft contact lens wear. His refraction has been stable for at least the past year. There is no history of prior ocular trauma, infection, or prior surgery. He takes no systemic or ocular medications, and has no known drug allergies.

W	OD −4.50 + 0.50 x 90° 20/25+ OS −4.75 + 0.75 x 90° 20/30	**Uncorrected Va** OD 20/400 OS 20/400
M	OD −4.75 + 0.50 x 90° 20/20 OS −5.25 + 0.75 x 85° 20/20	
C	OD −4.75 + 0.50 x 90° 20/20 OS 5.25 + 0.75 x 90° 20/20	
K	OD 43.5 x 90°/43.0 x 180° OS 43.5 x 90°/42.5 x 180°	

Pachymetry	Topography	Scotopic Pupils
OD 475 μm	Regular	OD 6.5 mm
OS 480 μm	astigmatism OU	OS 6.0 mm

Additional Examination

The patient does not have deep-set eyes. The palpebral fissure is wide OU. The slit-lamp examination reveals normal corneal structure without evidence of guttata or keratoconus. The lenses are clear, and the intraocular pressure is 13 mmHg OU by applanation tonometry. Dilated funduscopic examination is unremarkable. Orbscan evaluation reveals posterior elevations of 28 μm in the right eye and 33 μm in the left eye.

Discussion

With the exception of a thin cornea, this patient has no other contraindications to laser refractive surgery. There are those who believe that a cornea with central thickness of less than 500 μm is inherently abnormal. Even with an estimated residual stromal thickness of 270 μm, such as in this case, a better solution may be surface ablation. If the refractive error were significantly higher, a phakic intraocular lens could be considered.

Surface ablation may have a higher risk of corneal haze in those patients who have an ablation depth of 75 μm or greater. The prophylactic use of mitomycin-C (MMC) 0.02%, using the proscribed protocol (refer to Chapter 3), may help prevent such an outcome. In this patient, after careful discussion and informed consent regarding the use of MMC, surface ablation with MMC was performed.

When using MMC in the context of refractive surgery, several considerations are important. First and foremost is the accurate compounding of MMC. Since there is a fairly narrow therapeutic window, it is imperative that the correct concentration be used. In most series to date, 0.02% (0.2 mg/mL) of MMC is used.

When planning the entered refraction into the laser, it is important to reduce the spherical correction by approximately 10% in order to compensate for the effect of MMC in corneal wound healing, which may result in postoperative hyperopia. (See Chapter 3 for discussion on nomogram adjustment by age and refractive error.) A postulated mechanism for this is that MMC may prevent the compensatory wound healing that typically reverses the initial hyperopic "overshoot" after myopic surface ablation.

Another important concept is the meticulous adherence to the established protocol for the use of MMC. By doing so, the possible complication rate is dramatically reduced. This involves limiting the exposure of MMC to the central cornea, and away from the limbus, stem cells, sclera, and fornices. This is best accomplished by the use of a corneal light shield, a 6- to 8-mm disk-shaped Merocel sponge. Careful irrigation of any excess MMC from the surface of the eye with 30 mL of balanced salt solution will also help reduce the likelihood of complications.

A bandage contact lens is placed on the eye, and topical antibiotics and steroids are used qid for 1 week. Steroids are then tapered over the subsequent 3 weeks. With this technique, reepithelialization is not delayed, and is usually completed within 3 to 5 days, similar to cases of surface ablation in which MMC is not used.

Take-Home Points

1. Avoid LASIK on very thin corneas. Surface ablation may be a better long-term solution.
2. Consider MMC prophylaxis in higher myopic surface ablations, when the estimated ablation depth is 75 μm or greater.
3. Follow the MMC protocol for preparation and application very meticulously.
4. Adjust the entered refraction according to the nomogram (see Chapter 3) to take into account the effect of MMC on wound healing.

CASE 21

A 40-year-old woman with congenital nystagmus and mild amblyopia OU presented for LASIK consultation in the hopes that the surgery would improve her visual acuity. The patient had

W	OD −3.00 + 2.00 x 89° 20/40 OS −3.25 + 1.75 x 100° 20/40	**Uncorrected Va** 20/100 20/200
M	OD −3.25 + 2.25 x 91° 20/40 + 2 OS −3.00 + 2.00 x 95° 20/30 − 1	
WR	OD −2.22 + 2.19 x 91° OS −1.98 + 1.93 x 96°	
C	OD −2.75 + 2.25 x 90° 20/30− OS −2.50 + 2.00 x 95° 20/30−	
K	OD 42.00 x 180°/44.25 x 90° OS 41.75 x 188°/44.00 x 98°	

Pachymetry	Topography	Scotopic Pupils
OD 550 μm	No cone OU	OD 5.9 mm
OS 557 μm		OS 6.3 mm

become intolerant to the soft daily wear contact lenses she had used for the previous 15 years. Her past ocular history was otherwise noncontributory and her general health was excellent. The risks of LASIK surgery were explained in detail. It was explained that surgery was unlikely to improve her visual acuity beyond what she could do in glasses or contact lenses.

Additional Examination

Exposure is excellent. There is no detectable tropia. The slit-lamp examination, IOP, and dilated fundus examination was normal. WaveScan measurement showed HOA 8.8% and RMS 2.88 OD; and HOA 8.8% and RMS 2.89 OS.

Discussion

This case brings up two important issues for discussion. First is amblyopia or reduced best-corrected acuity. The nature of the reduced acuity must be elucidated. LASIK is a surgical procedure designed for a healthy eye. Any corneal abnormality causing reduced acuity would likely lead to an unpredictable result after LASIK surgery and would, therefore, be a contraindication. Decreased acuity due to a potentially progressive cataract would be another contraindication. However, mild amblyopia in an otherwise healthy eye is not a contraindication provided the patient has reasonable expectations. The limitations on postoperative acuity need to be carefully explained and understood before surgery. In most cases the reduced amblyopic target acuity is easier to achieve with LASIK. If, however, a significant tropia is associated with amblyopia, caution is advised. Improving the unaided acuity may affect suppression and result in diplopia.

The second issue is nystagmus. It is potentially difficult to obtain a WaveScan in a patient with a moving eye. Large-amplitude nystagmus might be difficult for the laser to track and it also may be difficult to center a microkeratome, because the eye is moving as suction is being applied. Finally, registration could be an issue. It is difficult to mark such a patient at the slit lamp, for alignment with the laser. Accurate registration is an important step in any custom LASIK surgery or in conventional surgery to correct significant astigmatism.

In this case the patient was marked, the WaveScan refraction was double-checked, and the tracker was tested with the patient before any treatment commenced. The flaps and ablations were well centered and the surgery proceeded without complication.

Surgical Plan

	Right Eye	Left Eye	Comments
Ring diameter	9.5 mm	9.5 mm	Hansatome
Plate thickness	160 μm	160 μm	Usually creates a 120-μm flap
Ablation zone	6.0 mm with transition to 8.0 mm	6.0 mm with transition to 8.0 mm	VISX STAR S4 CustomVue
No nomogram adjustment needed (enter into VISX)	$-2.22 + 2.19 \times 91°$ sphere increased -0.50 D $-2.72 + 2.19 \times 91°$	$-1.98 + 1.93 \times 96°$ sphere increased -0.50 D $-2.48 + 1.93 \times 96°$	Spherical portion can be adjusted ±0.75 D. Cylinder power and axis are fixed.
Ablation depth Residual stromal thickness (RST)	Low ablation depth with ample corneal thickness. RST adequate OU	Low ablation depth with ample corneal thickness. RST adequate OU	Ablation depth is calculated by WaveScan unit

At 2 months postoperatively, the patient had uncorrected acuity of 20/50 OD and 20/30 − 2 OS. The manifest refraction was OD $-0.50 + 0.25 \times 90$ and OS $+0.50 + 0.25 \times 105$ with best-corrected visual acuity (BCVA) of 20/30 − 2 and 20/25 − 2, respectively. Although the patient still has some residual refractive error, the BCVA showed a one-line improvement over the preoperative best-corrected visual acuity.

Take-Home Points

1. Mild amblyopia, in and of itself, is not a contraindication to LASIK surgery, provided the patient has reasonable expectations.
2. Nystagmus can pose a problem for marking and registration, WaveScan acquisition, microkeratome centration, and laser tracking.
3. The patient should be evaluated before surgery to determine if the laser can track the eyes. A robust tracker can increase the safety of LASIK in the nystagmus patient.

CASE 22

This 34-year-old man with myopic astigmatism desired LASIK so he could drive, play golf and tennis, and watch TV without glasses. He had no significant ocular history. He admitted to being very squeamish about his eyes, and had some difficulty focusing straight ahead during his LASIK consultation.

		Uncorrected Va
W	OD −4.75 + 1.50 x 90° 20/20 OS −5.50 + 1.75 x 90° 20/20	20/400 20/400
M	OD −5.00 + 1.50 x 90° 20/15 OS −6.00 + 2.00 x 90° 20/15	
C	OD −4.75 + 1.75 x 90° 20/20 OS −5.50 + 1.75 x 90° 20/20	
K	OD 43.50 x 180°/45.50 x 90° OS 43.75 x 178°/45.75 x 88°	

Pachymetry	Topography	Scotopic Pupils
OD 560 μm	With-the-rule	OD 6.0 mm
OS 557 μm	astigmatism OU	OS 6.0 mm

Additional Examination

There was nothing unusual about the slit-lamp exam of the anterior segment. His ability to cooperate for the eye examination was suboptimal. He was a "squeezer" who was photophobic and had difficulty maintaining fixation for the examination. There was concern about this patient's ability to cooperate for the laser ablation, especially maintaining fixation. In addition, he had a moderate amount of astigmatism so proper alignment of the laser on his cornea was critical for effective laser correction.

Discussion

This patient was an acceptable, although not ideal, candidate for LASIK surgery. He had a thick cornea and was expected to have a generous residual stromal thickness after myopic ablation. The main concern was about his ability to cooperate for the laser ablation. As usual, the 12 and 6 o' clock axes were marked at the slit lamp with a sterile marking pen, prior to bringing the patient into the LASIK suite to be prepped and draped. Despite the availability of the VISX S4 excimer laser tracking system, the Moria suction ring on a low-vacuum setting was used during laser ablation to help stabilize the globe. Proper alignment of the globe was important because of the dangers of a misaligned treatment of moderate astigmatism.

After making the cutting pass on high vacuum with the Moria CB microkeratome, the device was switched to low vacuum. The microkeratome was reversed and removed, but the suction ring remained on the eye. The low-vacuum setting enabled the suction ring to maintain a firm grasp on the globe, but at a much lower and safer level of IOP. While holding the metal suction ring handle with the left hand, the globe could be stabilized while performing the laser ablation. The ablation went smoothly, and the patient felt relieved that the potential fixation problem was overcome by using the low-vacuum technique.

Surgical Plan

	Right Eye	Left Eye	Comments
Ring size	0	0	Moria CB
Microkeratome head	130 μm	130 μm	Typically cuts 160-μm flap
Ablation zone	6.5 mm with blend zone	6.5 mm with blend zone	VISX STAR S4
Cycloplegic Rx	$-3.25 - 1.50 \times 180$	$-3.75 - 1.75 \times 180$	Minus cylinder form
Calculations using Dr. Rosenfeld's nomogram correction (VISX)	$-2.93 - 1.50 \times 180$	$-3.38 - 1.75 \times 180$	10% reduction of sphere using the cycloplegic examination in minus cylinder form
Flap thickness	160 μm	160 μm	
Ablation depth	56 μm	62 μm	
Residual stromal thickness	344 μm	335 μm	>250 μm OU

Take-Home Points

1. The low-vacuum setting on the Moria microkeratome permits exquisite control of the globe during laser ablation.
2. Proper alignment of the axis of astigmatism is critical for treating moderate to high levels of astigmatism.

7

CASE 23

A 46-year-old dental hygienist with a 30-year history of hard PMMA contact lens wear was seen for refractive consultation. She had early symptoms of presbyopia and had begun to wear near correction over her contact lenses. Her past ocular history was otherwise negative. Her past medical history was significant for medically controlled hypertension.

W	OD –6.50 + 0.50 x 72° OS –6.00 + 0.50 x 64°	**Uncorrected Va** 20/400– 20/400–
M	OD –6.75 + 0.50 x 110° 20/20 OS –6.00 + 1.00 x 70° 20/20 with + 1.25 add → 20/20 near OU	
C	OD –6.75 + 0.25 x 120° 20/20 OS –6.00 + 0.75 x 70° 20/20	
K	OD 45.50 x 90°/44.50 x 180° OS 46.50 x 77°/45.25 x 167°	

Pachymetry	**Topography**	**Scotopic Pupils**
OD 500 μm	+0.75 D x 90° OD	OD 6.5 mm
OS 495 μm	+1.00 D x 77° OS	OS 6.5 mm

Additional Examination

Her corneas, tear film, lids, and conjunctiva were normal. Her corneal maps were regular without signs of contact lens–induced warpage.

Discussion

This patient was a long-time rigid PMMA contact lens wearer. This type of patient represents a challenge in two ways. First, the surgeon must be sure that there are no signs of contact lens–induced effects on the cornea. These include contact lens warpage, which can induce irregular astigmatism, masked astigmatism, and/or myopia that is hidden by the flattening effects of the rigid contact lens. The corneal maps must look smooth and regular and the principal astigmatic axes must be 90° apart. The magnitude and direction of the topographic astigmatism should closely match the refractive astigmatism although there is usually 0.25 to 0.50 D more astigmatism seen on the maps compared to the refraction. Second, patients who are long-time rigid contact lens wearers have higher visual expectations than patients who wear soft lenses or spectacles. The rigid lenses mask any irregular astigmatism on the patient's cornea and produce an artificially regular surface. These patients should be counseled that their postoperative vision may never be as good as their vision with their rigid lenses.

This patient at age 46 is already experiencing presbyopic symptoms; therefore, careful and complete counseling about presbyopia should be undertaken. Monovision correction for this dental hygienist would be ill advised because of the effect on stereopsis.

Finally, this patient has thin corneas with a relatively high refractive error. Therefore, the corneas are too thin for LASIK. The risk of haze after surface ablation in this case is significant. This should be discussed with the patient. Consideration of adjunctive mitomycin-C treatment would be advisable. The techniques for surface ablation (PRK, Epi-LASIK, and LASEK) should be discussed.

7

Surgical Plan

	Right Eye	**Left Eye**	**Comments**
Considerations	Do not perform LASIK if the cornea is too thin. Be sure that there are no effects from the rigid contact lens		
Ring size	None in PRK	None in PRK	Cornea too thin

continued

	Right Eye	Left Eye	Comments
Plate size	None in PRK	None in PRK	Cornea too thin
Ablation zone	6.5 mm with blend	6.5 mm with blend	Pupil = 6.5 mm
Spherical equivalent	−7.50 D	−6.25 D	
Conventional surface treatment based on manifest and cycloplegic refractions Treatment is entered in minus cylinder form	−6.75 D sphere 0.50 D × 110° −6.25−0.50 × 20°	−5.75 D sphere 0.75 D × 70° −5.00 − 0.75 × 160°	There is no nomogram adjustment with PRK
Ablation depth	120 μm	98 μm	The Alcon software calculates the ablation depth
Residual stromal thickness	500 μm − 120 μm = 380 μm	495 μm − 98 μm = 397 μm	

Take-Home Points

1. Be sure the patient stays out of her rigid contact lenses until the refraction and topography become stable. The stable topography should be consistent with the refraction.
2. Warn patients in their mid-forties about the effect of myopic LASIK on presbyopia and discuss treatment options. Avoid monovision in patients who require excellent stereopsis to perform their jobs.
3. Avoid LASIK if the cornea is too thin.

CASE 24

A 46-year-old man presents for LASIK consultation. He is hoping to be less dependent on distance glasses and understands he will need to wear reading glasses. He is not interested in monovision. The patient explains he could never wear contact lenses because he is an intense "eyelid squeezer." He has a history of hypertension and hypercholesterolemia. He also has sleep apnea and wears a continuous positive airway pressure (CPAP) mask every night to assist his breathing during sleep (Case 24, Fig. 1).

W OD −8.25 + 1.00 x 72° 20/30+ OS −6.00 + 0.75 x 77° 20/30−	**Uncorrected Va** CF 3′ CF 3′

M OD −7.50 + 1.00 x 85° 20/25−   OS −5.50 + 0.75 x 85° 20/20−

C OD −7.50 + 1.00 x 90° 20/25+   OS −5.50 + 0.75 x 85° 20/20−

K OD 41.62 x 179°/43.25 x 89°   OS 42.00 x 180°/42.87 x 90°

Pachymetry	**Topography**	**Scotopic Pupils**
OD 556 μm	No evidence	OD 6 mm
OS 550 μm	of ectasia OU	OS 6 mm

7

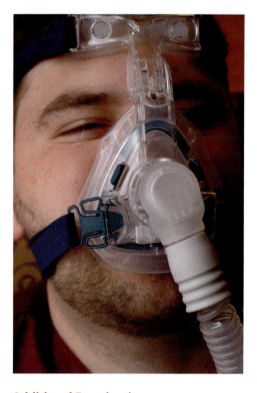

Case 24, Figure 1

Donning the CPAP mask risks bumping the eye and displacing the flap. Air flow over the flap may cause excessive dryness. (Courtesy Robert S. Feder, M.D.)

Additional Examination

Intense blepharospasm noted when attempting tonometry, but IOP is measured and is normal. A 12-Δ right exotropia is noted. The slit-lamp and fundus examinations are normal.

Discussion

Although this patient is highly motivated to have LASIK surgery, he is a poor candidate. Intense blepharospasm can be associated with an incomplete or partial flap intraoperatively. It can also be associated with a displaced flap. In addition this patient wears a CPAP mask at night (refer to Case 24, Fig. 1). The proximity of the mask edge to the eye may also increase the risk of flap displacement.

While LASIK is a poor choice, a surface ablation procedure is a viable option for this patient. The surgeon must carefully explain how surface ablation is different from LASIK. A patient expecting the rapid visual rehabilitation and minor irritation commonly experienced after LASIK surgery will be disappointed with the increased discomfort and slow return of vision after PRK. With the VISX STAR S4 laser and a 6.5-mm optical zone the estimated ablation depth would be 105 μm OD and 77 μm OS if the nonadjusted refraction is used for the calculation. Many surgeons feel that ablation depths of 75 μm or more are associated with significantly more postoperative haze and recommend using topical mitomycin-C (MMC) 0.2 mg/mL (0.02%) applied to the stromal bed with a 6.0-mm foam corneal protector to reduce the risk of haze. (Refer to Chapter 3 on MMC.) The exact amount of time the MMC is applied varies by the surgeon from 12 seconds to 2 minutes. If MMC is used, it is important to reduce the spherical portion of the treatment by 10% to 12%. It is also important to inform the patient that MMC has not been FDA approved for this purpose, MMC may permanently affect the healing ability of the cornea, and long-term studies on its use to prevent corneal haze have yet to be done.

Remember in any high myopia case to always check the keratometry readings. To estimate the expected postsurgical corneal curvature, multiply the spherical equivalent of the cycloplegic refraction by 0.7 or 0.8 (depending on how conservative the surgeon is) and subtract the product from the average of the presurgical keratometric values. If the result is less than 35.00 D there is an increased risk of poor visual function and keratorefractive surgery may not be advisable. In this case, the result of the curvature calculation is significantly greater than 35.00 D leaving room for retreatment if necessary. The small risk of postoperative diplopia related to the preexisting exotropia should be discussed. Finally, this presbyopic patient must be educated about monovision and the need for reading glasses if full correction is achieved.

Take-Home Points

1. Blepharospasm is a risk factor for partial or incomplete flap intraoperatively.
2. Wearing a nighttime CPAP mask may increase the risk of both flap displacement and dryness.
3. Surface ablations deeper than 75 μm are more likely to develop stromal haze postoperatively.
4. The use of topical MMC 0.2 mg/mL may reduce the risk of postoperative stromal haze, but requires a 10% to 12% reduction in spherical myopic power. The use of MMC requires significant patient education.
5. Do not forget to calculate the postoperative corneal curvature in any high myopia patient to be certain the new corneal contour will not be <35.00 D, possibly too flat to support good visual function.
6. Warn the patient with a tropia about the possibility of diplopia postoperatively, if the ability to suppress the wandering eye is disturbed.
7. Make sure the myopic patient of presbyopic age being treated in both eyes for distance really understands the impact this will have on unaided near vision.

CASE 25

A 32-year-old man presents for LASIK evaluation. His past medical history is negative. The past ocular history is significant for a 10-year history of disposable soft contact lens wear, but no history of prior ocular trauma, infection, or prior surgery. He takes no systemic or ocular medications, and has no known drug allergies. His refraction has been stable for more than 1 year.

		Uncorrected Va
W	OD −4.50 + 0.50 x 90° 20/25	20/400
	OS −4.75 + 0.75 x 90° 20/30	20/400
M	OD −4.75 + 0.50 x 90° 20/20	
	OS −5.25 + 0.75 x 85° 20/20	
C	OD −4.75 + 0.50 x 90° 20/20	
	OS −5.25 + 0.75 x 90° 20/20	
K	OD 43.00 x 180°/43.50 x 90°	
	OS 42.50 x 180°/43.50 x 90°	

Pachymetry	Topography	Scotopic Pupils
OD 475 μm	Regular	OD 6.5 mm
OS 480 μm	bow-tie OU	OS 6.5 mm

Additional Examination

The patient does not have deep-set eyes. The palpebral fissure is wide OU. The slit-lamp examination reveals normal corneas without evidence of guttata or keratoconus. The lenses are clear, and the intraocular pressure is 13 mmHg OU by applanation tonometry. The dilated funduscopic examination is unremarkable. Orbscan evaluation reveals posterior elevation of 47 μm in the right eye and 49 μm in the left eye. The anterior elevation, keratometry, and pachymetry maps of the Orbscan are normal. Specifically, there is no inferior steepening on the keratometry map, and although the overall pachymetry is low, there is no focal area of thinning on the pachymetry map, either centrally or inferiorly, corresponding to the area of highest posterior elevation.

Discussion

This patient is a good candidate for laser vision correction by surface ablation (PRK) except for the abnormal posterior elevation on Orbscan. The Orbscan uses a scanning slit to image the cornea, and by compiling the images, it can reconstruct the anterior and posterior curvature of the cornea. Analysis is made with reference to a "best-fit sphere" and, therefore, any curvature above or below that sphere is given a positive or negative elevation value. Some believe that the earliest corneal changes in ectasia occur in the posterior cornea; therefore, if a patient has significant posterior elevation of the cornea, it may be an early indicator of forme fruste keratoconus. Although no absolutes can be given, it is generally accepted that values above 50 μm (0.050 mm) of posterior elevation are highly suspicious, and values between 40 and 50 μm should at least prompt a discussion with the patient of the potential for ectasia.

Surface ablation techniques may be a safer alternative to LASIK in this setting. Although one cannot unequivocally state that the risk of ectasia after surface ablation is zero, the risk is probably much less than with LASIK. In the setting of high myopia or in cases of higher risk for the development of haze, the judicious use of prophylactic MMC may be beneficial. There are many good reasons to avoid any elective corneal surgery in patients with keratoconus (KC) or forme fruste keratoconus (FFKC). Even a relatively "safer" procedure such as PRK with MMC is not recommended at this time due to unknown effects of laser ablation on these corneas, and the unknown effect of MMC on keratocytes in patients with KC or FFKC. The procedure has the potential to cause acceleration of the ectatic process.

Take-Home Points

1. Analysis of the posterior corneal surface with the Orbscan may be beneficial in identifying patients with FFKC or KC.
2. Use caution in performing LASIK in patients with posterior elevation above 40 μm.
3. Avoid LASIK in patients with posterior elevation above 50 μm.

CASE 26

A 31-year-old woman with a history of soft contact lens wear for 15 years presents for LASIK consultation. The patient has a history of migraines. There is no history of other eye problems. The patient states she has not needed new glasses in past year. Medications include Imitrex and Prozac.

W	OD −5.75 20/20 OS −5.75 20/40+ (old Rx)	Uncorrected Va OD CF OS CF
M	OD −6.75 20/20 OS −6.25 + 1.50 x 35° 20/20−	
C	OD −6.25 20/15 OS −6.00 + 1.50 x 45° 20/15−	
K	OD 45.50 x 180°/45.50 x 90° OS 45.50 x 142°/46.50 x 52°	

Pachymetry	Topography	Scotopic Pupils
OD 529 μm OS 501 μm	Preoperative: Case 26 Figures 1, 2, and 3	OD 6.0 mm OS 6.0 mm

Additional Examination

After 3 weeks out of contact lenses, the cycloplegic refraction remained stable. IOP and fundus examinations were normal. Corneal topography was obtained at that time. See Case 26 Figures 1 and 2, OD and OS, respectively. Normal band view of OS is seen in Case 26, Figure 3.

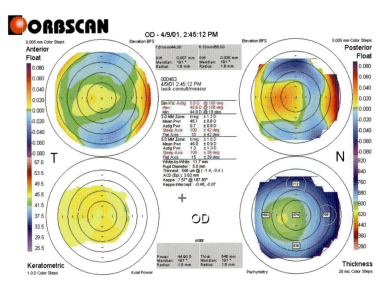

Case 26, Figure 1

Preoperative topography OD. (Courtesy Robert S. Feder, M.D.)

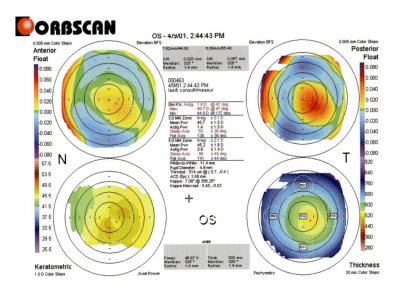

Case 26, Figure 2

Preoperative topography OS. (Courtesy Robert S. Feder, M.D.)

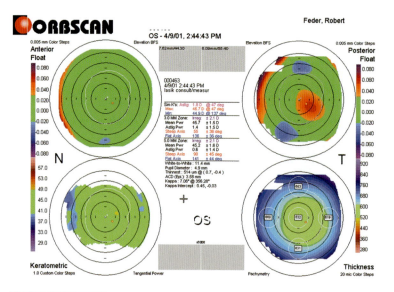

Preoperative normal band view OS. (Courtesy Robert S. Feder, M.D.)

Discussion

A critical review of the preoperative topography maps is essentially normal in the right eye (Case 26, Fig. 1); however, the power map of the left eye (Case 26, Fig. 2) in the lower left corner deserves special consideration. Notice the dumbbell appearance and particularly how the superior portion is skewed to the right. Rabinowitz refers to this finding as skewed radial axes and has suggested that a deviation greater than 21 degrees is an important index in screening patients for the diagnosis of keratoconus. Refer to the discussion on corneal topography in Chapter 2. In this patient the central corneal power value is less than the 47.2 D cutoff described by Rabinowitz, but the Sim-K astigmatism of 1.8 D is greater than the 1.5 D index.

Another way to look at this patient is to examine the Orbscan II topography using the normal band scale (Case 26, Fig. 3). This was discussed in the section on topography in Chapter 2. Remember that if orange is present in two maps, surface ablation would be a better option than LASIK, provided the risk of ectasia has been explained. Review of this map shows orange in the posterior elevation map upper right and a small orange spot in the power map on the lower left. The presence of orange in two maps is one indicator of a higher risk of ectasia with LASIK. PRK is the preferable choice provided the patient is informed of the ectasia risk.

Another useful index found on the Orbscan II unit is the posterior elevation difference with best-fit sphere. This value is found when the curser is placed on the highest part of the posterior elevation map. The value in the gray box to the left should ideally be <0.04 mm. In this case, which was treated prior to our awareness of this index, the value was >0.05 mm. Caution is also recommended when the irregularity at the 3.0-mm zone is >±2.0 D or the irregularity at the 5.0-mm zone is >±2.5 D. A more conservative approach would be to use ±1.5 D at 3.0 mm and ±2.0 D at 5.0 mm. The value in this case is ±2.1 D at both diameters. Finally, if the cornea is >20 μm thinner in the periphery than in the center, the postoperative ectasia risk may be increased. No set of indices is foolproof in preventing postoperative ectasia. It is recommended that several indices and analyses be used to determine whether a particular patient is suitable for keratorefractive surgery.

In this patient notice also that there is a significant difference in corneal thickness between the two eyes, with the eye suspicious for forme fruste keratoconus being 28 μm thinner than the fellow eye with ultrasonic pachymetry. The patient is eager to have LASIK surgery in both eyes despite the increased risk of postoperative ectasia in the left eye. The options in this case are to avoid corneal refractive surgery, consider PRK in the left eye, or proceed with LASIK. Because LASIK would involve ablation at a deeper layer of the cornea, PRK would be preferable. Conservative surgeons would avoid surgery particularly in the OS given a picture suggestive of forme fruste keratoconus. If surgery is considered, a detailed discussion of the ectasia risk and the implications for long-term postoperative visual function is essential. The consent form must be modified to indicate the discussion has taken place and the patient understands this specific and relevant risk.

Surgical Plan: LASIK OD and PRK OS

	Right Eye	Left Eye	Comments
Ring size	8.5 mm	N/A	K >45.50
Plate size	160 μm	N/A	Usually thinner flap occurs in thin corneas
Ablation zone	6.5 mm	6.5 mm	Pupils <6.0 mm
Spherical equivalent	−6.25 D	−5.25 D	
Calculations with nomogram correction (enter into VISX)	$-6.25 \times 6\% = 0.375$ $-6.25 + 0.38 = -5.87$ −5.87	−6.00 + 1.50 × 45°	Some surgeons prefer to use the axis from the manifest refraction
Ablation depth	6.25 D × 15 μm/D = 94 μm	5.25 D × 15 μm/D = 79 μm	The risk of haze may be increased, due to an ablation depth greater than 75 μm
Residual stromal thickness (RST)	529 μm − 160 μm − 94 μm = 275 μm >250 μm	501 μm − 79 μm = 422 μm	This patient may require an RST >300 or more to prevent ectasia

Postoperatively this patient achieved an uncorrected acuity of 20/20 OD and 20/30 OS. Her refraction 6 months after surgery was plano OD and −0.50 + 1.50 × 050 20/25 OS. She is aware than her acuity is better OD, but is overall quite happy with the refractive outcome. The postoperative topography map 6 months after surgery OS is shown in Case 26, Figure 4. The left eye shows further

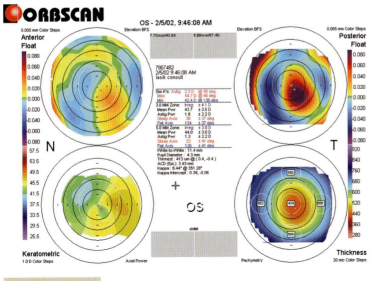

Case 26, Figure 4

Postoperative topography OS. (Courtesy Robert S. Feder, M.D.)

skewing of the radial axes with the development of superotemporal flattening. The posterior float, upper left, is much steeper OS (PRK eye) than it was OD despite the much greater RST OS. Whether there will be continued progression is not known, but further close follow-up is warranted.

Take-Home Points

1. Reduced best-corrected acuity and significantly decreased central thickness relative to the fellow eye are signs that may be present in association with forme fruste keratoconus.
2. Review preoperative topography carefully for signs of keratoconus or pellucid marginal degeneration (PMD). Different indices provided on most topography equipment can help determine the presence of subclinical keratoconus, but may not detect PMD.
3. If corneal ectasia is present, the patient should not have corneal refractive surgery. If a patient does not seem to understand the risk that may be present in any case, do not do refractive surgery.
4. In borderline cases PRK might be a better choice than LASIK to maximize the RST. If the ablation depth is greater than 75 μm, the use of topical mitomycin-C is a consideration to reduce the risk of haze. However, the long-term effects of mitomycin-C particularly in cases such as this are not known.
5. Even when PRK is performed and the RST is greater than 300 μm, progressive ectasia may occur.

CASE 27

A 35-year-old woman comes in for LASIK consultation. Her husband had successful LASIK surgery 1 year previously and she wondered if she could be a candidate.

She tried contact lenses, but could never wear them comfortably. If she had to she could see without glasses, but she would get a headache. She wears glasses full time at work and for leisure activities, both for near and distance.

		Uncorrected Va
W	OD+3.25 20/20–3 OS+3.50 20/25–	20/30 18 pt 20/80 24 pt
M	OD+3.75 20/15 OS+4.25 + 0.50 x 55° 20/20 +	
C	OD+4.50 20/15 OS+5.50 + 0.50 x 60° 20/15 slow	
K	OD 43.25 x 15°/44.00 x 105° OS 43.50 x 12°/44.00 x 102°	

Pachymetry	Topography	Scotopic Pupils
OD 544 μm	Regular with-the-rule	OD 5.0 mm
OS 537 μm	astigmatism	OS 5.0 mm

Additional Examination

The external examination shows good exposure with no evidence of dry eye. The motility examination does not reveal a tropia or phoria. The slit-lamp examination, IOP, and fundus are normal.

Discussion

The key finding in this case is the discrepancy between the spectacle correction and the cycloplegic correction. The difference is + 1.25 D OD and over +2.00 D OS. Given this degree of hyperopia, it is not a surprise that she has difficulty functioning without correction despite her prepresbyopic age. The question is on which refraction should the treatment be based? If you treat on the cycloplegic refraction, she will be quite myopic initially and this might be difficult for her to tolerate. Further, adding the required overcorrection of 25% of the spherical equivalent (see the hyperopia nomogram, Table 2.12, page 58, which is based on age and spherical equivalent) to the sphere portion of the treatment boosts the sphere to +7.19 D. This is well above the approved range for hyperopia with the VISX STAR S4. On the other hand, treating on the manifest refraction will leave her significantly undercorrected and symptomatic as she gets older. What to do? The first step with this easygoing individual is to explain the situation. Good communication, including the patient in the decision-making process, is especially helpful in situations such as this. The best approach is to gradually increase the glasses correction, allowing her sufficient time to adapt to a spectacle correction that is close to the cycloplegic refraction. This process may occur over several weeks or even months; therefore, patience on the part of the doctor and the patient will be required.

Once the patient is comfortable with the full correction, the question of how to deal with the large degree of hyperopia moves to the forefront. Treatment of the right eye is within the approved parameters for LASIK, while the left eye exceeds the upper limit. Because she cannot wear a contact lens, both eyes must be corrected. The options for the left eye include insertion of a phakic IOL (not yet approved in the United States for hyperopia) and clear lens exchange with insertion of an accommodating IOL or multifocal implant. The multifocal IOL is a less desirable option when used as a unilateral treatment. Another option is PRK. PRK for hyperopia does not require a nomogram adjustment and the treatment would, therefore, be within the approved range. It has the advantage of not being an intraocular procedure, but the disadvantage of postoperative discomfort and slower visual rehabilitation. Finally, with large hyperopic keratorefractive procedures, it is important to apply the keratometric conversion factor (0.7 or 0.8 times the spherical equivalent of the treatment) and add it to the preoperative average keratometry value to confirm that the proposed treatment will not induce corneal steepening greater than 50.00 D.

Surgical Plan

	Right Eye	Left Eye	Comments
Ring size	9.5 mm	None for PRK	
Plate size	160 μm	None for PRK	Hansatome flap usually thinner than 160 μm
Ablation zone	9.0 mm	9.0 mm	Hyperopic protocol
Calculations with nomogram correction (enter into VISX)	$+4.00 \times 25\% = 1.00$ $+4.00 + 1.00 = +5.00$ $+5.00$ D	$+5.50 + 0.50 \times 60°$	No nomogram adjustment for PRK OS
Ablation depth	$5 \text{ D} \times 8 \text{ μm/D}$ $= 40 \text{ μm}$	$5.75 \text{ D} \times 8 \text{ μm/D}$ $= 46 \text{ μm}$	
Residual stromal thickness	$544 \text{ μm} - 160 \text{ μm}$ $-40 \text{ μm} = 344 \text{ μm}$ $>250 \text{ μm}$	$537 \text{ μm} - 160 \text{ μm}$ $- 46 \text{ μm} = 331 \text{ μm}$ $>250 \text{ μm}$	Hyperopic ablation is not deepest centrally, so RST is significantly greater than 250 μm

Take-Home Points

1. If the manifest and cycloplegic refractions are significantly different, explain this to the patient and help the patient adapt to a correction similar to the cycloplegic before surgery.
2. PRK on the VISX STAR S4 does not require a nomogram adjustment and this can allow an appropriate large treatment to be done within the approved range.
3. Calculate an expected postsurgical keratometry value by using the conversion factor (0.7 or 0.8 times the spherical equivalent added to the average preoperative keratometry value). The postoperative keratometry allowing room for retreatment should ideally be >35.00 D and <50.00 D.

7

CASE 28

A 56-year-old man with a history of hyperopia presents for LASIK consultation. He states that he could not tolerate contact lens wear. He has a history of bipolar disorder and anemia. His current medications include Effexor, Buspar, Wellbutrin, and Xanax. He has fainted several times in the past when he has had a blood test.

W	OD+3.00 20/25+ Add +2.75 OU OS +2.75 + 0.50 × 90° 20/15	**Uncorrected Va** 20/100 18 pt @14" 20/100 18 pt @14"
M	OD+3.25 20/20– OS +3.50 20/15	
C	OD+3.00 20/20 OS +3.50 20/15	
K	OD 43.75 x 180°/43.75 x 90° OS 44.00 x 180°/44.25 x 90°	

Pachymetry	**Topography**	**Scotopic Pupils**
OD 551 µm OS 551 µm	Regular astigmatism	OD 4.0 mm OS 4.0 mm

Additional Examination

Exposure is excellent, the refraction is stable, and the rest of the examination is normal.

Discussion

The clinician must assess this patient's candidacy for LASIK. Is the patient's psychiatric illness stable and might he be expected to have difficulty adapting to the changes that will occur following surgery? LASIK for hyperopia is quite different than for myopia. Regression is expected and, therefore, a significant age-dependent overcorrection must be built into the treatment. It can take as long as 6 months for the refractive error to stabilize. Initial myopia requiring distance glasses with transition over time to a need for reading glasses must be carefully explained and understood. The history of anemia should be investigated and addressed if necessary. Significant anemia may be a risk factor for retinal ischemia during the application of suction. The history of vasovagal reaction should also not be overlooked. Whereas surgery with a patient in the supine position is beneficial, pretreatment with an intramuscular injection of 1 mL of atropine 0.4 mg/mL given 30 minutes prior to surgery can help block a vasovagal reaction. The hyperopic profile with the VISX laser requires a 9.0 mm ablation zone so a large flap is necessary. The maximum ablation depth of 8 µm per diopter of correction occurs at a 5-mm-diameter ring around the center of the ablation. Therefore the cornea would have to be quite thin before the ablation depth would make surgery unsafe.

Surgical Plan

	Right Eye	**Left Eye**	**Comments**
Ring size	9.5 mm	9.5 mm	Large flap required for hyperopic LASIK
Plate size	160 µm or 180 µm	160 µm or 180 µm	Hansatome
Ablation zone	Hyperopic LASIK profile	Hyperopic LASIK profile	VISX STAR S4
Cycloplegic refraction	+3.00 D	+3.50 D	Make sure full cycloplegia

continued

	Right Eye	Left Eye	Comments
Calculations using the hyperopic nomogram correction (see Table 2.12, page 58) (enter into VISX)	+3.00 × 30% = 0.90 +3.00 + 0.9 = +3.90 +3.90 D	+3.50 + 30% = 1.05 +3.50 + 1.05 = +4.55 +4.55 D	Increase the correction to compensate for the expected postoperative regression; +4.55 D is close to the maximum +5.00 D approved for VISX
Ablation depth	3.9 D × 8 μm/D = 31 μm	4.55 D × 8 μm/D = 36 μm	Deepest ablation, 8 μm/D, occurs in a 5-mm-diameter ring around the center of the ablation zone
Residual stromal thickness	551 μm − 160 μm −31 μm = 360 μm	551 μm − 160 μm −36 μm = 354 μm	Hyperopic ablation is not deepest centrally, so RST is significantly greater

Take-Home Points

1. Remember both the psychosocial as well as the anatomical criteria for LASIK surgery.
2. Pretreatment with 1 mL of atropine 0.4 mg/mL by intramuscular injection can help prevent a vasovagal reaction.
3. Overcorrection is necessary to compensate for the postoperative regression that often occurs with hyperopic LASIK.
4. Hyperopic patients need to be educated about the possible need for distance glasses after surgery and that it may take up to 6 months for the refraction to stabilize.

CASE 29

This 34-year-old woman presented for LASIK consultation. She had heard about customized treatment for correction of hyperopia and wondered if she was a candidate. She has become increasingly contact lens intolerant over the years and would like to decrease her dependence on

W	OD +3.50 sph 20/25− OS +3.75 sph 20/25−	Uncorrected Va 20/100 20/200
M	OD +4.00 + 0.55 x 60° 20/20−1 OS +4.00 + 0.75 x 127° 20/20	
WR	OD +4.17 + 0.65 x 55° OS +3.74 + 0.73 x 141°	
C	OD +4.25 + 0.50 x 60° 20/20 OS +4.00 + 0.62 x 130° 20/20	
K	OD 40.62 x 147°/41.12 x 57° OS 40.12 x 45°/40.87 x 135°	

Pachymetry	Topography	Scotopic Pupils
OD 562 μm OS 570 μm	Regular astigmatism	OD 7.5 mm OS 7.2 mm

glasses and contact lenses. She is in good health and has had no eye problems in the past. She takes birth control pills, but no other medication. Her grandmother had an attack of glaucoma in her 70s that was successfully treated with laser.

Additional Examination

The external, slit-lamp, and fundus examinations are normal. The angle is wide open and the IOP is 15 mmHg OU. WaveScan measurement showed 7.8% HOA and RMS 6.99 OD; and 6.4% HOA and RMS 7.73 OS.

Discussion

While pachymetry is a major concern in treating high myopia, it is somewhat less of a concern in high hyperopia, because the maximum ablation depth is less per diopter and the deepest ablation does not occur at the thinnest part of the cornea. For the high hyperopia treatment, corneal curvature becomes a more important concern. The resulting corneal curvature should ideally not exceed 50.00 D on keratometry. Multiplying the spherical equivalent of the correction by the conversion factor of 0.7 or 0.8 and adding it to the preoperative average keratometry value provides an estimate of this value.

In this case the cornea is flat so there is plenty of room to steepen the cornea without exceeding the limit just discussed. However, creating a flap with the microkeratome can be an issue in a patient with a flat cornea. There is increased risk of a free cap being created or a flap that is too small to accommodate the larger hyperopic ablation zone. A larger-diameter ring on the microkeratome should be used. The femtosecond laser is an excellent alternative because the flap diameter created is independent of corneal curvature.

Often patients who have a higher level of hyperopia can have a latent component. The key here, as in myopic patients, is clinical correlation with the manifest, the cycloplegic, and the WaveScan refractions. Patients who have significant deviation should not be treated with the CustomVue platform.

Surgical Plan

The manifest, cycloplegic, and WaveScan refractions were well matched so no physician adjustment was used. Surgery was planned using the Hansatome (160-μm head and 9.5-mm ring) and CustomVue with the VISX STAR 4 laser. There was no adjustment. The surgery proceeded in an uncomplicated fashion.

Follow-Up Evaluation

At 3 months postoperatively, the patient presented with some overcorrection (myopic shift) OD > OS resulting in compromised uncorrected acuity, although best-corrected acuity remained unchanged from preoperatively.

Manifest Refraction	Uncorrected Va
OD −1.25 + 0.25 × 90° 20/20	20/50
OS −0.75 + 0.50 × 75° 20/20	20/30

In general CustomVue hyperopic treatments tend to result in refractive errors near plano in the early postoperative period. The amount of overcorrection that resulted in this case occasionally occurs in high hyperopic corrections. This may be the result of the longer treatment time. Over time, the overcorrection tends to regress. If this persists at the 6-month postoperative visit and is stable, then a CustomVue enhancement can be considered in the same manner as a myopic enhancement case. In general, hyperopic CustomVue treatments tend to be closer to emmetropia earlier when compared with conventional treatments and therefore regress less.

Take-Home Points

1. Low hyperopia cases treated with CustomVue typically end up near plano postoperatively, but high hyperopic cases may be prone to overcorrection. This may be related to the longer treatment time.
2. Careful clinical correlation of manifest and wavefront refractions is extremely important in treating hyperopic patients.
3. Avoid cases when the estimated average postoperative keratometry is >50.00 D.
4. If the preoperative cornea is flat, use a large microkeratome ring or IntraLase.

CASE 30

A 49-year-old woman with a history of hyperopic astigmatism presents for consultation. She has worn toric soft contact lenses for many years and her refraction has been stable for more than 1 year. She had crossed eyes as a child and was treated with glasses only. Without glasses she currently is unable to see distance or near. She is right eye dominant.

		Uncorrected Va
W	OD+2.50 + 1.25 x 94° 20/25− OS +3.75 + 1.50 x 86° 20/30	CF distance; 18 pt near CF distance; 18 pt near
M	OD+3.00 + 1.25 x 90° 20/15 OS +4.75 + 2.00 x 85° 20/20	
C	OD+3.00 + 1.50 x 90° 20/15 OS +5.00 + 2.00 x 85° 20/20	
K	OD 46.50 x 6°/47.75 x 96° OS 45.75 x 178°/46.75 x 88°	

Pachymetry	Topography	Scotopic Pupils
OD 505 μm OS 501 μm	Regular astigmatism OU	OD 7.0 mm OS 7.0 mm

Additional Examination

The patient has a prominent brow, but lax lids and a wide palpebral fissure. The corneal diameter is 12 mm OU. The motility examination reveals an 8Δ esophoria at distance. The IOP and fundus examination are normal.

Discussion

Several useful teaching points are exemplified in this case. In the evaluation the pushed plus manifest refraction uncovered nearly all of the hyperopic correction noted in the cycloplegic refraction. The +3.75 D spherical equivalent and the +1.25 D of astigmatism in the right eye are well within the approved range for hyperopic LASIK even when 23% of the spherical equivalent is added to the sphere (per the nomogram for hyperopic LASIK, Table 2.12, page 58). This is not the case for the left eye. The nomogram percentage adjustment is 28% for a +6.00 D spherical equivalent in a 49-year-old, which would add 1.68 D to the spherical portion of the refraction. This would exceed the approved range for hyperopic correction with the VISX laser, which would require off-label use of the laser. Most surgeons would not advise off-label use of the laser and would instead look for alternatives. Some surgeons prefer to avoid keratorefractive surgery near the approved upper limits for myopia and hyperopia. The patient should be informed that at the upper extremes of approved treatment a loss of best-corrected acuity or reduced night vision might occur. Clear lens extraction with a toric IOL or limbal relaxing incision would be an alternative for the hyperopic patient, whereas a phakic IOL might be a better choice for the high myope due to the risk of retinal detachment. In this case a surface ablation procedure would be an alternative to LASIK for the left eye. PRK does not require a nomogram adjustment. The surgeon can use the cycloplegic refraction if it is close to the manifest refraction.

A large flap is required for hyperopic LASIK in order to accommodate the 9.0-mm treatment zone. In this case the keratometry values are >45.00 D so an 8.5-mm Hansatome ring would be an acceptable choice. Because of the prominent brow, the surgeon should be prepared to position the patient in the chin-up position to achieve better exposure. The corneas are somewhat thin, but this should not pose a problem for this hyperopic patient. Keep in mind that a thin flap is likely to occur with a microkeratome and with the same blade the flap in the second eye would be even thinner. The femtosecond laser is less dependent on corneal thickness in creating flaps of a desired thickness.

As with any hyperopic patient, it is important to discuss the slower visual rehabilitation and the possible need for distance glasses. If the PRK option is selected for the left eye, the rehabilitation will be even slower. The epithelial debridement will need to be large enough to accommodate the 9.0-mm ablation zone and will therefore take the surface longer to heal and stabilize. The final point is to explain in lay language to this esophoric patient that in the event of postoperative anisometropia, added strain on fusion might result in symptomatic diplopia.

Surgical Plan

	Right Eye	Left Eye	Comments
Ring size for LASIK	8.5 mm	9.0-mm epithelial debridement	Steep small cornea; 8.5-mm ring is the better choice OD
Plate size for LASIK	160 μm or 180 μm	Not applicable	Thin flaps result from mechanical microkeratome flaps in thin corneas
Ablation zone	9.0 mm	9.0 mm	VISX STAR S4
Spherical equivalent	+3.75 D	+6.00 D	
Calculations with nomogram correction	$+3.75 \times 23\% = 0.86$ $+3.00 + 0.86 = +3.86$	$+6.00 \times 28\% = +1.68$ $+5.00 + 1.68 = +6.68$ (see comment)	+6.68 (sphere + nomogram adjustment) exceeds the FDA-approved limit. With PRK treat on cycloplegic refraction
(enter into VISX)	$+3.86 + 1.50 \times 90°$	$+5.00 + 2.00 \times 85°$	
Ablation depth	$4.61 \text{ D} \times 8 \text{ μm/D}$ $= 37 \text{ μm}$	$6.00 \text{ D} \times 8 \text{ μm/D}$ $= 48 \text{ μm}$	
Residual stromal thickness	$505 \text{ μm} - 160 \text{ μm}$ $-37 \text{ μm} = 308 \text{ μm}$ $>250 \text{ μm}$	$501 \text{ μm} - 160 \text{ μm}$ $-48 \text{ μm} = 293 \text{ μm}$ $>250 \text{ μm}$	Hyperopic ablation is not deepest centrally, so RST is greater

Take-Home Points

1. If the spherical equivalent plus the nomogram adjustment exceeds the approved limit for the laser, consider using PRK, which does not require a nomogram adjustment.
2. Explain to patients that at the extremes of approved hyperopic treatment, a loss of best-corrected postoperative visual acuity can occur.
3. Clear lens extraction with a toric IOL to correct astigmatism, a multifocal IOL (provided both eyes will ultimately be treated), or an accommodating IOL with LRI are additional options when the amount of hyperopic correction is excessive.

A 66-year-old woman had 8-cut radial keratotomy in the left eye 10 years ago. She continued to wear a soft contact lens in the right eye. Over the years she developed decreasing vision in the left eye and symptoms of eyestrain. She wondered if laser surgery could improve her symptoms. She was not interested in monovision and was made aware she would need reading glasses following surgery. She understood the risks of surgery. After being out of her contact lens, her refraction was followed until stable. Old records were obtained and the refraction in the OS was stable over the previous 18 months.

W	OD–4.50 20/20–3 OS +3.00 + 1.25 x 30° 20/20+	**Uncorrected Va** OD CF OS 20/400
M	OD–4.75 20/15 OS +3.00 + 0.75 x 40° 20/20+	
C	OD–4.50 + 0.50 x 175° 20/15– OS +3.00 + 0.75 x 40° 20/20±	
K	OD 44.75 x 15°/45.00 x 175° OS 37.12 x 12°/38.50 x 102°	

Pachymetry	Topography	Scotopic Pupils
OD 510 μm OS 498 μm (≥537 μm in midperiphery)	Regular OD Central flattening OS	OD 5 mm OS 5 mm

Additional Examination

The keratometry reading OS prior to RK was 44.00 D ✕ 44.25 D @ 180°. The RK incisions are thin without noticeable epithelial plugs. There is no corneal neovascularization. The cornea is otherwise clear. There is no cataract. The IOP and fundus are normal.

Discussion

LASIK surgery can be safely performed following radial keratotomy provided the conditions are optimal. The RK scars should be thin and free of large epithelial plugs. Ideally, there should be at most only minimal irregular astigmatism; that is, the patient should be correctable to 20/20. If the best-corrected visual acuity (BCVA) is <20/20, the postoperative LASIK result is less predictable.

The cornea is somewhat thin centrally. This was presumably present preoperatively, because RK would not thin the uninvolved central cornea. The thin cornea does not preclude hyperopic LASIK, because the deepest ablation is at 5 mm and is only 8 μm/D. Although the central cornea is flat, the microkeratome will engage the cornea in the periphery where the cornea is not so flat. The risk of a free flap is small. Base the ring diameter on the preoperative keratometry. When the flap made with the microkeratome is lifted, care is required to avoid disrupting the incisions. A thicker flap is usually an advantage to avoid separation. If the incisions do separate, the excimer procedure can still be done, but the pieces should be meticulously replaced at the end of the procedure and a bandage soft contact lens placed. The risk of epithelial ingrowth is probably increased if this occurs. IntraLase should not be done following RK because the required flap dissection could potentially disrupt the RK incisions. In addition, the waste gases from photodisruption can push through the RK incisions and form a small buttonhole.

The hyperopic nomogram adjustment is different following RK (see Table 2.12, page 58) and in a 66-year-old woman a 2% addition is suggested. For patients under age 50, in contrast to standard hyperopia, a reduction in the hyperopic correction is suggested. The hyperopic nomogram is also different for treatment of consecutive hyperopia following LASIK.

Because the right cornea is somewhat thin, the femtosecond laser might be a better choice than the microkeratome. The laser is capable of greater precision with regard to flap thickness. The microkeratome usually will create a thinner flap in a thinner cornea.

Given the patient's age, a discussion of monovision is warranted. If desired, determine the nondominant eye and either reduce the myopic correction or increase the hyperopic correction appropriately.

Surgical Plan

	Right Eye	Left Eye	Comments
Ring size	IntraLase 9.0-mm flap diameter in case retreatment needed	9.5 mm	Preoperative K <45.00 D
Plate size	IntraLase 110-μm flap depth, usually creates a flap no greater than 120 μm	180 μm	Hansatome flap in a thin cornea can be quite thin. Very thin flap after RK is a disadvantage.
Ablation zone	6.0 mm	9.0 mm	Hyperopic protocol OS
Calculations with nomogram correction (enter into VISX)	$4.25\ D \times 9\% = 0.38$ $-4.50 + 0.38 = -4.12$ $-4.12 + 0.50 \times 175$	$+3.00 + 0.75 \times 40°$ See Table 2.12 for nomogram adjustment $+3.375 \times 2\% = 0.07$ $+3.07 + 0.75 \times 40°$	+2% nomogram adjustment for a 66-year-old with consecutive hyperopia after RK
Ablation depth	$4.25\ D \times 12\ \mu m/D$ $= 51\ \mu m$	$3.445\ D \times 8\ \mu m/D$ $= 28\ \mu m$	
Residual stromal thickness	$510\ \mu m - 120\ \mu m$ $-51\ \mu m = 339\ \mu m$ $>250\ \mu m$	$498\ \mu m - 180\ \mu m$ $-28\ \mu m = 290\ \mu m$ $>250\ \mu m$	RST OS likely >291 μm because flap likely to be thinner than 180 μm and hyperopic treatment is not deepest centrally

Take-Home Points

1. LASIK can safely be done following RK if there is no more than minimal irregular astigmatism, thin well-healed scars, and no large epithelial plugs.
2. The microkeratome should be used rather than the femtosecond laser, with the ring size based on the preoperative keratometry.
3. Should the flap separate, carefully replace the pieces after the excimer ablation has been completed and place a bandage contact lens on the eye.
4. The suggested nomogram adjustment for consecutive hyperopia following RK is considerably different than for treatment of primary hyperopia (see Table 2.12). A reduction rather than an addition to treatment may be required for patients under 50.

CASE 32

A 58-year-old woman was referred for management of painful recurrent corneal erosions, which had occurred in both eyes over a 2-year period. The pain would always begin in the early morning and last from a few hours to a few days. The episodes occurred at least once a week and she could never predict when an erosion would occur. Her mother had similar problems for years before she died of heart disease. She had tried tear supplements, hypertonic sodium chloride ointment and drops, as well as a bandage soft contact lens without relief of her symptoms. Epithelial debridement was tried in the left eye, but the symptoms recurred. Fortunately, her vision in spectacles remains

W OD +2.25 20/25 OS +2.00 20/25	**Uncorrected Va** 20/200 20/200
M OD +2.25 + 1.00 x 25° 20/20– OS +2.00 + 1.00 x 160° 20/20–	
C OD +2.25 + 1.00 x 30° 20/20– OS +2.25 + 1.00 x 164° 20/20–	
K OD 41.00 x 112°/41.75 x 22° OS 40.87 x 70°/41.50 x 160°	

Pachymetry	**Topography**	**Scotopic Pupils**
OD 534 μm OS 536 μm	Regular astigmatism OU	OD 5.0 mm OS 5.0 mm

excellent at distance and near. She is amenable to any suggestion that would allow her life to return to normal. She has heard about LASIK surgery from a friend and wonders if it would help her.

Additional Examination

The slit-lamp examination was significant for dots and fingerprints on the surface of the paracentral and midperipheral cornea OU. There was no evidence of corneal scarring or corneal neovascularization; and no staining with fluorescein. The anterior segment was otherwise completely normal. The IOP and fundus examinations were normal.

Discussion

This patient suffers from epithelial basement membrane dystrophy, which she likely inherited from her mother. Conventional treatments with lubricants, hypertonic NaCl, bandage soft contact lens, and debridement have failed to control the patient's symptoms. Anterior stromal puncture is a treatment that has not been tried. In the absence of a frank erosion, it might be difficult to know exactly where to apply the punctures. The patients with this dystrophy often have diffuse involvement. This patient is a poor candidate for LASIK surgery because of the high risk of epithelial sloughing. The corneal hypoesthesia associated with LASIK might afford some pain relief, but cutting the corneal nerves to relieve corneal erosions symptoms is not a practical solution.

Photorefractive keratectomy (PRK) is a practical solution, which would ultimately relieve symptoms, stabilize the cornea, and correct the hyperopic astigmatism with one procedure. Phototherapeutic keratectomy has been described as a remedy for recurrent corneal erosion. The hyperopic ablation would treat all but an 0.8-mm central area within a 9.0-mm ablation zone. No nomogram adjustment is needed with hyperopic PRK. Her cornea has ample thickness and would not become abnormally steep after the treatment. Provided the patient understands the risk of surgery, PRK is an excellent therapeutic option for this patient.

Surgical Plan

	Right Eye	**Left Eye**	**Comments**
PRK OU			
Ablation zone	9.0 mm	9.0 mm	VISX STAR S4
Enter into VISX	+2.25 + 1.00 × 25°	+2.25 + 1.00 × 160°	No nomogram adjustment needed for hyperopic treatment
Ablation depth	+2.75 D × 8 μm/D = 22 μm	+2.75 D × 8 μm/D = 22 μm	Low risk of central haze

7

Take-Home Points

1. LASIK surgery should be avoided in patients with epithelial basement membrane dystrophy.
2. PRK is an excellent option for treating the hyperopic patient suffering from recurrent corneal erosion, because the laser treatment of the surface will correct the refractive error; once the eye has healed it will help prevent erosions from occurring postoperatively.
3. In some basement dystrophy cases the surface is too irregular to get an accurate refraction. This can complicate performing PRK. Phototherapeutic keratectomy can reduce the risk of erosions, but may increase the degree of hyperopia.

CASE 33

A 60-year-old woman who successfully wore monovision contact lenses is interested in having LASIK surgery because her contact lenses become uncomfortable in the evening. The patient is planning to retire and travel extensively; and she has concerns about hygiene conditions in developing nations where she will be doing volunteer work. She has a basic fear that should she lose her glasses or be caught in a fire, she would not be able to find her way without visual correction.

		Uncorrected Va
W	OD –5.00 + 1.00 x 180° 20/20 OS –6.50 + 1.75 x 180° 20/20	20/400 20/400
M	OD –5.25 + 1.25 x 180° 20/20 OS –6.75 + 1.75 x 180° 20/20	
C	OD –5.00 + 1.00 x 180° 20/20 OS –6.50 + 1.75 x 180° 20/20	
K	OD 44.00 x 180°/43.00 x 90° OS 44.50 x 180°/43.00 x 90°	

Pachymetry	Topography	Scotopic Pupils
OD 564 μm OS 554 μm	Regular astigmatism OU	OD 6.0 mm OS 6.0 mm

Additional Examination

The patient has a normal external examination with no evidence of blepharitis or conjunctivitis. The corneas are clear. There is no evidence of epithelial basement membrane dystrophy and Schirmer testing reveals 8 mm of wetting at 5 minutes with anesthesia in each eye. The IOP and fundus examinations are normal. The right eye is dominant.

Discussion

This 60-year-old woman requesting monovision LASIK surgery has good reasons to undergo LASIK. Her advanced age does increase the risk for an epithelial defect during flap creation. This risk may be significantly reduced if the surgeon chooses to use the IntraLase to create the flap; however, there may be an increased risk of diffuse lamellar keratitis (DLK). If the Hansatome is used, the Zero Compression head will reduce the risk of epithelial damage. If the surgeon chooses to use the Nidek MK-2000 with a 160-μm plate and an epithelial defect occurs, then the best treatment for this would be to smooth the epithelium back into position and place a bandage contact lens over the flap at the end of the case. The presence of an epithelial defect and the use of a bandage contact lens may both increase the risk of DLK postoperatively. Therefore, the surgeon may choose to increase the strength or frequency of topical steroids used in the early postoperative period to avoid DLK.

Another important discussion point is the use of punctal plugs in this patient. Placement of punctal plugs at the end of LASIK surgery while the surgeon is waiting for the cornea to dry is advantageous in patients who are placed in bandage contact lenses, have an intraoperative epithelial defect, or have any risk for a dry eye postoperatively. A 60-year-old woman with a preoperative Schirmer test of 8 mm would be at risk for postoperative dry eye. Placement of silicone punctal plugs in the lower punctum preoperatively, intraoperatively, or postoperatively may help decrease this risk.

In calculating the parameters to enter into the laser for this patient, ocular dominance must be determined. In this patient, the right eye is dominant, therefore the full cycloplegic refraction is treated. This refraction is converted into negative cylinder, $-4.00 -1.00 \times 90°$. The Nidek LASIK look-up table (see discussion of the Nidek laser in Chapter 2) is used to identify a treatment of $-2.816 - 0.911$. The cylinder is treated fully, because the patient has less than a 1.25 D cylinder, and the sphere is reduced by 12% as an optical zone of 6.5 mm and transition zone of 7.5 mm are utilized. The parameters entered into the laser for the right eye are -2.478 D sphere -1.00 D cylinder axis 90°.

Monovision correction should be discussed with the patient preoperatively. The determination is made to leave the patient with a correction of -2.25 D OS. If the patient has her contact lens prescription, an attempt to duplicate the degree of undercorrection of the near eye can be made. If the patient is not aware of the correction or is not certain about the use of monovision, a trial of contact lenses to use at home, work, or during leisure activities should be provided.

The reading correction is created by converting the cycloplegic refraction into negative cylinder form, -4.75 D $- 1.75$ D $\times 90°$, and adding $+ 2.25$ D to the sphere. The resultant refraction is -2.50 D $- 1.75$ D $\times 90°$. Using the nomogram in Table 2.18, an optical zone of 6.5 mm and a transition zone of 7.5 mm are selected. The Nidek LASIK look-up table is utilized and the desired correction is identified as -0.930 D sphere, -1.85 D cylinder. The full cylinder is treated and the sphere is reduced by 12%. The parameters entered into the laser are -0.818 D sphere, -1.858 D $\times 90°$.

Surgical Plan

	Right Eye	Left Eye	Comments
Treatment: cyclorefraction in negative cylinder	$-4.00 - 1.00 \times 90°$	$-4.75 - 1.75 \times 90°$ Reducing sphere by $+ 2.25$ yields $-2.50 - 1.75 \times 90°$	OD dominant. OS should be near eye
Ring size	9.5 mm	9.5 mm	
Plate size	160 μm	160 μm	
Optical zone (OZ)	6.5 mm	6.5 mm	Could use standard 5.5
Transition zone (TZ)	7.5 mm	7.5 mm	Could use standard 7.0
Calculations with nomogram	Find the negative cylinder desired correction in the Nidek LASIK look-up table: $-2.816 - 0.911$ and reduce sphere by 12%	Find the negative cylinder desired correction in the Nidek LASIK look-up table: $-0.930 -1.858$ and reduce sphere by 12%	Do not reduce if using 5.5/7.0 OZ/TZ
Spherical treatment	-2.478 D	-0.818 D	
Cylinder treatment	$-1.00 \times 90°$	$-1.858 \times 90°$	
Approximate ablation depth	65 μm	42 μm	
Residual stromal thickness	554 μm $-$ 160 μm -65 μm $= 339$ μm >250 μm	564 μm $-$ 160 μm -42 μm $= 362$ μm	

Take-Home Points

1. In a 60-year-old woman there is an increased risk of epithelial defects during creation of the LASIK flap. As a result, the surgeon should be prepared either to use the IntraLase or to manage the epithelial defect, either of which will increase the risk of DLK postoperatively. The Hansatome with a Zero Compression head may reduce the risk without increasing the chance of DLK. Should an epithelial defect occur, a bandage contact lens is indicated and the frequency or concentration of topical steroids may be increased during the early postoperative period.
2. In a patient 60 years of age, the risk of postoperative dry eyes is increased and the use of silicone punctal plugs in the inferior punctum is recommended. An alternative may be the use of topical cyclosporine.
3. The possibility of treating monovision should be discussed with the patient preoperatively and careful calculations should be made after the dominant eye and the amount of monovision are determined. The contact lens prescription or a trial of monovision preoperatively can be helpful.

CASE 34

A 26-year-old graduate student is interested in LASIK. She wears glasses full time and wishes to be less dependent on glasses. She enjoys scuba diving and snorkeling and has been unable to get a diving mask that adequately corrects her vision. She is in good health, has a negative past ocular history, and has a stable refraction.

		Uncorrected Va
W	OD –3.00 + 4.00 x 94° 20/20– OS –2.00 + 2.25 x 86° 20/30	OD CF dist; 12 pt near OS CF dist; 12 pt near
M	OD –2.75 + 3.75 x 97° 20/20 OS –2.75 + 3.00 x 85° 20/20	
C	OD –2.50 + 3.25 x 95° 20/20+ OS –3.00 + 3.50 x 85° 20/20	
K	OD 40.50 x 6°/43.75 x 96° OS 41.00 x 178°/43.00 x 88°	

Pachymetry	Topography	Scotopic Pupils
OD 560 μm OS 559 μm	OD +3.5 D at 94°, regular astigmatism OS +3.0 D at 89°, regular astigmatism	OD 8.0 mm OS 8.0 mm

Additional Examination

Excellent exposure with normal slit-lamp, IOP, and fundus examinations.

Discussion

This patient has mixed astigmatism in both eyes. Note that the spherical portion of the refraction is less than the astigmatic portion and they are of opposite signs. The VISX laser is FDA approved for treatment of mixed astigmatism, allowing a single laser treatment to correct the refractive error. Patients with higher levels of astigmatism generally have difficulty with unaided distance and near vision even prior to presbyopic age. The laser correction will benefit both distance and near visual function. If the patient does not correct to 20/20, refractive amblyopia may be present.

However, it is also possible the refraction is inadequate. Wavefront technology can be helpful in this situation even if custom laser surgery is not being done. The WaveScan will generate a refraction that may be more accurate than was done with subjective refraction or retinoscopy. The manifest and cycloplegic refractions can be based on the wavefront-assisted manifest refraction (WAMR).

The mixed astigmatism profile requires a 9.0-mm treatment zone. This is ideal for this patient with 8.0-mm pupils. The patient should still be warned about the possibility of nighttime glare or haloes. A large flap will be needed to accommodate the large treatment zone.

Given the high degree of astigmatism, registration of the patient with the laser is critically important. The patient should be marked at the slit lamp at the 3 and 9 o'clock meridians and just prior to laser ablation the form-fit pillow should be adjusted to align the marks with the reticle in the laser microscope. Simply moving the head may be inadequate to ensure that the patient's head will not slip back into the same unwanted position.

Surgical Plan

	Right Eye	Left Eye	Comments
Ring size	9.5 mm	9.5 mm	Need larger flap for mixed astigmatism
Plate size	160 or 180 μm	160 or 180 μm	Hansatome
Ablation zone	9.0 mm	9.0 mm	Standard ablation profile for mixed astigmatism
Spherical equivalent	Treat on the cycloplegic refraction	Treat on the cycloplegic refraction	Mixed astigmatism profile; VISX STAR S4
Enter into VISX	No calculations needed $-2.50 + 3.25 \times 095$	No calculations needed $-3.00 + 3.50 \times 085$	
Ablation depth (from VISX computer)	560 μm $-$ 160 μm -21 μm $= 379$ μm >250 μm	559 μm $-$ 160 μm -27 μm $= 372$ μm >250 μm	High astigmatism correction reduces the ablation depth in mixed astigmatism treatment

Take-Home Points

1. Treating astigmatism will improve reading function even in young people.
2. Do not assume the patient has refractive amblyopia unless a careful refraction has been done. Wavefront technology can help with refraction even if custom surgery is not being done.
3. No nomogram adjustment is required with the VISX mixed astigmatism profile.
4. Use a larger flap when treating a patient with mixed astigmatism.
5. The larger treatment zone of 9.0 mm is helpful for large-pupil patients, but it is important to discuss the risk of glare and haloes with the patient.
6. Do not forget to mark the eye at the slit lamp for registration of the patient with the laser.

7

CASE 35

A 27-year-old marketing director with a long history of wearing spectacles because he was unable to see well in contact lenses comes for a LASIK evaluation. He is an avid sports enthusiast who would like to do all his sports without glasses. He has tried soft lenses without achieving adequate visual function and was unable to tolerate hard lenses. He is currently using no ocular medications and has no significant medical history.

W	OD −1.00 + 3.00 x 90° 20/20 OS −3.00 + 1.50 x 90° 20/20	**Uncorrected Va** 20/70 20/400
M	OD −1.00 + 3.25 x 90° 20/20 OS −2.75 + 1.25 x 90° 20/20	
C	OD −1.00 + 3.00 x 90° 20/20 OS −3.00 + 1.25 x 90° 20/20	
K	OD 43.00 x 180°/45.75 x 90° OS 43.50 x 180°/44.75 x 90°	

Pachymetry	**Topography**	**Scotopic Pupils**
OD 549 μm	OD regular astigmatism	OD 5.0 mm
OS 528 μm	OS regular astigmatism	OS 5.0 mm

Additional Examination

There is a normal external examination with adequate tear film. His corneal topography reveals asymmetry in the astigmatism between the two eyes, but the topography pattern reveals regular astigmatism in each eye. The IOP and fundus examinations were normal.

Discussion

This patient is an acceptable candidate for LASIK surgery, but in his right eye he presents with mixed astigmatism. In the left eye, he presents with myopic astigmatism. Calculation of a treatment plan for the right eye with mixed astigmatism requires a multistage, multizone approach (see Nidek laser section, Chapter 2). To do so, the cycloplegic refraction is converted to negative cylinder +2.00 − 3.00 axis 180°. The first stage of the treatment is plano minus one-half the cylinder at the negative cylinder refraction axis with a 6.5-mm optical zone and 7.5-mm transition zone. This equates to plano −1.50 × 180°. The second stage is plano plus one-half the cylinder at the positive cylinder refraction axis with a 5.5-mm optical zone and a 9-mm transition zone. Therefore, treatment 2 is plano +1.50 axis 90°, optical zone is 5.5 mm, and transition zone is 9.0 mm. For the third stage of treatment, the sphere must be calculated. The negative cylinder (−3.00) is multiplied by 0.35 to determine the hyperopic shift or A. In this case it is −1.05 D. The hyperopic shift is subtracted from the spherical equivalent (+0.50). The result is +0.50 − (1.05) = −0.55 D sphere. This is multiplied by a correction factor of 0.85 to equal −0.4675. Therefore, the treatment is −0.468 sphere with a 6.5-mm optical zone and 7.5-mm transition zone. To perform multistage, multizone treatments with the Nidek laser, each treatment is programmed into the laser, the flap is lifted, and each treatment is performed sequentially.

For the left eye, when converted to minus cylinder, the desired correction is −1.75 − 1.25 × 180°. To treat at a 6.5-mm optical zone with a 7.5-mm transition zone, you must find −1.75 − 1.25 on the Nidek LASIK look-up table (provided by Nidek): −0.73 sphere and −1.22 cylinder. According to the nomogram in Table 2.18, the cylinder is treated fully because it is ≤1.25 D and the sphere is reduced by 12%; therefore, the actual amount of treatment is −0.64 sphere. For the left eye, the following data would be entered into the Nidek EC-5000: −0.64 sphere, +1.25 cylinder, 6.5-mm optical zone, 7.5-mm transition zone.

Surgical Plan

	Right Eye	**Left Eye**	**Comments**
Treatment cyclorefraction in negative cylinder	+2.00 − 3.00 × 180	−1.75 − 1.25 × 180	Mixed astigmatism OD requires multistage, multizone treatment

continued

	Right Eye	Left Eye	Comments
Ring size	9.0 mm	9.5 mm	A larger flap allows for adequate exposure if a hyperopic enhancement is required
Plate size	160 μm	160 μm	
Optical zone		6.5 mm	
Transitional zone		7.5 mm	
Calculations with nomogram	Plano −1.50 × 180° (6.5/7.5) Plano +1.50 × 90° (5.5/9.0)	−0.73 (12%) = −0.09 reduction	
Spherical treatment	−0.468 sphere (6.5/7.5)	−0.64 D	
Cylinder treatment	Treat full cylinder OD	−1.25 D × 180°	
Approximate ablation depth	20 μm	30 μm	
Residual stromal thickness	369 μm 549 μm − 160 μm − 20 μm = 369 μm	338 μm 528 μm − 160 μm − 30 μm = 338 μm	
Considerations	Multistage multizone ablation results in less tissue removal		

Take-Home Points

1. Treat mixed astigmatism using multistage, multizone ablation profile following the nomogram in Table 2.20.
2. When expanding the optical zone and treatment zone, follow the myopic astigmatism nomogram in Table 2.18.

CASE 36

A 26-year-old man works in sales and requests LASIK surgery. He has not worn contact lenses for a year, because he cannot see as well with them. Without his glasses he cannot see distance or near. He is healthy and has no other significant past ocular history.

W	OD −4.75 + 4.75 x 106° 20/30+ OS −5.00 + 5.00 x 80° 20/25	Uncorrected Va OD 20/200 Near 18 pt OS 20/200 Near 8 pt
M	OD −5.25 + 5.00 x 100° 20/20+ OS −4.75 + 4.50 x 80° 20/15−	
C	OD −3.75 + 4.75 x 100° 20/15 OS −4.00 + 4.50 x 85° 20/15−	
K	OD 41.25 x 6°/44.87 x 96° OS 41.00 x 175°/45.00 x 82°	

Pachymetry	Topography	Scotopic Pupils
OD 602 μm OS 597 μm	Regular with-the-rule astigmatism OU	OD 6.5 mm OS 6.5 mm

7

Additional Examination

There is a heavy brow, but lax lids and a wide fissure. The slit-lamp examination, IOP, and fundus examinations are normal.

Discussion

The refractive error in this case would be classified as mixed astigmatism, because the myopic sphere in the cycloplegic refraction is less than the cylindrical correction and has an opposite sign. This patient has surprisingly good visual acuity for an individual with this much astigmatism. Notice that the unaided near acuity is measured here and should be measured in any case of hyperopia and in patients with significant astigmatism. The perceived improvement in the prepresbyopic patient is at near as well as in the distance.

The fact that this patient is comfortable in glasses with visual acuity in the 20/25 to 20/30 range is a favorable sign because his vision expectations would be less than someone who is accustomed to 20/15 visual acuity. It is imperative to educate this patient that at the upper levels of astigmatism correction 20/30 acuity is a more realistic expectation. The likelihood of retreatment is greater in this patient and this should also be discussed preoperatively. In addition, with conventional LASIK night vision issues may arise because the astigmatism treatment area is smaller than the pupil diameter in the dark. The treatment zone in the VISX mixed astigmatism profile is 9.0 mm, which should adequately cover the pupil. The flap will need to be large enough to accommodate this large treatment zone.

The new mixed astigmatism profile for CustomVue LASIK with the VISX STAR S4 laser can treat up to 5 D of astigmatism, but was not available at the time this patient was treated.

When treating large degrees of astigmatism, careful preoperative marking is essential to avoid the effect of cyclotorsion on astigmatism correction. Iris registration software will hopefully lessen alignment inaccuracies.

Some surgeons will reduce the spherical power of the correction by 0.2 D for each diopter of astigmatic correction. The logic behind this is that for each diopter of flattening in the steep meridian there is 0.2 D of steepening in the flat meridian. Therefore, it is necessary to back off from the full spherical correction. Many surgeons have not found it necessary to make this adjustment.

For VISX laser treatment of mixed astigmatism, no nomogram adjustment to the cycloplegic refraction is needed. Multistage treatments are unnecessary. The patient is treated using the mixed astigmatism profile on the cycloplegic refraction. Surgeons vary on how the axis of astigmatism is handled. Some will use the axis in the cycloplegic refraction, while others use the axis from the manifest refraction. Still others will split the difference between the two.

Surgical Plan

	Right Eye	Left Eye	Comments
Ring size	9.5 mm	9.5 mm	
Plate size	160 μm	160 μm	Hansatome
Ablation zone	Mixed astigmatism profile 9.0 mm	Mixed astigmatism profile 9.0 mm	Pupils size should not be a problem
Enter into VISX	No nomogram adjustment needed here $-3.75 + 4.75 \times 100°$	No nomogram adjustment needed here $-4.00 + 4.50 \times 80°$	The axis of cylinder matches the manifest refraction; see text
Ablation depth taken from laser computer; RST well above 300 μm	32 μm	34 μm	Cylindrical correction reduces impact of the myopic correction on ablation depth

7

At 1 year after surgery this patient has unaided acuity of 20/15− and 4 pt OD and 20/20± and 4 pt OS with no symptoms of nighttime glare or haloes. This result exceeded the expectations of the patient and the surgeon.

Take-Home Points
1. Mixed astigmatism is present when the myopic sphere is less than the plus cylinder. This should be treated with a mixed astigmatism profile, if possible.
2. Expectations should be lower in patients with high astigmatism. UCVA of 20/30 or better after retreatment is reasonable. Retreatment is more likely. Counsel younger patients that near vision may improve after surgery. Night vision may be more problematic.
3. Registration (aligning the patient marks made at the slit lamp with the laser microscope reticle) is crucial in patients with high astigmatism due to the potential negative effects of cyclotorsion.
4. With current mixed astigmatism profiles even patients with high astigmatism may achieve surprisingly good visual acuity after surgery.

CASE 37

A 38-year-old man is interested in LASIK surgery to correct his vision. He currently uses a contact lens OS when he drives otherwise he prefers to go with no correction. He does not have a pair of glasses and has never liked wearing them. His contact lenses bother him. For as long as he can remember, his left eye has been extremely nearsighted. He denies ever having double vision even when his contact lens is in place OS. He has no family history of eye disease and is otherwise healthy. He has read a lot about LASIK and is familiar with the risks of surgery.

W	No contact lens OD With soft contact lens OS 20/30	Uncorrected Va OD 20/40+ OS CF 3′
M	OD −1.25 + 1.50 x 4° 20/15 OS −13.75 + 0.75 x 150° 20/20	
C	OD −1.00 + 1.25 x 4° 20/15− OS −13.25 + 0.75 x 150° 20/20− Vertex distance 12 mm	
K	OD 44.00 x 90°/ 44.00 x 180° OS 45.87 x 60°/46.50 x 150°	

Pachymetry	Topography	Scotopic Pupils
OD 584 μm OS 585 μm	Against-the-rule astigmatism OU; no cone OU	OD 5.0 mm OS 5.0 mm

Additional Examination
The external examination shows lax lids and a wide palpebral fissure. No tropia or phoria was detected while the patient was wearing the contact lens. The slit-lamp examination, IOP, and dilated fundus examinations were completely normal.

Discussion
Marked anisometropia can usually be corrected with keratorefractive surgery. A careful motility examination with the patient wearing full contact lens correction is important to reduce the risk of postoperative diplopia. In this case a full correction with LASIK is not recommended. While

Surgical Plan

After considerable discussion of the various options, the patient chose to have clear lens exchange with the STAAR Toric lens implant. The 2.0 D astigmatic lens was used for the right eye because it gives 1.5 D of cylinder correction. The lens was implanted with the long axis at 145 degrees. The left eye was corrected with the 3.5 D STAAR Toric lens implant because it gives 2.25 D of correction. This lens was aligned at 40 degrees. Postoperatively the patient had 20/30 uncorrected acuity without fluctuation. Reading glasses were prescribed.

Take-Home Points

1. Progressive hyperopic shifts after RK are becoming more common as time passes from the RK era. When stable, it is possible to obtain a good refractive correction.
2. Refractive procedures will not eliminate the glare from the RK incisions.
3. Surface ablation may be safer than LASIK by avoiding problems of flap segmentation and stretching of incisions caused by the suction ring.
4. Phakic IOL or clear lens exchange avoids manipulation of a stable cornea and provides a wide range of refractive correction. Accuracy with IOL power calculations requires advanced biometric techniques.
5. These previously myopic patients may be at increased risk of retinal detachment with clear lens exchange.

CASE 40

A 45-year-old business executive has never worn glasses and always had good vision until the last 2 years when he started with reading glasses and now finds that he needs them even when driving. He hates wearing glasses and wants laser vision correction to allow him to drive the car and read without glasses. He plays ice hockey without wearing his glasses, but needs them for golf. He has hypertension controlled with a diuretic, but is otherwise in good health. He has never had a complete eye examination and is not aware of any eye problems in family members.

W	Uses +2.00 readers for driving as well as reading	**Uncorrected Va** 20/60 OU	
M	OD+2.00 20/40 OS +2.00 20/40		
C	OD+4.75 20/20 OS+4.50 20/20		
K	OD 45.50 x 180°/45.75 x 90° OS 45.50 x 180°/45.50 x 90°		

Pachymetry	Topography	Scotopic Pupils
OD 555 µm OS 547 µm	Mild inferior steepening OU; posterior elevations are normal OU	OD 5.2 mm OS 5.2 mm

Additional Examination

The eyelid fissures are adequate for the microkeratome suction ring. The corneal diameter is 10.3 mm for each eye. The eyes are orthotropic. The slit-lamp examination reveals clear corneas and normal anterior segments. The angles are open to the top half of the trabecular meshwork and the lenses are clear. There is no posterior segment pathology.

Discussion

This man demonstrates some typical findings for patients with uncorrected hyperopia. Most of these patients believe that they have excellent distance vision even though their acuity is poor. They know that they need glasses for reading and try to go without glasses for as many activities as possible. This patient just uses his +2.00 over-the-counter reading glasses to help drive at night and see road signs. Sports that do not require acuity or near vision (e.g., ice hockey, football) are not a problem for them. These patients often are unhappy after correction of their refractive error unless the presbyopia is addressed as well.

The examination uncovers three issues that need to be considered in order to determine what procedure will best help this patient:

1. The cycloplegic refraction falls within the range of hyperopic LASIK, but the accuracy of laser correction tends to fall off with treatment above +4.00 D. To achieve a monovision near correction, he will need more than 6 D of correction and this exceeds the limit for most lasers.
2. The keratometry readings are somewhat steep for a hyperope and the amount of steepening needed to correct his refractive error and presbyopia will exceed the 50.00 D upper limit used by most surgeons.
3. The corneal diameter is rather small. Hyperopic LASIK requires a large-diameter treatment zone and, therefore, a large flap to accommodate the ablation. His corneal diameter may be too small and the flap may extend into the limbus with bleeding that might complicate the laser ablation. While a surface ablation can avoid this problem, care must be taken to avoid damage to the limbal stem cells with alcohol-assisted epithelial removal.

Treatment Plan

The patient was informed that laser vision correction would not provide the best results for his vision problems. When he had the full cycloplegic correction in a trial frame he felt that the correction was too strong and he would be satisfied with just the laser correction in the amount of his current +2.00 reading glasses. Clear lens exchange with an accommodative lens implant was discussed as the best option for his vision problems. While phakic lens implants are available outside of the United States to correct this amount of hyperopia, they will not correct presbyopia. Conductive keratoplasty is not powerful enough for this degree of correction. The patient elected to seek laser vision correction from two other providers, but was told again that this would not be appropriate for his needs. He returned and was given a progressive course of disposable contact lenses increasing as tolerated until he achieved his full cycloplegic correction for distance and maintained his current reading glasses as needed. He insisted that the contact lenses were making his vision worse since he could not see clearly when he removed them, and he believed that he was seeing clearly before he started to wear them. After 6 weeks he was comfortable with his full cycloplegic correction and underwent clear lens exchange with ReSTOR lens implants in both eyes targeted for a final refraction of +0.50. Following surgery, he was 20/20 in both eyes at distance and J2 for reading.

Take-Home Points

1. The latent hyperope should be allowed to adapt into the cycloplegic correction to allow the full amount of hyperopia to be treated.
2. The corneal diameter must be considered when a large flap is required.
3. The preoperative corneal contour must be assessed to ensure that it will not become too steep (>50.00 D) after surgery.
4. Clear lens exchange with an accommodating IOL is a viable option for correcting the hyperopic patient in the presbyopic age group.

7

4. Manage active bleeding during the case by applying light pressure at the limbus with a sponge for 1 to 2 minutes before lifting the flap. Interrupt the ablation as needed to swab blood out of the treatment zone; irrigate blood from beneath the flap to reduce the risk of diffuse lamellar keratitis.

CASE 42

This 60-year-old hyperopic man with 1+ nuclear sclerotic cataracts and 20/20 best spectacle-corrected vision OU desired LASIK to be able to play golf and drive and see the dashboard of his car without glasses.

W OD+2.75 − 0.50 × 93° 20/20 OS +3.00 − 0.50 × 82° 20/20	**Uncorrected Va** OD 20/400 OS 20/400	
M OD+3.25 − 0.50 × 92° 20/20 Note: minus cylinder form OS +3.25 − 0.50 × 83° 20/20		
C OD+3.25 − 0.50 × 92° 20/20 OS +3.25 − 0.50 x 83° 20/20		
K OD 42.75 × 142°/43.25 × 52° OS 42.25 × 101°/42.50 × 110°		

Pachymetry	**Topography**	**Scotopic Pupils**
OD 531 µm	OD spherical	OD 6.0 mm
OS 535 µm	OS spherical	OS 6.0 mm

Original Surgical Plan

	Right Eye	Left Eye	Comments
Ring size	−1	−1	Hyperopia
Microkeratome head	130 µm	130 µm	See Moria microkeratome discussion in Chapter 2
Ablation zone	9.0 mm	9.0 mm	VISX
Cycloplegic Rx	+3.25 − 0.50 × 092	+3.25 − 0.50 × 083	
Calculations with nomogram adjustment (enter into VISX)	No adjustment +3.25 − 0.50 × 092	No adjustment +3.25 − 0.50 × 083	Before we knew the need to overcorrect hyperopia
Flap thickness	160 µm	160 µm	Assumed
Ablation depth	22 µm	22 µm	Hyperopic Rx in midperiphery
Estimated residual stromal thickness	531 µm − 160 µm −22 µm = 349 µm (if Rx were central)	535 µm − 160 µm −22 µm = 353 µm (if Rx were central)	Hyperopic ablation is not deepest centrally, so RST is significantly greater

The case was aborted after the microkeratome created a truncated superiorly hinged flap OD. The truncated flap was repositioned in its stromal bed, a bandage contact lens was placed, and the laser ablation was canceled. Fortunately, the inferior edge of the flap was just above the superior edge of the pupil OD. The truncated flap healed and the patient was counseled about his options for refractive surgery including a repeat attempt at LASIK, PRK over the truncated flap, contact lenses, or living with his eyeglasses. One month later his visual acuity returned to baseline OD, with a mild change in refraction of $+3.50 - 1.00 \times 77°$ resulting in 20/20 visual acuity. Two months after the initial attempt, the patient elected to have LASIK performed OU using the same Moria CB microkeratome with a -1 suction ring. His LASIK went uneventfully, and he obtained 20/30 vision OU on the first postoperative day, and 20/20 vision OU at 1-month postoperatively. A faint scar persists above the visual axis OD, near the superior hinge of the flap.

	Right Eye	Left Eye	Comments
Ring size	-1	-1	Hyperopia
Microkeratome head	130 μm	130 μm	Moria
Ablation zone	9.0 mm	9.0 mm	
Cycloplegic Rx	$+3.50 - 1.00 \times 92°$	$+3.25 - 0.50 \times 83°$	
Enter into VISX	No nomogram adjustment $+3.50 - 1.00 \times 92°$	No nomogram adjustment $+3.25 - 0.50 \times 83°$	Before we knew the need to overcorrect hyperopia
Flap thickness	160 μm	160 μm	Assumed
Ablation depth	20 μm	22 μm	Hyperopic Rx in midperiphery
Estimated residual stromal thickness	531 μm $-$ 160 μm -20 μm = 351 μm (if deepest ablation were central)	535 μm $-$ 160 μm -22 μm = 353 (if deepest ablation were central)	Hyperopic Rx in midperiphery RST >250 μm

Take-Home Points

1. Abort the laser ablation if there is a problem with creation of the flap, particularly when the flap cannot accommodate the LASIK ablation.
2. Wait at least 3 months before attempting to make a new flap. Some surgeons wait 6 months. The surgical options are to consider a repeat attempt at LASIK or PRK.
3. If the inferior edge of the original LASIK flap had been more inferior, one might have considered creating a slightly larger and thicker flap, in order to be sure that the microkeratome cut begins outside the original flap edge and proceeds beneath the original cut.
4. Given the superior location of the inferior edge of the truncated flap, we could use the same microkeratome settings we attempted to utilize initially.

CASE 43

A 61-year-old woman complained of persistent decreased vision 24 years after having undergone radial keratotomy (RK) in each eye. She denied any fluctuation of vision, glare problems, or discomfort. She wore spectacles full time.

Examination showed a 4-cut RK with an optical zone of 4.5 mm. The incisions were generally thin with no gaping or prominent epithelial plugs, although slightly irregular. Visual acuity with her current 4-year-old glasses was 20/40 OD and 20/30 OS. The spherical equivalent of her glasses prescription was +3.25 OD and +3.50 OS. Cycloplegic refraction resulted in visual acuity of 20/20 in each eye. Scotopic pupils were 4 mm.

	Right eye	**Left eye**
Post-RK cycloplegic refraction	+3.75 + 0.50 × 160°	+4.00 + 0.50 × 5°
Post-RK keratometry	37.50 × 38.25 @ 105°	38.00 × 38.00
Post-RK pachymetry	572 μm	574 μm
Post-RK BSCVA	20/20	20/20

The preoperative discussion with the patient emphasized that a realistic expectation for post-operative UCVA was 20/40. The patient was told she might continue to need spectacles for distance for some tasks, and that she might lose a line of vision and have a BSCVA of about 20/25. A +3.25 trial lens was placed over each eye in the cycloplegic state to simulate the expected post-operative results.

LASIK was performed in the usual manner using a Bausch & Lomb Hansatome with a 180-μm head. No nomogram adjustment was made. No mitomycin-C was used. In the left eye there was some instability at the inferior RK incision with slight splaying of the inferior segments. These were carefully repositioned, and a bandage contact lens was placed on the eye to be removed the next day. The patient developed +1 to +2 haze OU postoperatively that gradually cleared. The patient was maintained on topical steroids four times a day for 3 months. Despite a persistent refractive error in the left eye, the UCVA remained good and patient was able to see reasonably well at near without spectacles for a significant number of tasks.

	Right eye	**Left eye**
Post-retreatment UCVA	20/25	20/30
Post-retreatment cycloplegic refraction	−0.50	−2.00 + 3.25 × 160°
Post-retreatment keratometry	40.50 × 40.50	42.00 × 39.75 @ 90°

Discussion

This case is an example of the ideal RK patient for retreatment. The absence of fluctuating vision suggests maintenance of adequate corneal stability. Peripheral treatment for hyperopia may cause progressive symptoms that may be more likely in patients with poor corneal stability. Patients should be warned that it is not possible to determine how much glare and night vision issues are coming from irregular astigmatism associated with the original incisions and how much from the refractive error induced by the original RK procedure. Even a surface retreatment may not reduce glare, and as in any refractive procedure, may result in increased problems. Nevertheless, patients who are hyperopic after prior RK surgery are usually gratified by a significant if not complete correction of their refractive error.

Take-Home Points

1. Careful evaluation of the corneal incisions in patients having had RK will dictate the decision regarding the type of hyperopic procedure to be done, surface ablation or LASIK.
2. The surgeon should be prepared to deal with potential segment instability in the corneal flap.

7

CASE 44

A 45-year-old-man presented for LASIK consultation. This patient is quite apprehensive about the procedure and gets nervous when anyone gets close to his eyes. As such, he has never been able to wear contact lenses. After a complete history and evaluation it was determined that he would be a satisfactory candidate for surgery. He chose to have the IntraLase procedure, because he perceives it to be a safer alternative for creating the flap.

			Uncorrected Va
W	OD −5.00 −1.00 × 90° 20/20		OD 20/200
	OS −5.00 − 0.50 × 90° 20/20		OS 20/200
M	OD −5.00 −1.25 × 90° 20/20 Note: minus cylinder form		
	OS −4.75 − 0.75 × 90° 20/20		
C	OD −5.00 −1.25 × 90° 20/20		
	OS −4.75 − 0.75 × 90° 20/20		
K	OD 43.00 × 90°/44.50° × 180°		
	OS 42.75 × 90°/43.50° × 180°		

Pachymetry	Topography	Scotopic Pupils
OD 550 μm	Regular astigmatism	OD 6.5 mm
OS 560 μm	OU	OS 6.5 mm

On the day of treatment he was even more anxious than when examined in the office. He was given twice the normal amount of oral diazepam, 10 mg, 30 minutes preoperatively.

In particular, he disliked the insertion of the speculum just prior to placing the suction ring on the eye, and a strong Bell's reflex was observed. He was encouraged to look straight ahead, suction was applied to the fixation ring, and the applanating lens was brought down on to the cornea. About halfway through the raster pattern ablation, suction was lost and the cone lost contact with the cornea.

Discussion

Suction loss most likely occurred in this patient due to squeezing eye movement during creation of the flap. Other possibilities include a faulty suction ring with a slow leak or the formation of conjunctival chemosis. Suction loss with a microkeratome can result in an incomplete flap, free cap, or no cap at all with a large epithelial defect. When this occurs with a blade keratome, there is typically a time lag of 3 to 6 months before any excimer treatment can be considered, whether it be a repeat LASIK or PRK with adjunctive mitomycin-C to reduce the risk of haze. In contrast, loss of suction during the creation of a laser-made flap is an easier complication to handle.

If suction loss occurs during creation of the flap, the surgeon should first assess the status of the bulbar conjunctiva. If it is fairly chemotic and the likelihood of obtaining good suction is not favorable, the patient should return for treatment another day. If treating on another day, a new applanating cone is used and the flap depth should be set at least 20 μm deeper to avoid creating a wedge of corneal stroma by cutting in two planes of tissue.

If the conjunctiva is not chemotic, the surgeon can reapply the same suction ring (or a new suction ring if the device is felt to be faulty) to the eye. The same applanating lens should be used with the same settings for flap thickness and diameter. The previously treated stromal bed will not be damaged by relasering immediately at the same stromal depth.

If suction is lost during the initial creation of the side cut, the laser can be reprogrammed to make only the side cut. This flap diameter should be reset 0.2 mm smaller to avoid any wedges of stroma being created from the intersection of two side cuts. If suction is lost with 5 or fewer seconds to go during the side cut, only the epithelium remains and the flap edge can be cut with a Vannas scissors at the time the flap is lifted to perform the excimer treatment.

Take-Home Points

1. Suction loss, while rare with the IntraLase, can still occur.
2. Watch the entire treatment carefully in order to recognize a problem and quickly stop the femtosecond laser ablation, if necessary.
3. Retreatment with the IntraLase is possible immediately if suction can be reobtained; otherwise, it is best to return on another day.

7

A 55-year-old man is interested in refractive surgery to decrease his dependence on distance correction. He doesn't wear contact lenses and has no history of ocular trauma or recurrent erosions. He understands he will need reading glasses after surgery.

W	OD−5.00 +1.00 × 90° 20/20 OS −5.25 +1.25 × 90° 20/20 3 years old	**Uncorrected Va** 20/400 OU
M	OD−5.00 +1.00 × 90° 20/20 OS −5.25 +1.25 × 90° 20/20	
C	OD−5.00 +1.00 × 90° 20/20 OS −5.25 +1.25 × 90° 20/20	
K	OD 43.50 × 180°/44.25 × 90° OS 43.50 × 180°/44.50 × 90°	

Pachymetry	**Topography**	**Scotopic Pupils**
OD 540 μm	OD regular bow-tie	OD 6.5 mm
OS 540 μm	OS regular bow-tie	OS 6.5 mm

Additional Examination

The anterior and posterior segment examinations were normal.

The patient undergoes LASIK on the right eye first. After the microkeratome pass, there is an obvious 4 × 3 mm central corneal irregularity. How would you proceed?

The surgeon uses a dry cellulose sponge to try to determine whether it is simply epithelial loosening or whether the stromal aspect of the flap is also irregular. It is felt that the flap stroma is normal. The surgeon then gently lifts the flap, taking care not to traumatize the epithelium, and inspects the underside of the flap and the stromal bed for evidence of irregularity, for example, a buttonhole. Once it is determined that the underside of the flap appears regular and the size of the stromal bed is large enough to fit the planned laser ablation, the laser treatment is applied. The flap is floated into position and the interface irrigated. Once the flap rests in good position, the epithelium is very delicately moved with a moist cellulose sponge into as normal an anatomic configuration as possible. The flap is left to adhere for several minutes. A bandage soft contact lens (BSCL), Focus Night & Day, 8.6/−0.50, is placed on the eye. Due to the potential problems of a large area of epithelial loosening, such as delayed visual rehabilitation and increased risk of DLK and epithelial ingrowth, it is decided not to proceed with surgery on the fellow eye that day. The patient is placed on a fluoroquinolone and prednisolone 1% drops four times a day, and frequent preservative-free artificial tears.

The patient is seen the following day. The uncorrected and best-corrected vision is 20/400 OD. Slit-lamp examination reveals that the BSCL is in good position. There is a central oval area of epithelial whitening measuring approximately 3 × 4 mm (Case 45, Figs. 1 and 2). There is minimal stromal inflammation, no stromal infiltrate and the anterior chamber is deep and quiet. The patient is followed every 1 to 2 days for a week at which time the BSCL was removed. Over that time, the size of the whitened epithelium becomes smaller and smaller and eventually disappears. The uncorrected vision reaches 20/30 and with a correction of −1.00 + 0.50 × 90, the visual acuity improves to 20/20−2. Slit-lamp examination reveals mild microstriae and trace interface haze.

Discussion

Risk factors for epithelial loosening/defect include a history of recurrent erosions, anterior basement membrane dystrophy, and increased age. Patients at higher risk for epithelial loosening/defect should be informed of this risk preoperatively. Some patients might select a surface ablation procedure instead of LASIK. Many surgeons consider anterior basement membrane dystrophy as a contraindication to LASIK.

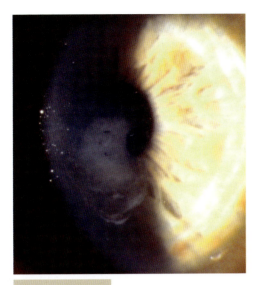

Case 45, Figure 1

Epithelial slippage. (Courtesy Christopher J. Rapuano, M.D.)

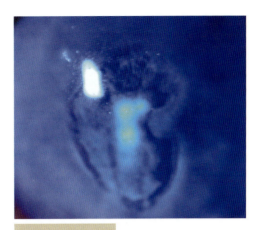

Case 45, Figure 2

Same cornea as Fig. 1 with fluorescein instilled and cobalt blue illumination. (Courtesy Christopher J. Rapuano, M.D.)

Prior to proceeding with LASIK in such patients, several precautions should be taken to decrease the risk of epithelial problems. Preoperative dry eye syndrome and blepharitis should be treated. A microkeratome with a lower risk of epithelial trauma (e.g., a Hansatome with a Zero Compression head or a femtosecond laser) should be selected when available. The eye should be anesthetized with the smallest effective dose of topical anesthetic, just prior to the procedure. The cornea should be well lubricated just before the microkeratome pass.

Once an area of loosening or defect is noted after the flap is created, it is critical to determine whether the flap stroma and the interface are normal. If so, the laser ablation can be performed. If not, the laser treatment should probably be deferred. If the epithelium is loose, the surgeon must decide whether to attempt to replace it in its original location or remove it and allow new epithelium to grow in. Generally, if the epithelium appears viable (i.e., not shredded), it is reasonable to attempt to replace it. Either way a BSCL is usually placed. With any epithelial irregularity, there is an increased risk of DLK and microstriae. If the epithelial irregularity involves the flap edge, there is also an increased risk of epithelial ingrowth. When properly managed, these eyes can do very well. Remember, when there is an untoward event in the first eye, it is often best not to proceed with surgery on the fellow eye on the same day.

Surgical Plan

	Right Eye	**Left Eye**	**Comments**
Treat cycloplegic refraction in negative cylinder	$-4.00 - 1.00 \times 180$	$-4.25 - 1.25 \times 180$	
Ring size (Amadeus microkeratome)	9.0 or 9.5 mm	9.0 or 9.5 mm	A larger flap allows for adequate exposure if a hyperopic enhancement is required

continued

	Right Eye	Left Eye	Comments
Plate size	140 μm	140 μm	Amadeus microkeratome
Optical zone (VISX laser)	6.5 mm	6.5 mm	Larger treatment zone decreases risk of visual aberrations
Transition zone	8.0 mm	8.0 mm	A blend zone decreases risk of visual aberrations
Calculations (see Chapter 2 for alternative nomogram)	−4.00 D (−15%) = −3.40 D sphere	−4.00 D (−15%) = −3.40 D sphere	Subtract 15% as over age 40
Spherical treatment Cylinder treatment	−3.40 D −0.90 D × 180	−3.40 D −1.17 D × 180	Subtract 10% of cylinder
Approximate ablation depth	54 μm	54 μm	
Residual stromal thickness	540 μm − 140 μm −54 μm = 346 μm >250 μm	540 μm − 140 μm −54 μm = 346 μm >250 μm	

Take-Home Points

1. Corneas need to be examined carefully preoperatively. If anterior basement membrane dystrophy is present, think twice about proceeding with LASIK.
2. Loose epithelium should be replaced in its original location at the end of the procedure.
3. When there is an untoward event in the first eye, it often best not to proceed with surgery on the fellow eye the same day, because there may be delayed visual rehabilitation with suboptimal final results, and there is a higher risk of a similar problem in the fellow eye.

CASE 46

A 26-year-old man with a stable refraction desires improved uncorrected vision. He has been out of his DWSCL for 2 weeks. He has no history of ocular trauma or recurrent erosions.

		Uncorrected Va
W	OD−5.00 20/20 OS −5.00 20/20 3 years old	20/400 20/400
M	OD−5.00 20/20 OS −5.00 20/20	
C	OD−5.00 20/20 OS −5.00 20/20	
K	OD 40.00 × 180°/40.50 × 90° OS 40.50 × 180°/41.00 × 90°	

Pachymetry	Topography	Scotopic Pupils
OD 550 μm OS 550 μm	OD regular bow-tie OS regular bow-tie	OD 6.5 mm OS 6.5 mm

Additional Examination

The anterior and posterior segment examinations are normal.

Surgical Plan

	Right Eye	Left Eye	Comments
Treat cycloplegic refraction	−5.00 D	−5.00 D	
Ring size (Amadeus microkeratome)	9.5 mm	9.5 mm	Flat K's increase the risk of a free cap. Use a larger suction ring and larger hinge
Hinge size	0.9 mm	0.9 mm	
Plate size	160 μm	160 μm	Amadeus microkeratome
Optical zone VISX STAR S4	6.5 mm	6.5 mm	Larger treatment zone decreases risk of visual aberrations
Transition zone	8.0 mm	8.0 mm	A blend zone decreases risk of visual aberrations
Calculations	−5.00 (−10%) = −4.50 D sphere	−5.00 (−10%) = −4.50 D sphere	Subtract 10% as under age 30 years
Spherical treatment	−4.50 D	−4.50 D	
Approximate ablation depth	60 μm	60 μm	
Residual stromal thickness	550 μm − 160 μm −60 μm = 330 μm >250 μm	550 μm −160 μm −60 μm = 330 μm >250 μm	

Discussion

Due to the flat keratometry readings, the patient was warned he had a higher risk of a free cap with LASIK. The option of a surface ablation procedure was discussed, but the patient wanted to proceed with LASIK. What adjustments would you make in this case?

A large suction ring, 9.5 mm, and a large hinge width, 0.9 mm, are selected based on the nomogram provided by the microkeratome manufacturer. Additionally, a 160-μm rather than a 140-μm plate is selected, to give a little more thickness to the hinge. Heavy, asymmetric gentian violet marks are made on the right cornea, so they do not wash away during the procedure. Suction is obtained without difficulty. The pupil dilates, the tonometry is >65 mmHg, and the patient notes the light dim. The flap is created. As the blade retracts, the surgeon watches the ink marks on the flap to make sure the flap remains on the cornea and not in the microkeratome. The flap is slowly lifted and moved to the side, taking great care to place minimal stress on the hinge. The hinge is noted to be small, but intact. The ablation is performed without difficulty and the interface is irrigated and the flap replaced, aligning the ink marks. Again, minimal stress is placed on the hinge. The flap is allowed to adhere for 4 minutes, 1.5 minutes longer than average. Would you proceed with surgery on the left eye and, if so, would you make any changes to the treatment plan?

The decision is made to proceed with LASIK on the left. The microkeratome hinge width is adjusted to 1.0 mm for the left eye. Because the keratometry readings are slightly steeper on the left, along with a larger programmed hinge, the surgeon felt the risk of a free cap was small. Again, the cornea is marked, suction obtained, the microkeratome pass performed, and the blade retracted with the flap in place. However, as the flap is moved to the side, it is clearly a perfectly circular free cap. It is placed epithelial side down on the nasal conjunctiva. The stromal bed is inspected and is felt to be uniform and large enough for the planned ablation, which is then performed without difficulty. The free cap is then replaced, right side up, on the stromal bed. Holding the edge gently with fine forceps, the interface is gently irrigated and then the free cap positioned, taking great care to line up the ink marks. The gutter is dried to make sure it is uniform for 360 degrees. The cap is allowed to adhere for 5 minutes after which a BSCL, Focus Night & Day 8.6/−0.50, is placed. He is placed on topical fluoroquinolone, prednisolone 1%, and preservative-free tears OU. The patient is told about the free cap and the danger of rubbing or touching his eye and to contact the surgeon immediately with any increase in pain or should the contact lens come out.

He is seen the following day. The flap on the right and the free cap on the left are in excellent position. He is seen 2 days later and 2 days after that at which time the BSCL is carefully removed without difficulty. The patient ends up happy with very good uncorrected vision. He is told that a future LASIK enhancement would be more difficult due to the free cap and, if necessary, a surface ablation might be a better option.

Flat corneas increase the risk of smaller flaps and free caps with mechanical microkeratomes. Adjustments for flap corneas include larger suction rings and larger hinge widths. However, these adjustments are not always successful. A free cap is less likely when a femtosecond laser is used to make the flap provided care is taken to dissect the flap after it has been created. The femtosecond laser flap is not dependent on corneal curvature.

In retrospect, what else could have been done to prevent the small hinge on the right and the free cap on the left? Certainly, a surface ablation procedure could have been performed. With LASIK, an even thicker flap, for example, a 180-μm flap could have been used. For the second eye, when there is a small hinge on the first, a new microkeratome blade might result in a thicker flap with a slightly more substantial hinge. Once the free cap occurred, another option would have been to place one or four interrupted 10-0 nylon sutures to secure the cap for a few days or weeks.

Once a free cap is noted, it must be located and protected. It may remain in the microkeratome and be damaged or discarded by the technician. Once it is safely stored (typically epithelial side down on a moist surface such as conjunctiva or a wet 4 × 4 gauze pad) the stromal bed needs to be inspected for uniformity and size to determine whether the laser ablation can be done. The cap then needs to be replaced in its original position using the ink marks and checking the gutter. If a free cap is small, the marks may not reach the edge of the cap. Extra care must be taken to align the flap properly in this challenging situation. Managed properly, eyes with free caps can end up with excellent visual results. In fact, prior to the advent of the flap hinge, LASIK procedures were performed with intentional free caps.

Take-Home Points

1. Pay attention to the corneal curvature during the preoperative evaluation to appropriately inform the patient of the surgical risks.
2. Adjust the microkeratome settings to decrease the chance of suboptimal flaps.
3. Mark the cornea to aid in proper replacement of the flap or free cap.
4. When removing the microkeratome from the eye, make sure the flap is on the cornea.

CASE 47

A 45-year-old woman with a stable refraction of −6.00 D, normal anterior and posterior segment examinations, normal topography, pachymetry, and pupil size undergoes LASIK. Asymmetric gentian violet marks are made temporally and superiorly. A Chiron (now Bausch & Lomb) Automated Corneal Shaper (ACS) microkeratome is used to make the LASIK flap. The technician alerts the surgeon that suction is achieved according to the machine. The patient tells the surgeon that the light has dimmed. The Barraquer tonometer does not demonstrate a consistently small circle. How would you proceed?

Because the tonometer did not confirm proper suction, the surgeon should have released the suction ring, checked the microkeratome, and reattempted to achieve adequate suction. Instead the surgeon proceeds with creation of the flap. After the pass is made and the microkeratome is removed from the eye, the corneal surface appears irregular. The surgeon makes sure the technician does not clean the microkeratome until he checks the cornea and makes certain there are no missing pieces of cornea. The surgeon then carefully examines the cornea to figure out whether the flap epithelium and/or stroma are abnormal. It is clear that a shredded flap stroma is present. The temporal edge of the flap is relatively normal appearing, although the flap in that area is definitely thinner than usual. Approximately one-third of the way across the cornea, the flap becomes very irregular and becomes a completely free cap with jagged edges about two-thirds of the way across the cornea. How would you proceed?

The best option at this point is to attempt to replace all the pieces of cornea into their original orientation. This maneuver can be achieved with fine forceps and dry and moist cellulose sponges. If any pieces are missing, the microkeratome needs to be inspected again searching for any lost tissue. Once the epithelium and stroma are pieced back together, and allowed to adhere for several minutes, a BSCL is placed, fluoroquinolone and prednisolone 1% drops are instilled, and the eyelid speculum carefully removed. The patient is examined at the slit lamp immediately and again 30 minutes later. The patient is placed on a topical fluoroquinolone and prednisolone 1% drops four times daily and seen the following morning.

The patient's best-corrected visual acuity (BCVA) is 20/25 with approximately the same refraction as preoperatively. The BSCL is removed on postoperative day 4; the epithelial surface is intact and the stroma quite smooth. Over the next several months the BCVA returns to 20/20. Treatment options, including repeat LASIK with a microkeratome or femtosecond laser and transepithelial PRK with or without mitomycin-C, are discussed with the patient. The patient elects not to proceed with refractive surgery and to continue with contact lens wear.

Discussion

One of the worst intraoperative complications during LASIK is a shredded flap. It is unlikely to occur (1) if the machine registers good suction, (2) the patient says the light has dimmed, and (3) the IOP measures >65 mmHg. Most surgeons use a Barraquer tonometer or pneumotonometer to check the pressure. If these three conditions are not met, it is often best to stop. Release suction and recheck the machinery and try again. Occasionally "pseudosuction" is achieved, meaning that the suction ports are occluded with conjunctiva, so the machine senses adequate suction, but the IOP is not adequately elevated. Suction may be adequate as the microkeratome pass is started, but can be lost during creation of the flap (often related to patient movement or squeezing), which can shred or amputate a flap. Future treatment options include repeat LASIK with a microkeratome or laser and transepithelial PRK with or without mitomycin-C.

Take-Home Points

1. Use multiple methods to make sure the IOP is adequate to safely create the flap.
2. Whatever the cause, if the stromal component of the flap is not perfect, the pieces should be replaced in their original position (as best as possible), a BSCL placed, and no laser treatment applied.
3. When there is an untoward event in the first eye, it often best not to proceed with surgery on the fellow eye the same day.

POSTOPERATIVE DECISION MAKING

The cases presented in this section cover postoperative management issues such as enhancement, dry eye, striae, epithelial ingrowth, buttonhole, flap displacement, diffuse lamellar keratitis (DLK), and infection. While there are some simple cases, many of the cases are fairly complex. The indexes for these cases are combined with the intraoperative decision-making cases. The cases are arranged according to issue as much as is practical. The format may vary depending on the nature of the case and the author.

Intraoperative and Postoperative Planning Index			
Patient Characteristic	**Case Number**	**Page Number**	**Contributor**
Anisometropia	57	227	Steven Rosenfeld
Astigmatism	54	224	Michael Rosenberg
	57	227	Steven Rosenfeld
Astigmatism mixed	55	224	Colman Kraff
Bandage contact lens	45	208	Christopher J. Rapuano
	46	210	Christopher J. Rapuano
Basement membrane dystrophy	45	208	Christopher J. Rapuano
Bleeding under flap or on stromal bed	41	202	Robert S. Feder
Blepharospasm	66	238	Steven Rosenfeld
Buttonhole	62	234	Robert S. Feder
	67	239	Parag Majmudar
	68	241	Robert S. Feder
Cataract	58	229	Christopher J. Rapuano
Conductive keratoplasty	56	225	Lawrence Gans
Cornea transplant	57	227	Steven Rosenfeld
Custom ablation	49	218	Michael Rosenberg
	50	219	Colman Kraff
Diabetes	41	202	Robert S. Feder
Diffuse lamellar keratitis (DLK)	71	246	Christopher J. Rapuano
	72	247	Michael Vrabec
	73	249	Christopher J. Rapuano
	74	249	Robert S. Feder
Dry eye	41	202	Robert S. Feder
	59	230	Christopher J. Rapuano
Enhancement	48	217	Michael Rosenberg
	49	218	Michael Rosenberg
	50	219	Colman Kraff
	52	222	Parag Majmudar
	53	223	Michael Rosenberg
	54	224	Michael Rosenberg
	55	224	Colman Kraff
	56	225	Lawrence Gans
	57	227	Steven Rosenfeld
	65	237	Michael Rosenberg
	66	238	Steven Rosenfeld

continued

continued

4. Anytime there is a significant discrepancy between the manifest and WaveScan refraction, it is best to err on the side of the manifest refraction and not perform the CustomVue treatment.

CASE 51

After 3 months, the patient in Case 23 had stabilized. The corneal surface was smooth and the minimal corneal haze had faded. The patient's uncorrected Va was 20/15 OD and 20/50 OS. The refractive error was plano OD and +1.50 + 0.50 × 155° OS. Therefore, the patient was overcorrected and hyperopic OS. Because the postoperative refractions were stable and the residual corneal thickness was adequate, a repeat treatment OS was planned.

W	OD none OS none	**Uncorrected Va** 20/15 20/50–
M	OD Plano OS +1.00 + 0.50 x 155°	
C	OD Plano 20/20 OS +1.50 + 0.50 x 155° 20/20	
K	OD not tested OS 41.00 x 132°/40.50 x 42°	

Pachymetry	**Topography**	**Scotopic Pupils**
OD not tested OS 380 μm	Normal central flattening S/P PRK OS	OD 6.5 mm OS 6.5 mm

Discussion

Because the 46-year-old patient was unhappy with her hyperopic refractive error OS, a retreatment was performed.

Surgical Plan: First Retreatment

	Left Eye	**Comments**
Do not perform further laser if the cornea is too thin. Make sure postoperative refractive error is stable.		
Ring size	None—PRK	Too thin for LASIK
Plate size	None—PRK	
Ablation zone	6.5 mm with 8.0-mm blend	Pupil = 6.5 mm
Spherical equivalent	+1.75 D	
Conventional surface treatment based on manifest and cycloplegic refractions Treatment is entered in minus cylinder form	+1.75 D sphere 0.50 D × 155° +1.75 − 0.50 × 65°	There is no nomogram adjustment with PRK
Ablation depth	32 μm	The Alcon software calculates the ablation depth
Residual stromal thickness	380 μm − 32 μm = 348 μm	Must be >250 μm

W	OD none OS none	**Uncorrected Va** 20/20 20/30
M	OD – 0.50 20/20 OS –1.00 20/25	
C	OD Plano 20/20 OS –1.00 20/25	
K	OD Not tested OS 40.90 x 132/40.50 x 042	

Pachymetry	**Topography**	**Scotopic Pupils**
OD not tested OS 345 μm	Expected central flattening and depression OS	OD 6.5 mm OS 6.5 mm

The patient's original PRK was performed in February 2002; the enhancement charted above was performed in July 2002. By June 2004, the patient's uncorrected Va was 20/20 OD and 20/30 OS (see data chart above). There was a refractive error of −0.50 OD and −1.00 OS. The patient complained of poor night vision and poor contrast sensitivity OS. Wavefront testing revealed a RMS of 0.76 μm OS with high horizontal coma, spherical aberration, trefoil, and tetrafoil OS. It was decided to enhance the left eye with a wavefront-guided custom PRK in March 2005.

Second Discussion

Alcon wavefront testing was performed twice in the left eye with consistent results. An Alcon wavefront-guided custom PRK was performed in March 2005 because of poor visual acuity from residual myopic refractive error and pronounced higher order aberrations. Corneal thickness was determined and found to be adequate at 345 μm. The refractive error and corneal healing were stable from the retreatment almost 3 years previously. Four months after the wavefront-guided custom PRK OS the patient is extremely happy with 20/20 uncorrected Va OS, a plano refraction OS, and a reduction of the higher order aberrations with a RMS of 0.32 μm.

Surgical Plan: Second Retreatment

	Right Eye	**Left Eye**	**Comments**
	Test the patient vision with the wavefront-derived refraction in phoropter before committing her to treatment.		
Ring size	None—PRK	None—PRK	Too thin for LASIK
Plate size	None—PRK	None—PRK	
Ablation zone		6.5 mm with blend	Standard for custom ablation
Spherical equivalent		−1.00 D	
CustomCornea treatment based on Alcon wavefront measurements	No treatment performed OD	−0.50 D sphere 0.55 D × 175°	There is no nomogram adjustment with PRK. An offset of +0.25 D was programmed to reduce the spherical treatment
Ablation depth		30 μm	The Alcon software calculates the ablation depth
Residual stromal thickness		345 μm − 30 μm = 315 μm	>250 μm

7

2. Any haze or keratitis associated with the primary treatment must be treated or allowed to clear prior to retreatment.

CASE 54

A 44-year-old man had LASIK in both eyes. Three months after the procedure he continued to complain of difficulty with intermittent blurry vision, and persistent haloes and star-bursting phenomenon at night. The LASIK flaps were without striae, keratitis, epithelial in-growth, or fluorescein staining. Topography confirmed well-centered ablations OU. Essential data are shown in the following table. Limbal relaxing incisions (LRIs) were performed in each eye using paired 30-degree arcs in the right eye, and paired 45-degree arcs in the left eye. See Chapters 4 and 6, respectively, on retreatment and alternatives to LASIK for more information on the LRI technique.

	Right Eye	Left Eye
Original cycloplegic refraction	−9.50 + 1.25 × 105°	−9.75 + 1.50 × 70°
Original keratometry	44.25 × 45.25 @ 60°	44.25 × 46.00 @ 70°
Original pachymetry	629 μm	619 μm
Scotopic pupil	6.5 mm	6.5 mm
UCVA before LRI	20/25−	20/40
Cycloplegic refraction before LRI	−0.25 + 0.75 × 30° 20/20	−1.25 + 1.00 × 40° 20/20
Keratometry before LRI	39.25 × 40.00 @ 30°	38.75 × 39.25 @ 45°
Pachymetry before LRI	498 μm central 670 μm peripheral	485 μm central 672 μm peripheral
UCVA after LRI	20/20−	20/20−

Discussion

The patient had a residual refractive error in each eye, with oblique astigmatism as the primary abnormality. The spherical equivalent in each eye was about +0.25. Patients with residual "with-the-rule" or "against-the-rule" astigmatism have fewer subjective complaints than patients with oblique astigmatism. Because our general environment is oriented primarily vertically and horizontally, for most patients with astigmatism, at least one of these orientations is in relatively good focus, and patients are able to interpret what they are seeing accurately. Patients with oblique astigmatism have a blur for both vertically and horizontally oriented borders and, therefore, have more subjective complaints.

Take-Home Points

1. The elimination of oblique astigmatism frequently results in a subjective improvement out of proportion to any modest improvement in visual acuity.
2. Limbal relaxing incisions are an easy and safe way to reduce or eliminate residual astigmatism in patients with a spherical equivalent close to zero.

CASE 55

This 45-year-old man was originally treated with conventional LASIK for mixed astigmatism. His preoperative refraction was OD −1.00 + 4.00 × 120° 20/20 and OS −0.75 + 4.25 × 88° 20/20. Six months postoperatively the patient had an UCVA of 20/20 OU, but was lost to follow up until 4 years later. He then presented with complaints of decreased vision and was found to have residual refractive error OD.

W	No correction	**Uncorrected Va** 20/30−2 20/20
M	OD +0.25 + 1.50 x 100° 20/20 OS Plano	
C	OD +0.50 + 1.00 x 95° 20/20 OS +0.25	
WR	OD +1.32 + 0.85 x 95° RMS 2.09 19.9% HOA	
K	OD 43.12 x 175°/44.00 x 85°	

Pachymetry	**Topography**	**Scotopic Pupils**
OD 550 μm OS 550 μm	No cone	OD 6.5 mm OS 7.0 mm

Discussion

Following a complete examination, enhancement of the right eye using CustomVue was recommended. The difference between manifest and WaveScan refraction prompted an adjustment of −0.75 D toward an intended postoperative goal of plano. The standard 6.0-mm optical zone and 9.0-mm ablation zone were set. The patient was originally treated with the Hansatome (160-μm head and 9.5-mm ring). The maximum retreatment depth calculated by the CustomVue software was 23 μm. The patient would still be left with an RST of at least 367 μm postoperatively. The flap was marked at the slit lamp and lifted with the patient under the laser. Flaps can still be lifted even several years postoperatively. After several years flaps will occasionally demonstrate a prominent edge or a fibrotic appearance. These flaps can be a little more difficult to lift and care must be taken to carefully break the edge adhesions with a blunt fine-tipped spatula. The surgeon needs to be aware of where the original hinge location was in order not to tear it. In this case treatment proceeded in an uncomplicated fashion.

At 1-week postoperatively the patient had a plano refraction and a UCVA of 20/20−2. He was quite satisfied.

Take-Home Points

1. Custom enhancements can be performed after prior conventional LASIK.
2. The surgeon should be careful to make sure that the correlation between the subjective refraction and WaveScan refraction is close.
3. If a significant deviation exists between the two, then it might be best not to perform a WaveScan enhancement and to instead stick with a conventional treatment.
4. Adequate residual stromal bed thickness is extremely important.
5. Even years after LASIK surgery it may be possible to lift the flap.

CASE 56

A 44-year-old woman had LASIK performed 6 years previously to correct myopic astigmatism, and until 2 years ago she was happy with her uncorrected vision. At that time she began to notice the increasing need for reading glasses; and now she finds that she cannot dial her cell phone or even read her watch without them. Review of her previous surgery indicates that her preoperative correction was −5.00 D OD and −5.50 D OS. Her flaps were created with an 8.5-mm microkeratome ring. She is OS dominant.

7

	OD	OS
Uncorrected near vision	J8	J8
Near correction	+2.00 add J2	+1.00 add J4
Manifest refraction	+0.50 20/20	Plano 20/20
Cycloplegic refraction	+1.00 20/20	+0.75 20/20
Keratometry	39.50 × 39.50 @ 90°	39.00 × 39.50 @ 90°
Pachymetry	480 μm	477 μm
Scotopic pupil	6.4 mm	6.5 mm

The flap margins are difficult to see but are 7.0 mm in diameter with a nasal hinge in each eye. The rest of the anterior and posterior segment examination is normal.

Discussion

Presbyopia may become an increasingly common complaint as previously well-corrected LASIK patients get older. It presents earlier in myopic patients who were overcorrected. Even though prepared for this eventuality by counseling and informed consents, when the reality hits, patients express dissatisfaction and seek some remedy. There are three reasonable surgical options to present. LASIK enhancement can be performed to produce monovision with near correction in the nondominant eye. A contact lens trial will help define the amount of correction that gives comfortable monovision. The nondominant eye is generally felt to be the best choice for monovision near correction, but there are some people who are more comfortable the other way.

Near vision conductive keratoplasty (NVCK) has been used to correct presbyopia in previously unoperated eyes. It can be used to induce myopia in eyes after LASIK, but there are significant differences in the effect produced by the surgery in these eyes. There is an exaggerated response to the CK such that minimal treatment can produce a dramatic refractive correction. Thus only one ring of eight applications is typically applied and it can be performed with a 9.0-mm optical zone and still provide a robust correction. Because this probably depends on how much thinning the previous LASIK created, it is difficult to get a precise refractive correction in these cases. When NVCK is performed on post-LASIK eyes, the refractive effect is more like monovision with contact lens wear. These patients do not typically get back good distance vision in the operated eye and tend to rely on one eye for distance and the other for near vision rather than the blended effect produced by CK surgery in natural presbyopes.

The last option is clear lens exchange with an accommodative or multifocal implant. This can produce excellent distance and near vision and eliminates any future concerns of cataract development. This choice requires intraocular surgery for both eyes. With these lens implants, the precise refractive outcome is crucial to success, and it may be difficult to calculate the precise implant power in some patients after LASIK.

Surgical Plan

The patient decided to have NVCK surgery and wore a +2.50 corrective contact lens for a week in her nondominant right eye to be sure that she would tolerate the correction. After a week, she felt that a stronger correction was needed and this lens power was increased to +3.00. She tolerated this well and had an 8-spot Light Touch CK performed at an 8.5-mm-diameter. All the spots were outside of her flap and the flap remained secure. She had a 1-week correction of −2.75 − 0.50 × 65° that gradually regressed to a 6-week refraction of −2.00 − 0.50 × 50° for an UCNV of J2.

Take-Home Points

1. True monovision may not be comfortable for some patients, and a contact lens trial will help determine the eye and the appropriate lens power. Do not just assume that the nondominant eye is the best eye for reading correction.

2. Consider clear lens exchange with an accommodative or multifocal IOL for people who cannot tolerate monovision. Use sophisticated techniques to determine the proper lens power because an accurate refractive result is critical to success with these lenses.
3. CK after laser vision correction produces true monovision rather than blended vision. Prepare patients for the fact that their uncorrected distance vision will not come back in the treated eye.
4. CK after laser vision correction produces a more dramatic refractive change than in eyes that have not had prior surgery. A minimal treatment can produce an exaggerated effect.

CASE 57

This 77-year-old woman had long-standing Fuchs corneal dystrophy and had previously undergone cataract extraction with posterior chamber IOLs in both eyes. She subsequently developed pseudophakic bullous keratopathy and underwent a penetrating keratoplasty (PK) OD. She was left with significant postkeratoplasty astigmatism OD after all the sutures had been removed, measuring 7 D by keratometry and 8 D on refraction. Her best spectacle-corrected vision was 20/200. Although a rigid gas-permeable (RGP) contact lens trial improved her vision to 20/25 OD, she could not manipulate the contact lens.

W	OD Plano	Uncorrected Va: OD 20/400
M	OD −1.50 − 8.00 x 73°	
C	OD −1.50 − 8.00 x 73° 20/20	
K	OD: 44.50 x 84°/55.00 x 174°	

Pachymetry	Topography	Scotopic Pupil
586 μm	OD asymmetric ATR astigmatism	OD 3.5 mm

Myopic LASIK was performed OD in an effort to improve her best spectacle corrected vision and restore binocular vision.

Surgical Plan

	Right Eye	Comments
Ring size	+2	
Microkeratome head	130 μm	Moria usually cuts a 160-μm flap
Ablation zone	6.5 mm	
Cycloplegic Rx	−1.50 − 8.00 × 73°	
Calculations with nomogram correction (VISX)	95% factor for −1.23 − 4.00 × 73°	VISX could only treat 4 D of astigmatism
Flap thickness	160 μm	Assumed
Ablation depth (from tables)	68 μm	Deliberate under correction
Residual stromal thickness	586 μm − 160 μm −68 μm = 358 μm	Estimated >250 μm

The VISX laser was only approved to treat astigmatism of ≤4.0 D. We deliberately attempted to keep her mildly myopic, knowing that she would need an enhancement to further reduce her astigmatism. Four and one-half months later, her preoperative refraction of −1.50 − 8.00 × 75° had improved to $-2.25 - 5.00 \times 90°$ correcting her to 20/40, but the anisometropia still contributed to discomfort wearing this eyeglass prescription. Her keratometry measured $46.0 \times 52.6 @ 177°$. A pair of corneal relaxing incisions was placed along the horizontal meridian to try to reduce the postkeratoplasty astigmatism further. Four months after the relaxing incisions, her refraction improved to $-6.00 - 2.00 \times 100$ giving 20/30 vision, and her keratometry readings were 47.00 D $\times$ 48.75 D @ 27°.

Because we had successfully reduced the astigmatism, but increased the spherical myopia because of the coupling effect, we needed further manipulations to reduce the anisometropia. A repeat LASIK finally succeeded in reducing her refractive error to a level of 20/30 uncorrected. Finally, 4½ years after her penetrating keratoplasty, we had achieved excellent uncorrected vision OD and comfortable binocular vision.

Retreatment Plan after Relaxing Incisions

	Right Eye	Comments
Ring size	+2	
Microkeratome head	130 μm	Moria cuts a 160-μm flap
Ablation zone	6.5 mm	
Cycloplegic Rx	$-6.00 -2.00 \times 100$	
Calculations with nomogram correction (VISX)	90% factor for $-5.40 - 2.00 \times 100$	
Flap thickness	160 μm	Assumed
Ablation depth	89 μm	Pachymetry 558 μm prior to this LASIK
Residual stromal thickness	309 μm	

This case illustrates the difficulty of trying to treat large amounts of astigmatism with LASIK. LASIK will often not eliminate more than 4 D of astigmatism. Corneal relaxing incisions with or without compression sutures are more reliable at reducing high degrees of postkeratoplasty astigmatism than LASIK. One must always take into account the coupling effect of corneal surgery. Based on spherical equivalents, every 2 D of astigmatism reduced by tissue sparing corneal surgery (such as relaxing incisions or radial keratometry) will result in 1–2 D of increased steepening in the flat meridian. In retrospect, the relaxing incisions could probably have been performed before the LASIK. Note, however, that LASIK performed in the presence of deep keratotomy incisions increases the risk of wound rupture from increased IOP during flap creation.

LASIK flaps should generally be made larger than the graft diameter to reduce the chance of disrupting the keratoplasty wound. Some surgeons do not perform the excimer treatment immediately after the flap is cut, because significant changes in refractive error can result from simply creating a flap. The laser is later applied as a retreatment. In this case a second LASIK flap was cut at the same depth as the first. This increased the likelihood of an irregular stromal bed. If possible a second flap should be cut at a deeper level to avoid partially cutting into the first flap. Perhaps better alternatives to a second flap cut would be relifting the first flap or performing PRK with adjunctive MMC to prevent haze.

Finally, pachymetry should be carefully considered as an indicator of the health of the graft endothelium. If the cornea is somewhat thick, the endothelium may no longer be robust and flap adherence following LASIK may be an issue.

Take-Home Points
1. LASIK is an excellent procedure for correcting postoperative refractive error following intraocular surgery such as cataract surgery and penetrating keratoplasty.
2. The potential advantages of LASIK include the ability to relift the flap and perform enhancements if the desired refractive results are not obtained. The potential disadvantages of LASIK over a penetrating keratoplasty include the risk of rupturing the PK wound from the elevated

intraocular pressure during attachment of the suction ring, a risk of rejection of the corneal transplant, and a less reliable refractive response compared to pristine corneas.

3. Corneal relaxing incisions with or without augmentation sutures are more reliable than LASIK for reducing high degrees of postkeratoplasty astigmatism.

CASE 58

A 62-year-old man who underwent bilateral myopic LASIK 8 years previously complains of slowly progressive decreased vision starting about 1 year ago. He says his uncorrected distance vision was very good after his LASIK, although he did need reading glasses. During the past year he feels he is somewhat less dependent on his reading glasses.

Manifest refraction reveals mild myopia but does not improve his vision to a satisfactory level. Slit-lamp examination demonstrates a clear cornea with well-healed LASIK flaps and nasal hinges. The rest of the anterior and posterior segment examinations are unremarkable except for moderate nuclear sclerotic cataracts OU.

W +2.75 readers J3 OU	**Uncorrected Va** OD 20/50 OS 20/50	
M OD –1.00 + 0.50 x 90° 20/40 OS –1.00 + 0.50 x 90° 20/40		
C OD –1.00 + 0.50 x 90° 20/40 OS –1.00 + 0.50 x 90° 20/40		
K OD 39.5 x 180°/40.50 x 90° OS 39.5 x 180°/40.50 x 90°		

Pachymetry	Topography	Scotopic Pupils
OD 480 μm	Central symmetrical	OD 5.5 mm
OS 480 μm	flattening OU	OS 5.5 mm

The patient is unhappy with both his uncorrected and best-corrected visual function, and wants to discuss cataract surgery. What are the important issues with cataract surgery after LASIK?

Discussion

The most important issue is that intraocular lens (IOL) calculations are not as accurate after keratorefractive surgery. To make this problem worse, these patients generally expect to see well without correction following cataract surgery.

It is challenging to determine the actual corneal power after keratorefractive surgery. Multiple factors contribute to this difficulty. Small optical zones, especially after radial keratotomy, lead to inaccurate keratometry measurements since keratometers and most corneal topography machines measure the corneal curvature from data points several millimeters away from the center of the cornea. In addition, the anterior and posterior corneal curvatures do not resemble each other, especially after excimer laser surgery, which can lead to inaccurate results. Because the measured keratometry and simulated K readings are higher than the real central corneal power, the pseudophakic refractive result will be hyperopic. The converse is true for eyes after refractive surgery for hyperopia. Therefore, more accurate assessment of the corneal power must be obtained.

A variety of techniques are available for improving the accuracy of IOL calculations after keratorefractive surgery. One of the most reliable is the "clinical history method." This method can only be used if the preoperative keratometry and the pre- and postoperative refractive measurements are known. The preoperative keratometry is adjusted by the refractive effect of the surgery (adjusted to the corneal plane). For example, if the preoperative average keratometry reading is 45.00 D and the preoperative refraction was −5.00 D (vertex distance 12 mm) and the postoperative refractive was plano, the change in keratometry reading would be $-5/(1-(0.012x-5)) = 4.7$ so the new keratometry reading would be $45 - 4.7 = 40.3$ D.

Other methods depend on how much preoperative information is available. If only the pre- and postoperative refractions are known, another method involves adding 20% of the change in refraction to the current keratometry reading. For example, if the preoperative refraction was −5.50 D and the stable postoperative refraction (prior to any myopic shift from cataract) was −0.5 D, then the change in refraction was −5.00 D; and 20% of −5 D is −1. The current measured keratometry reading is 40 D so the "new" keratometry reading would be $40 + -1$ D $= 39$ D.

When no preoperative information is available, a "hard contact lens method" can be used, but the visual acuity must be adequate for this method to work. A hard contact lens of known base curve and power is placed on the eye. The eye is then refracted. The new refraction is compared to the refraction without the contact lens. The difference is subtracted from the curvature of the contact lens.

The modern third-generation theoretical optical formulas (e.g., Holladay 2, Hoffer Q, SRK/T, Haigis) are generally thought to be more accurate after keratorefractive surgery than the empirical regression formulas (e.g., SRK I, SRK II). Several methods should be used and the results compared. Usually the lowest keratometry reading and the highest IOL power generated are used.

None of these methods is perfect. These patients need to be told prior to cataract surgery that the refractive outcome may not be plano and further surgery—for example, IOL exchange, piggyback IOL, or even refractive surgery—may be needed to get the refraction closer to plano.

Take-Home Points

1. IOL calculations after keratorefractive surgery are not as accurate as prior to corneal surgery.
2. The more preoperative information you have, the better your chances are of accurately calculating the IOL power for cataract surgery.
3. Patients need to be told that they may need corrective lenses or additional surgery in order to achieve their best vision after cataract surgery.

CASE 59

A 50-year-old myopic woman seeks a refractive surgery consultation for her −3.50 D correction. One of the reasons she is interested in LASIK is that she is becoming increasingly contact lens intolerant. She understands that she will need reading glasses after surgery. The preoperative evaluation is unremarkable. There is no punctate fluorescein staining on the cornea or conjunctiva of either eye. The Schirmer test after topical anesthesia measured 7 mm of wetting OU. How would you proceed?

After appropriate informed consent, stressing the fact that her eyes would feel drier for weeks to months after surgery but they would most likely return to baseline after 3 to 6 months, she underwent uncomplicated LASIK OU. Postoperatively she is treated with a topical fluoroquinolone, prednisolone 1%, and preservative-free tears each four times daily. On the day after surgery her uncorrected visual acuity is 20/50, and 20/30 with −0.75 D sphere OU. She has significant central and superior SPK. How would you proceed?

Numerous options were discussed with the patient including punctal occlusion, use of tear gels and ointments, and cyclosporine drops. The patient opts for 90-day dissolvable collagen plugs and one was placed in the lower punctum OU. She was also started on cyclosporine 0.05% (Restasis) twice daily OU. Her preservative-free artificial tears were increased to every 2 hours while awake once the antibiotics and steroids were discontinued 5 days after surgery.

During the next several weeks her symptoms and punctate staining slowly improved. At 1 month postoperatively, her uncorrected vision had improved to 20/25, correcting to 20/20 with −0.25 D sphere OU. At 3 months postoperatively she had minimal dry eye symptoms, minimal inferior SPK, and her uncorrected vision improved to 20/20. She was still using the cyclosporine 0.05% twice daily, but had decreased the artificial tear use to two to three times a day.

Discussion

The incidence of tear deficiency increases with age, especially in women. Long-term contact lens use also probably increases dryness due to decreased corneal sensation and diminished blink rate. Consequently, as long-term contact lens users get older, they may have increasing contact lens intolerance and, hence, an increasing interest in refractive surgery.

During the consultation it is important to determine whether the patient has a significant dry eye condition, not to prevent refractive surgery, but rather to give appropriate informed consent and plan for optimal preoperative and postoperative management. Anterior and posterior blepharitis are both commonly associated with dry eyes, so the lids should also be carefully evaluated preoperatively and treated.

An important component of ocular surface health is corneal innervation. Many of the central nerves are severed during LASIK. Although corneal innervation tends to recover, it may take between 3 and 12 months. During this period, many patients experience increased symptoms of dry eye including reduced and/or fluctuating vision, foreign body sensation, and reflex tearing due to irritation. Fortunately these symptoms improve with time in the majority of patients. The major trunks of nerves enter the cornea at the 3 and 9 o' clock meridians. Some surgeons feel that a nasal-hinged flap preserves more of the nerves than a superior-hinged flap. The hypoesthesia induced from bilateral surgery may decrease the blink rate. This in turn increases exposure and contributes to an evaporative dry eye. Sequential surgery waiting for the first eye to recover before the second eye is done may be a consideration. The ambient humidity should always be considered in dry eye patients. The season and the geographical region may have an impact on the outcome in these patients.

Numerous treatment options are available pre- and postoperatively to treat dry eyes including minimally preserved and preservative-free artificial tears, tear gels and ointments, cyclosporine 0.05% (Restasis), and temporary and permanent punctal plugs. When the doctor and patient are considering starting cyclosporine 0.05%, several issues need to be discussed. The patient should know that it may take several weeks to have an effect, the drops may burn temporarily, and it is an expensive medication without a prescription insurance plan. Blepharitis should be treated with warm compresses, eyelid hygiene, and antibiotic ointment.

Take-Home Points

1. The patient should be evaluated by history and examination for evidence of dry eye. If present, the condition should be discussed with the patient and treated preoperatively.
2. Dry eye symptoms after LASIK are common, generally respond to treatment, and usually return to the preoperative state by 3 to 6 months postoperatively.

CASE 60

A 52-year-old woman presents for LASIK consultation. After evaluation she is found to be a candidate for surgery. She has realistic expectations and understands the risks. She does not want monovision treatment. A contact lens trial was offered, but she declined.

W	OD –4.00 20/20 OS –4.50 20/20	**Uncorrected Va** OD 20/400 OS 20/400
M	OD –4.25 + 0.25 x 180° 20/20 OS –4.50 20/20	
C	OD –4.25 + 0.25 x 180° 20/20 OS –4.50 20/20	
K	OD 43.75 x 90°/44.00 x 180° OS 44.00 x 180°/44.00 x 90°	

Pachymetry	**Topography**	**Scotopic Pupils**
OD 550 μm OS 550 μm	Spherical OU	OD 5.5 mm OS 5.5 mm

Additional Examination

The patient elects to undergo the procedure using the femtosecond laser to create the flap. A drop of brimonidine HCl 0.15% (Alphagan) is instilled 30 minutes prior to treatment in order to blanch the conjunctiva, making it easier to obtain suction with the suction ring. A drop of ketorolac tromethamine 0.5% (Acular) is used immediately postoperatively to help keep the eye comfortable. On examination the next morning, the flap of the right eye is noted to have slipped and the uncorrected visual acuity OD is 20/200 compared to 20/20 OS, where the flap is noted to be in good position.

The flap is refloated immediately once it is noted to be displaced. The patient is taken back to the laser suite and the eye carefully prepped and draped. A topical anesthetic and antibiotic is placed on the eye and the flap is completely retracted. The underlying bed is carefully observed for any encroachment of epithelium. If noted, the epithelium is wiped away from the bed. A drop of topical antibiotic is placed on the bed as well as a topical steroid before the flap is floated back into place with sterile balanced salt solution. An ironing-like motion may be required to smooth out any wrinkles that may have formed. The flap is left to dry in place for 10 minutes while the surface of the flap is moistened with balanced salt solution. A bandage contact lens is placed on the eye overnight and the patient given instructions to frequently lubricate the eye and not to touch it.

Discussion

Despite the presence of a steeper side cut angle in a laser-prepared flap (laser 70 degrees versus microkeratome 20 degrees), flap displacement can still occur after IntraLase. Flap slippage tends to occur more commonly in postmenopausal women. Such patients have a higher incidence of keratitis sicca, and it is thought that the movement of the eyelid over a dry cornea surface can pull the flap out of position. Therefore, added care to avoid direct trauma to the flap is warranted, as is added lubrication in the form of artificial teardrops or gels to reduce the likelihood of displacement. Hinge location can also play a role, because superior flaps are less likely to slip than nasal flaps. Topical brimonidine can also play a role in flap slippage and should be avoided perioperatively. Finally, adjusting the side cut angle to 70 degrees will make slippage of the flap less likely.

Take-Home Points

1. Flap displacement is possible with the IntraLase, but perhaps less likely than with a microkeratome.
2. A superior hinge, 70-degree side cut angle, frequent postoperative lubrication, and avoidance of brimonidine (Alphagan) perioperatively may reduce the incidence of this complication.
3. A displaced flap should be repositioned as soon as possible once it is recognized.
4. Brush back epithelium that has grown onto the stromal bed to reduce the risk of epithelial ingrowth.

CASE 61

A 38-year-old police detective underwent uneventful LASIK treatment (Case 4) achieving a post-operative uncorrected visual acuity of 20/20 in both eyes. Three months after surgery, while helping a friend move furniture, a wooden dowel rod struck him in the right eye. He presents in the office the next day complaining of pain and blurred vision OD.

Examination

Visual acuity without correction:	OD 20/400− OS 20/20
External examination OD:	1+ lid edema and erythema, 1+ conjunctival injection
Pupils:	Briskly reactive without APD
Slit-lamp examination:	See Case 61, Figure 1.

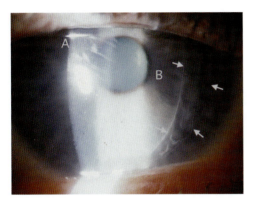

Case 61, Figure 1

Partial flap displacement/macrofolds. Arrows on the right indicate margin of the flap bed. Arrows on the left delineate the displaced flap edge. *A* indicates Descemet's folds due to stromal edema. *B* indicates macrofolds related to the displaced flap. (Courtesy Robert S. Feder, M.D.)

Discussion

This patient's symptoms of pain and decreased vision are consistent with the finding of a flap displacement OD that occurred as a result of the blunt injury. It is worth noting that this occurred 3 months postoperatively and is a reminder of the fragility of the flap even months after surgery. The findings of macrofolds in the flap and the presence of a gap between the flap edge and the peripheral cornea are typical. This flap should be repositioned as soon as possible. Most affected patients will seek attention soon after the injury so the macrofolds will be relatively easy to smooth out. Unless the area of flap slip is small, it is generally preferable to unseal the remainder of the flap edge and reflect the whole flap rather than working only on the part that has been displaced.

After a flap displacement, corneal epithelium will begin to grow over the gap. The epithelium appears as a smooth sheet and is relatively easy to differentiate from the rougher appearing stromal bed. It is very important to recognize the presence of this epithelium and clear it from the stromal bed in order to reduce the chance of epithelial ingrowth.

The epithelium is often irregular at the flap edge and a bandage contact lens should be placed on the eye. Depending on the extent of the injury, a traumatic iritis may be present. The patient should be treated with topical prednisolone 1% and a topical fluoroquinolone each four times daily. The patient should be watched closely for signs of DLK, iritis, and infection, as well as epithelial ingrowth.

The patient in this case recovered 20/20 unaided acuity.

Take-Home Points

1. Traumatic flap displacement can occur long after LASIK surgery.
2. The flap should be repositioned as soon as possible.

7

3. Macrofolds should smooth out as the flap is repositioned.
4. Reduce the risk of ingrowth by recognizing and removing overgrown epithelium from the flap bed before the flap is laid down.

CASE 62

A 38-year-old police detective (see Cases 4 and 61) had uncomplicated LASIK surgery to correct myopia with astigmatism. Three months postoperatively he suffered a traumatic flap displacement OD. The flap was repositioned and he had recovered 20/20 unaided acuity. Two months later he presented with the onset of irritation and blurred vision OD.

Examination

Visual acuity without correction: OD 20/25− OS 20/15−

External examination: No inflammation

Slit-lamp evaluation: OD See Case 62, Figure 1. The flaps OU are without striae or epithelial ingrowth.

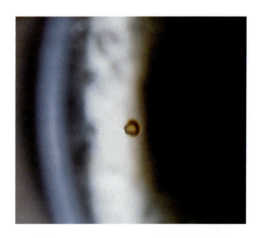

Case 62, Figure 1

Rust ring on a LASIK flap. (Courtesy Robert S. Feder, M.D.)

Discussion

This patient appears to have a rust ring in the LASIK flap. The consequence of aggressive removal would be a buttonhole in the flap, which conceivably could lead to epithelial ingrowth. Creating an epithelial defect in a LASIK flap could result in DLK and the epithelium may be slow to heal due to the neurotrophic nature of a LASIK flap. The consequence of leaving the rust ring would be chronic irritation and possibly the risk of infection. The decision was made to judiciously remove the retained foreign material. This was accomplished using a 25-gauge needle after topical anesthetic was instilled. The epithelium was slow to heal despite the use of a bandage soft contact lens. No DLK or epithelial ingrowth occurred, but a small scar developed at the site. The unaided visual acuity OD was 20/25−, which improved to 20/20+ with a −0.50 D sphere.

Take-Home Points

1. The possible consequences of corneal foreign body removal in a LASIK flap are persistent epithelial defect, DLK, buttonhole with or without epithelial ingrowth, and infection.
2. Epithelial healing may be slower in a neurotrophic LASIK flap.

7

CASE 63

A 58-year-old woman had undergone uncomplicated LASIK OU 3 years prior to correct −4.00 D. She was doing well with very good uncorrected distance vision in both eyes. She used reading glasses for near tasks. While gardening one morning (without glasses), she was poked in the left eye by a tree branch. She developed immediate pain and decreased vision in that eye. She went immediately to the Emergency Department where an ophthalmologist was called in to treat her.

In this case, the flap was dehisced, just attached at its hinge (Case 63, Fig. 1). The decision was made to replace it in the minor surgery suite using an operating microscope. After informed consent was obtained, the eye was prepped and draped, topical antibiotic and anesthetic were placed, and an eyelid speculum inserted. A blade (e.g., Alcon 67 or Beaver #15) was used to remove all debris and cells from the underside of the flap and from the stromal bed. Epithelium that had migrated onto the stromal bed was pushed peripherally. Once this was completed, the flap was replaced and the interface irrigated. There was a crease in the flap, where it has been folded prior to presentation at the hospital. The flap was stretched in an attempt to flatten the crease with a cyclodialysis spatula and dry and moist cellulose sponges. While the stretching helped the fold somewhat, it also damaged the flap epithelium slightly. The gutters were examined and felt to be even. A BSCL (Focus Night & Day 8.6/−0.50) was placed on the eye and the patient placed on a topical fluoroquinolone, prednisolone 1%, and preservative-free tears. The patient was seen daily and the BSCL was removed on the third postoperative day. The flap remained in excellent position with no significant striae and the uncorrected vision returned to baseline.

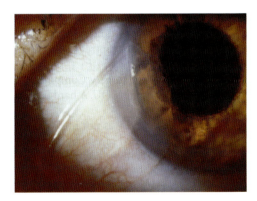

Case 63, Figure 1

Flap displacement. (Courtesy Christopher J. Rapuano, M.D.)

Discussion

What are the important issues to address in cases of trauma after LASIK? First, the extent of ocular injury needs to be evaluated, making sure there is not a ruptured globe, ocular foreign body, hyphema, and so forth. Second, check on the status of the LASIK flap, making sure it is intact and in good position. Third, if the LASIK flap is not in perfect position, decide how to best correct its position.

Trauma to a LASIK flap, even years postoperatively, can cause a partial or total flap dehiscence. In such cases the flap needs to be replaced in its original location. Both the bed and underside of the flap need to be cleaned of epithelium and debris. It is critical to debride the stromal bed of all epithelium, which begins to cover the periphery quickly after such an injury. Surface corneal epithelial cells migrate onto the stromal bed within an hour or two after such an injury. If these cells are not removed, epithelial ingrowth will occur. In fact, many surgeons will remove the epithelium 0.5 to 1.0 mm away from the flap edge to help prevent epithelial growth under the flap. After the flap is repositioned, the flap interface should be irrigated. Flap folds are

Cycloplegic refractive error before initial treatment	−7.00
Original keratometry	Not available
Original pachymetry	Not available
Cycloplegic refraction prior to retreatment	−1.75 + 2.00 × 10°
Pachymetry prior to retreatment	495 μm
Keratometry prior to retreatment	38.12 × 110°/39.25 × 20° (irregular)
Postoperative UCVA at 1 month	20/60
Postoperative cycloplegic refraction at 1 month	−1.75 + 1.75 × 80°
Postoperative UCVA at 2 months	20/30−
Postoperative cycloplegic refraction at 5 months	−1.00 + 1.00 × 95°
Postoperative UCVA at 10 months following LRI	20/25

circumstance, there are numerous reports of patients doing equally well after retreatment without the use of the medication.

Take-Home Points

1. Complicated cases require extended periods of observation before the final results become evident.
2. Visual rehabilitation after complicated LASIK may require multiple or different procedures performed sequentially, each after stabilization occurs.
3. Surface retreatment is usually a better alternative than recutting when working with poor-quality flaps and no information about the original LASIK surgery.

CASE 66

This 49-year-old woman had myopic astigmatism and small palpebral fissures. The ophthalmologist who performed her LASIK commented on the difficulty seating the microkeratome on her left eye due to the small interpalpebral fissures and intraoperative blepharospasm. The surgeon inadvertently created a free cap OS, and he proceeded with the refractive ablation because he felt there was an adequate stromal bed.

The patient was referred 5 months postoperatively for evaluation and management of undercorrected myopia OS. The initial examination revealed a small free cap (Case 66, Fig. 1). Her uncorrected visual acuity was 20/60, and the residual refractive error was −1.00 −0.75 × 30° OS correcting to 20/20.

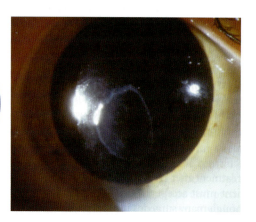

Case 66, Figure 1

Illustration of a small free cap from a different patient. BSCVA will depend on the degree of surface irregularity and stromal opacity near the visual axis. BSCVA in this patient would not be 20/20. (Courtesy Christopher J. Rapuano, M.D.)

		Uncorrected Va
W	OD −0.25 20/20 OS −1.75 −1.25 x 38° 20/20	OD 20/25 OS 20/70
M	OD −0.25 20/20 OS −1.75 −1.25 x 40° 20/20	
C	OD plano 20/20 OS −1.50 −1.50 x 40° 20/20	
K	OD 41.25 x 178°/41.75 x 88° OS 41.00 x 42°/42.75 x 132°	

Pachymetry	Topography	Scotopic Pupils
OD 510 μm OS 502 μm	Central flattening OD Regular astigmatism OS	OD 5.5 mm OS 6.0 mm

Given the potential instability of a free cap (e.g., the risk of a recurrent free cap with any attempt at relifting) and the small potential ablation zone, we elected to perform an excimer laser PRK to enhance her refractive result. To minimize the risk of dislodging the free cap, we elected to perform a "no touch" technique consisting of a laser epithelial removal, followed by the refractive keratectomy.

	Left Eye	Comments
Ablation zone	6.5 mm with 8.0-mm blend	
Cycloplegic Rx	−1.50 − 1.50 × 40°	
Calculations with nomogram correction (VISX)	10% reduction for mitomycin-C −1.35 − 1.50 × 40°	Reduce risk of post-PRK haze
Flap thickness	N/A	
Ablation depth (from tables)	40 μm	
Residual stromal thickness	502 μm − 40 μm = 462 μm	

There is a significant risk of post-PRK haze in a post-LASIK eye. We applied prophylactic mitomycin-C 0.02% on a Merocel circular sponge for 2 minutes after the laser ablation, and irrigated the cornea with 30 mL of chilled balanced salt solution. We reduced the cycloplegic refraction by 10% before entering the desired treatment into the laser, because the mitomycin-C inhibits the normal healing response. Her postoperative visual acuity was 20/25 uncorrected.

Take-Home Points

1. This case illustrates the risk of a free cap in a LASIK case, especially one in which there are problems getting the suction ring seated properly. Risk factors include a small interpalpebral fissure and poor patient cooperation.
2. Because of the potential instability of the free cap, LASIK enhancement is often best accomplished using surface PRK.
3. The prophylactic use of mitomycin-C is often desirable to reduce the risk of postoperative corneal haze in these cases.

7

CASE 67

A 20-year-old woman presents for a refractive surgery consultation. Her past ocular history is significant for attempted LASIK 6 weeks earlier, complicated by a buttonhole flap in the right eye. She is inquiring about visual rehabilitation for her right eye.

		Uncorrected Va
W	OD –4.50 + 0.50 x 90° 20/25 OS –4.75 + 0.75 x 90° 20/30	20/400 20/400
M	OD –3.00 20/20 OS –2.50 20/20	
C	OD –2.75 + 0.25 x 95° 20/20 OS –2.25 + 0.50 x 85° 20/20	
K	OD: 44.75 x 90°/44.75 x 180° OS: 44.75 x 90°/45.12 x 180°	

Pachymetry	Keratome	Dominant Eye
OD 554 μm OS 557 μm	ACS 180-μm flap 8.5-mm ring	OD

Additional Information

After identification of the buttonhole flap, the flap was repositioned carefully without application of the excimer laser. A bandage contact lens was placed, and the postoperative course was closely monitored for development of epithelial ingrowth or scarring. The patient's refraction and topographic examination were stable at 6 weeks, with BSCVA equivalent to preoperative levels. On slit-lamp examination, the corneal flap was well healed with a faint central buttonhole scar present (Case 67, Fig. 1).

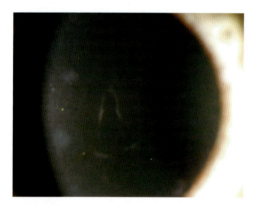

Case 67, Figure 1

Buttonhole flap. (Courtesy Christopher J. Rapuano, M.D.)

Discussion

In this patient who has already sustained a buttonhole flap, attempting to create another flap with a mechanical microkeratome is risky for several reasons. If the proximate cause of the first buttonhole flap is unknown, there is a higher likelihood that a second buttonhole may occur. Indeed, this patient's cornea was not excessively steep, and the surgeon was experienced in using the ACS microkeratome. In addition, the use of a mechanical microkeratome for the second surgery may also create a flap that intersects with the first, possibly resulting in irregular astigmatism. The femtosecond laser may be beneficial in recutting buttonholed flaps. However, another option is transepithelial PTK/PRK with adjunctive mitomycin-C (MMC). It has been reported that surface ablation over LASIK flaps, especially buttonholed flaps, may put the patient at increased risk for significant corneal haze. The use of MMC may prevent this.

This patient requested laser vision correction without the use of a microkeratome. The VISX STAR S4 was used to remove the epithelium with a 6.5-mm diameter and 50-μm depth PTK setting. PRK treatment, reduced due to the use of MMC, with a 6.0-mm optical zone and an ablation depth of 33 μm, was then applied. A 6-mm-diameter corneal light shield that had been soaked in mitomycin-C 0.02% was then placed on the stromal bed and left in position for 2 minutes. Following removal of the shield, the cornea was irrigated with 30 mL of balanced salt solution. A Soflens 66 bandage contact lens was then applied to the right eye. Standard PRK without MMC was then performed on the left eye.

Postoperatively, the patient had an uneventful course. Both corneas were well healed without any evidence of scarring or haze in either eye. At 16 weeks postoperatively, both corneas remained clear and the uncorrected visual acuity was 20/20 in both eyes. Manifest refraction was −0.25 D OD and plano OS.

Take-Home Points

1. Know your microkeratome and the typical flap thickness produced for each plate.
2. To minimize the potential for buttonholes, avoid LASIK with mechanical microkeratomes in steep corneas with an average keratometry value of >48 D.
3. If a buttonhole is created, do not apply the excimer laser treatment. Replace the flap carefully and place a bandage contact lens.
4. Recutting another flap should be avoided. Consider surface ablation with MMC prophylaxis.

CASE 68

A 56-year-old man had undergone LASIK surgery 3 years previously. Retreatment was performed twice OD and once OS. The original treatment data were unavailable. He was now being followed by his general ophthalmologist, who noted a white opacity in the superficial stroma OS that had not been seen previously. The patient was pain free, but he had noted a gradual decrease in vision OU since the surgery. The ophthalmologist suspected infectious keratitis and began treatment with frequent topical moxifloxacin. The opacity remained unchanged after 3 days of therapy. He now suspected fungal keratitis and sent him for consultation.

M	OD −1.50 + 1.50 x 123° 20 / 25− OS −0.75 + 1.25 x 70° 20/20−	**Uncorrected Va** 20/50 20/30−

K	OD 40.75 x 30°/42.25 x 120° Slightly irregular mires OU OS 40.50 x 160°/41.75 x 70°

External Examination
Lids without edema or erythema; no discharge; bulbar conjunctiva white and quiet

Slit-Lamp Examination
An 8.0-mm nasal hinged flap was present OU. There was scattered debris in the interface OU. A dense, white opacity was noted at the inferotemporal flap interface OS (Case 68, Fig. 1). There was no surrounding keratitis. There was a pinpoint area in the center of this lesion that appeared to be possible flap necrosis. The area showed negative staining. There was no vascularization or stromal edema. The anterior segment was otherwise normal in each eye.

Pachymetry	**IOP and Fundus**	**Dominant Eye**
OD 502 μm OS 510 μm	Normal OU	OD

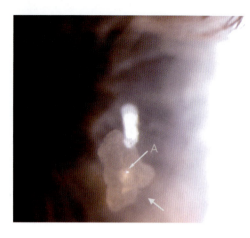

Case 68, Figure 1

A arrow points to area of suspected flap necrosis within a patch of dense epithelial ingrowth. Heavier arrow delineates the flap edge. (Courtesy Robert S. Feder, M.D.)

Given the lack of inflammation it seemed clear that this opacity did not represent infectious keratitis, bacterial or fungal. The dense, white opacity had the appearance of epithelial ingrowth with possible early flap necrosis. The lesion was not particularly large; however, the small central necrotic area was worrisome. The risk of further necrosis was explained to the patient and he agreed to a flap lift OS for removal of this material. He was not interested in further laser surgery and was content to wear glasses.

The patient was taken to the laser suite where, after instillation of topical anesthetic and appropriate prep and drape, the flap was partially lifted. A smooth patch of epithelium was adherent to the stromal bed. There was also some material on the underside of the flap. All of the epithelium was gently removed. The interface was irrigated, but the flap was not sutured. A bandage soft contact lens was placed. It could not be determined intraoperatively if the flap was intact; however, postoperatively a small buttonhole could be seen in the area that had appeared necrotic (Case 68, Fig. 2). After 8 months of follow-up, the epithelial ingrowth has not recurred and the vision is stable.

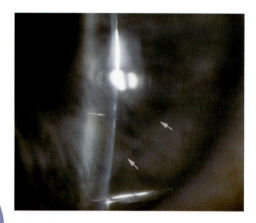

Case 68, Figure 2

Fine arrow indicates buttonhole caused by flap necrosis confirmed after flap lift and ingrowth removed. Heavier arrows delineate the flap edge. (Courtesy Robert S. Feder, M.D.)

Discussion

The risk of epithelial ingrowth is increased with multiple flap lifts for retreatment or in patients who have had a flap slip postoperatively. The adherence of the corneal epithelium is reduced in patients over the age of 50, in diabetics, and in patients with basement membrane dystrophy. Irrigating the interface after the flap is replaced can remove epithelial cells that have been trapped. This patient had moderate debris in the interface, suggesting inadequate irrigation. Ingrowth can

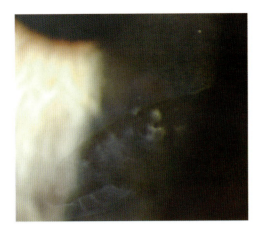

Case 68, Figure 3

Peripheral flap necrosis caused by epithelial ingrowth. (Courtesy Robert S. Feder, M.D.)

present contiguous with the flap edge or as an isolated lesion not connected with the flap edge. It can affect vision by causing irregular astigmatism or by blocking the visual axis. A dense patch of epithelium can prevent nutrients from reaching the overlying flap and therefore result in necrosis at the flap edge or within the flap (Case 68, Fig. 3). Occasionally even a dense lesion can resolve spontaneously (Case 68, Figs. 4A and B); therefore, a compliant patient can be watched carefully if the lesion is relatively small and out of the visual axis. The indications for treatment are ingrowth extending ≥2 mm from the flap edge, an opalescent patch that may threaten flap necrosis, or decreased vision due to opacity or irregular astigmatism.

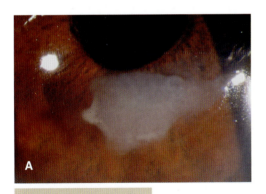
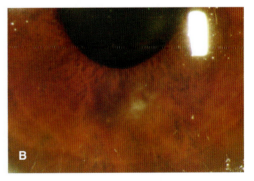

Case 68, Figure 4A, 4B

A: Dense epithelial ingrowth with no overlying flap necrosis. **B:** Same cornea 3 months later shows nearly complete resolution of ingrowth without treatment. (Courtesy Robert S. Feder, M.D.)

Take-Home Points

1. The risk of epithelial ingrowth is greater after flap displacement or retreatments, if epithelium is poorly adherent, or if the interface is not properly irrigated.
2. Ingrowth can affect vision by invading the visual axis or by inducing irregular astigmatism.
3. The indications for removal are extension ≥2 mm from the flap edge, increasing density of the lesion with threatened flap necrosis, or decreased vision.

The 55-year-old man from Case 45 returns 3 months after LASIK OD, which was complicated by a large area of central epithelial loosening that was treated and resolved. He now notes some ocular irritation and decline in his vision on the right.

M OD –1.50 + 0.75 x 90° (20/30)	**Uncorrected Va:** OD 20/50
C OD –1.25 + 0.75 x 90° (20/30)	
K OD 39.50 D x 180°/40.00 D x 90°	

Pachymetry	**Topography**	**Scotopic Pupil**
586 μm	OD asymmetric ATR astigmatism	OD 3.5 mm

Additional Examination

Slit-lamp examination reveals a well-healed epithelium OD with some mild peripheral anterior basement membrane dystrophy (ABMD) changes and a completely normal OS. There is an area of epithelial ingrowth inferiorly OD, from 5 to 8 o' clock reaching approximately 2 to 3 mm centrally from the flap edge. There is mild elevation of the flap and corresponding topographic flattening producing irregular astigmatism. Mild punctate fluorescein staining of the epithelium is present over the area of epithelial ingrowth. There is no stromal inflammation or vascularization and the anterior chamber is deep and quiet (Case 69, Fig. 1). How would you proceed?

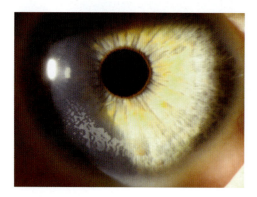

Case 69, Figure 1

Epithelial ingrowth beneath LASIK flap inferiorly. (Courtesy Christopher J. Rapuano, M.D.)

Discussion

A patient with epithelial ingrowth can usually be followed unless the condition is affecting vision or the health of the flap. Generally, small amounts of epithelial ingrowth, for example, less than 2 mm from the flap margin, do not cause trouble. When epithelial ingrowth extends greater than 2 mm toward the center of the cornea, it may begin to cause decreased vision from irregular astigmatism. Also large or dense areas of epithelial ingrowth can prevent proper nutrients from getting to the overlying flap and can lead to superficial punctate staining, epithelial defect, and even flap melting. In cases of decreased vision and a "sick" flap, as in this patient, the epithelial ingrowth should be removed. Patients need to understand the benefits and risks of this procedure, including recurrent epithelial ingrowth, decreased vision, infection, DLK, and the potential need for additional surgery.

Removal is typically performed with topical anesthesia using an operating microscope. The area may be outlined lightly with a marking pen to be able to identify exactly where it is under the operating microscope. Ink marks can also be made at the flap edge to aid in repositioning at the end of the procedure. The flap edge is opened with an instrument such as a Sinskey hook. Depending on the size and location of the epithelial ingrowth, a small area or the entire flap can be lifted with an instrument such as a cyclodialysis spatula. The stromal bed and the underside of the flap need to be scraped carefully but effectively with a sharp blade (e.g., an Alcon #67 blade or Beaver #15 blade) or semisharp knife (e.g., Tooke knife). While care does need to be taken not to damage the flap or stromal bed while scraping, no residual epithelium should remain. The epithelium often comes off as a sheet of tissue. The epithelium peripheral to the edge of the flap may also be also removed or pushed back from the flap margin for about 1 mm to prevent recurrent ingrowth. Once all the interface epithelium has been removed, the flap is replaced, the interface irrigated, and the flap allowed to adhere for several minutes. A BSCL may be placed for several days. The patient should be treated with topical antibiotics and steroids.

This patient underwent an uncomplicated flap lift and scrape procedure. The patient received topical fluoroquinolone and prednisolone 1% qid for 7 days and frequent preservative-free tears for a month. The BSCL was removed after 5 days. The uncorrected vision improved to 20/30 and with a −1.00 + 0.50 × 90°, the vision achieved 20/25+2 and the patient was happy.

Recurrent epithelial ingrowth can be treated in an identical manner if the surgeon believes this procedure is more likely to be successful a second time. Additional treatment options include flap suturing and placement of fibrin glue. Flap suturing involves the exact same initial procedure as the flap lift and scrape. Once the flap interface is cleared of epithelium and the interface irrigated, either interrupted sutures or a running 10-0 nylon suture is placed to secure the flap edge to the stroma. If fluorescein staining is noted at the flap edge preoperatively, this may be the origin of epithelial ingrowth. This site should be marked and a suture should be placed at this site to secure the flap at this location. Typically 7 to 14 interrupted sutures are placed if the entire flap is lifted (in all areas except the hinge) or fewer if just part of the flap is lifted. The knots are buried peripherally so as not to disrupt the flap when the sutures are removed. The sutures are usually kept in place for 4 to 6 weeks (Case 69, Fig. 2). Fibrin glue, for example, Tisseel (Baxter), can also be used to secure the flap edge in attempt to prevent recurrent epithelial ingrowth. It is placed on the flap edge once the flap interface is cleared of epithelium, irrigated, and repositioned. The glue dissolves over days to weeks.

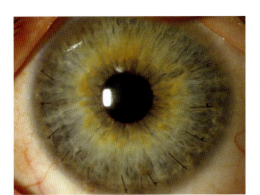

Case 69, Figure 2

Following a flap lift and removal of epithelium, the flap is sutured to reduce the risk of recurrence. (Courtesy Christopher J. Rapuano, M.D.)

7

Take-Home Points

1. Small degrees of epithelial ingrowth at the edge of the flap are common and do not require removal.
2. Larger degrees of epithelial ingrowth (e.g., >2-mm central growth) tend to cause problems such as irregular astigmatism and decreased vision and even damage to the health of the flap, and they require treatment.
3. When epithelial ingrowth is removed, both the underside of the flap and the stromal bed need to be scraped.
4. Recurrent epithelial ingrowth can be managed by suturing the flap or using fibrin glue to seal the flap edge after the offending epithelium has been removed.

CASE 70

A 45-year-old man with a refraction of −8.50 D OU and thin corneas measuring 487 μm OD and 472 μm OS desired LASIK. Computation of his residual stromal thickness (RST) showed results of 217 μm OD and 202 μm OS. Although there are no controlled studies to confirm the safe level of RST, we believe that ≥250 μm is a desirable threshold. Therefore, we elected not to perform LASIK and instead recommended PRK.

Given the high level of myopia, and the 115 μm of estimated stromal ablation, we elected to treat the ablated corneas with prophylactic mitomycin-C 0.02% on a Merocel sponge (corneal protector) for 2 minutes, and then rinse thoroughly with 30 mL of chilled balanced salt solution (BSS) per eye. His uncorrected visual acuity improved to 20/20 OU at 2 months postoperatively.

Nine months following the PRK, he developed late-onset corneal haze in an arcuate pattern OD, associated with a decrease in visual acuity to 20/30. He was treated with a corneal scraping and repeated application of mitomycin-C 0.02% on a Merocel corneal protector for 2 minutes. This was followed by a rinse with 30 mL of chilled BSS. Six weeks later, his uncorrected vision improved to 20/25 and his cornea was clear.

Four months after this treatment, the corneal haze recurred. This time he was treated with prednisolone acetate 1% drops (Pred Forte) every 2 hours while awake, and vitamin C 1,000 mg orally each day, which was then tapered gradually over 4 months. The corneal haze has not recurred.

Take-Home Points

1. PRK is an excellent alternative for corneas that are too thin for LASIK.
2. Late-onset corneal haze may occur after PRK, even in a patient who was treated with prophylactic mitomycin-C to try and prevent such an occurrence. This case demonstrates the benefit of topical steroids to treat corneal haze, rather than a repeat application of mitomycin-C.
3. Vitamin C, a potent antioxidant, may be of benefit in preventing post-PRK corneal haze.

CASE 71

A 48-year-old woman undergoes uncomplicated LASIK for −3.50 D myopia in both eyes using a mechanical microkeratome. On the first postoperative day, her uncorrected vision is 20/25 OU and other than mild subconjunctival hemorrhages OU, the examination is unremarkable. She is told to continue her antibiotic and steroid drops four times daily and to return in 1 week. However, on postoperative day 3 she notes more photophobia and is told to come in and be examined. Based on this information, what are you thinking about prior to examining her?

On examination, her uncorrected visual acuity is 20/30 OD and 20/25 OS. The slit-lamp examination OS is stable, but there is mild inflammation at the level of the flap interface in the midperiphery and centrally OD. The cornea has a granular appearance with a slight undulating pattern. There is no epithelial defect, cellular clumping, focal infiltration, or anterior chamber reaction; the iris details are clearly visible. The diagnosis of diffuse lamellar keratitis (DLK) is made and the patient is treated with topical prednisolone acetate 1% every 2 hours while awake and is seen the following day. The examination is unchanged, but the patient feels slightly worse. The prednisolone is increased to every hour while awake. The patient is seen daily and slowly improves over the next week and the steroid drops are slowly tapered and stopped over 3 weeks. The inflammation resolves over several weeks and the uncorrected vision improves and is equal to the left eye.

Discussion

The two biggest concerns prior to seeing this patient are infection and sterile inflammation (DLK). DLK is a sterile inflammatory reaction that typically occurs within a few days after LASIK. The exact etiology is often unknown. It most commonly occurs in a sporadic fashion but occasionally occurs in epidemics, often due to bacterial toxins resulting from contaminated sterilization equipment. It is associated with epithelial defects, both at the time of LASIK and months or years later (so-called late-onset DLK). A sterile inflammatory reaction that looks identical to DLK can also occur with other corneal surface problems such as recurrent corneal erosions and HSV dendritic keratitis. There may be an increased incidence of DLK with use of a bandage soft contact lens, although it is difficult to separate the lens as a cause from the reason the lens is being used. The differential diagnosis of both classic DLK and especially late-onset DLK also must include infection. If there is a high index of suspicion for infection, the flap needs to be lifted and the stromal bed and underside of the flap scraped for smears and cultures.

DLK is graded from 1 through 4 depending on location and severity (see illustrations in Chapter 5, pages 103–104). Milder forms of DLK involving only the periphery are treated with moderate dose topical prednisolone 1% and follow-up within 2 days. More severe forms are treated with hourly steroids or even oral prednisone and patient follow-up in 1 day. For more severe forms, such as when there is a dense accumulation of white blood cells in the interface centrally, the flap may need to be lifted and the interface debris removed. Scrapings can be sent for smears and cultures since the specimen is easily accessible. Ideally, the severe form is prevented by appropriate treatment and follow-up. The main danger of DLK is that the severe inflammation causes tissue loss and scarring. The tissue loss can lead to localized central thinning and flattening, causing irregular astigmatism and poor vision. Scarring can also reduce vision.

Take-Home Points

1. Patients need to be examined carefully on the first postoperative day for signs of DLK and, if present, they should be treated with an increased frequency of topical steroids and followed closely.
2. Late-onset DLK can occur from ocular surface problems such as corneal abrasions, recurrent erosions, and HSV dendritic keratitis, but it can also be a sign of indolent flap interface infection, such as with atypical mycobacteria or fungus.

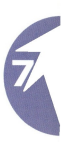

CASE 72

This 28-year-old man presents to the clinic expressing an interest in refractive surgery. He enjoys windsurfing and downhill skiing, which he cannot do in his glasses. He has not been able to wear contact lenses, because it is difficult for him to insert the lenses.

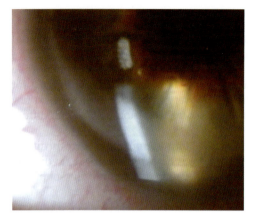

Case 74, Figure 1

Initial presentation diagnosed as DLK. (Courtesy Robert S. Feder, M.D.)

The topical steroid was increased to every hour. The patient returned the next day with increased irritation and watering in the OD. The unaided acuity was 20/25− OD and 20/15 OS. The infiltrate in the OD had increased in density, making the view of iris detail difficult. The area of inflammation extended 1.5 mm circumferentially and 1.0 mm centrally beneath the flap. A small epithelial defect was noted. There was no anterior chamber reaction. Mild peripheral flap inflammation was noted in the OS extending 1 mm from the flap edge superotemporally. What action should be taken at this point?

The flap OD was partially lifted and irrigated. The bed was gently scraped and the undersurface of the flap scraped. Topical fluoroquinotone was placed in the interface. A bandage contact lens was placed on the right eye. Oral prednisone 40 mg was added. The next day the patient felt 40% improved. The visual acuity OD was 20/40−. There was no discharge. The epithelial defect OD was nearly healed. There was a DLK-like picture extending from 10 to 2 o'clock inferiorly and about 2 mm centrally (Case 74, Fig. 2). The DLK OS looked better superiorly, but a new infiltrate was present inferotemporally. With worsening DLK OD despite adding oral prednisone and a new infiltrate OS, what action should be taken?

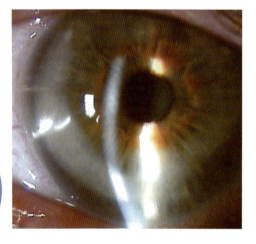

Case 74, Figure 2

Progression of DLK-like inflammation despite treatment. (Courtesy Robert S. Feder, M.D.)

The decision was made to relift the flap for culture and scraping. Scrapings were plated on blood, chocolate, and Sabouraud's agar, along with Lowenstein-Jensen slant and a second agar for atypical mycobacteria. The interface was swabbed with a lightly moistened Merocel sponge. Oral prednisone was boosted to 80 mg per day and oral doxycycline 100 mg was added to reduce the risk of keratolysis.

On day 3 the visual acuity was 20/100 OD and 20/20+ OS. The infiltrate OD was receding. The cultures were negative. The infiltrate OS was slowly increasing. By 6 days after LASIK surgery, the infiltrates were being replaced with stromal haze. There was 20% thinning of the stroma inferiorly with no epithelial defect. There was no anterior chamber reaction. By 2 weeks post-LASIK the prednisone had been reduced to 40 mg and the doxycycline 50 mg twice daily. Topical steroid was reduced to four times daily.

The visual acuity was 20/20 OD with −2.50 D and 20/20− OS with −0.75 D. The prednisone was tapered off during the next week.

After 7 months the central corneal was clear in both eyes but haze and thinning was noted in the periphery of the flap OD > OS. The visual acuity was OD 20/15 with −3.25 D and OS 20/15− with −1.25 + 0.50 × 120° on cycloplegic refraction. Did the patient have regression or was the change in refraction due to the inflammation and subsequent scarring? What action should be taken now to improve her visual acuity? What are the options and what are the consequences of each option?

Discussion

This case illustrates the management of postoperative inflammation after LASIK. The cause of inflammation after surgery is often not found. No risk factors, such as lid margin disease, epithelial defect, or improper sterilization techniques, were identified at the start of the inflammation that occurred in this case. She did have a scar in the OS noted preoperatively (see Case 2) without a corresponding history or record of erosion, ulceration, or keratitis. Inflammation after LASIK often gets worse before improving despite frequent topical prednisolone and oral prednisone. The surgeon managing this case had a low threshold for relifting the flap for both culture and the removal of inflammatory material in the interface. The risk of relifting the flap is relatively low; however, the risk of continued inflammation—that is, corneal thinning and scarring—is significant. In this case the inflammation was contained in the periphery preserving the BCVA, however thinning did occur in the periphery OD. This may have contributed to the large regression that occurred in that eye. Should retreatment be considered?

Because of the peripheral thinning, relifting the flap, especially in the OD, would be hazardous. PRK over the flap could be done provided there is sufficient residual stromal thickness. Haze is more likely to occur when ablating a LASIK flap, and a recurrence of inflammation could occur. Adjunctive mitomycin-C could be considered to reduce the risk of haze, but its long-term effects in this setting have not been well studied. Intacs could also be inserted to correct low myopia, but the risk of unexpected inflammation would be higher in this patient.

Because of the high preoperative myopia the patient is able to appreciate the significant improvement in visual function despite the regression. Glasses and/or contact lenses are always an option that should be presented as a nonsurgical approach to dealing with regression.

Take-Home Points

1. The etiology of postoperative inflammation is often not found, but infectious keratitis should always be considered.
2. Close observation with aggressive use of topical and oral steroids early on is important to prevent significant central progression with associated thinning and scarring.
3. A low threshold for lifting the flap for removal of inflammatory debris and possible culture is advised.

CASE 75

A 35-year-old woman undergoes hyperopic LASIK in order to correct a refractive error of +2.50 D in both eyes. The surgery is uncomplicated. Her initial postoperative course is unremarkable. Approximately 2 weeks after surgery the patient notes some mild light sensitivity in the right eye.

On slit-lamp examination at that time the surgeon notes multiple tiny white "dots" scattered in the flap interface OD (Case 75, Fig. 1). The left cornea is clear. There is no epithelial defect, no interface or stromal inflammation, and no anterior chamber reaction. How would you proceed?

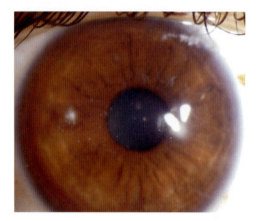

Case 75, Figure 1

Multiple fine infiltrates within the flap interface. (Courtesy Christopher J. Rapuano, M.D.)

The surgeon feels these "dots" are likely reactions to interface debris and decides to reexamine the patient in 1 week. Over the next week, the patient's symptoms are unchanged. On examination the "dots" are slightly larger than 1 week prior, but no other findings are noted. How would you proceed?

The surgeon places the patient on ofloxacin 0.3% every 2 hours while awake. Fourth-generation fluoroquinolones were not available at the time. The "dots" become small infiltrates at the level of the flap interface over the next week and symptoms gradually worsen. How would you proceed?

The surgeon decides to lift the flap and scrape the stromal bed for smears and cultures. Slides are sent for Gram, Giemsa, Calcofluor white, and Ziehl-Nielsen acid-fast stains. Culture media are chocolate, blood, Sabouraud's agar, and a Lowenstein-Jensen slant. Topical fortified amikacin (50 mg/mL) and vancomycin (25 mg/mL) are placed on the stromal bed. The flap is replaced and the patient started on hourly amikacin and vancomycin around the clock, 5 minutes apart. The smears are negative. The cultures are negative initially. The infiltrates worsen significantly during the following 2 weeks. The patient develops increased pain, redness, light sensitivity, and decreased vision. On examination the flap is diffusely infiltrated and edematous (Case 75, Fig. 2). There is a full-thickness hole in the flap in an area of epithelial erosion. There is a large hypopyon. The surgeon decides it is best to remove the flap to debulk the infection and allow better penetration of antibiotic. This procedure is performed with the operating microscope by lifting the flap and amputating the superior hinge with Vannas scissors. The flap is bisected and half is sent for histopathology and half is sent for culture. The stromal bed is again scraped for smears and cultures and to debulk the infection and inflammatory debris. At this time the original culture is determined to be atypical mycobacteria. The second stromal bed culture confirms this finding. The patient is continued on the amikacin and topical clarithromycin (10 mg/mL) is used in place of the vancomycin. The infection resolves during the next several weeks and the antibiotics are slowly tapered. The eye heals with significant central corneal scarring and a best-corrected vision of 20/400.

Discussion

Many different pathogens have been reported to cause post-LASIK infection. Most infections early after LASIK are due to Gram-positive organisms, especially staphylococcus and streptococcus. Most infections with onset after the first few weeks are due to atypical mycobacteria and less

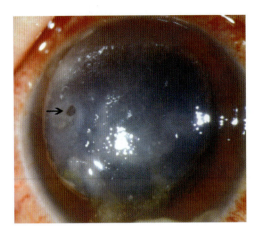

Case 75, Figure 2

Flap edema and infiltration with a focal area of necrosis (*arrow*). (Courtesy Christopher J. Rapuano, M.D.)

commonly to fungi. Small, white inflammatory reactions to debris in the flap interface can occur and need to be distinguished from infections. Typically a foreign body can be identified in the center of a sterile inflammatory reaction. Additionally, there is no surrounding edema or anterior chamber reaction and they cause no symptoms. If unsure, they can be followed closely to make sure they resolve.

When an infectious infiltrate is suspected after LASIK, scrapings for smears and cultures should be performed. If the infiltrate is superficial (often associated with an epithelial defect), surface scrapings can be done with no need to lift the flap. If the infiltrate is in the interface, the flap needs to be lifted and the interface scraped. Multiple smears and cultures should be obtained, as described earlier. Intensive broad-spectrum antibiotics should be started in order to cover Gram-positive bacteria, Gram-negative bacteria, and atypical mycobacteria, until specific culture and sensitivity results are available. Currently, other medications are available for the treatment of atypical mycobacteria infections including a topical fourth-generation fluoroquinolone (gatifloxacin 0.3% or moxifloxacin 0.5%) and oral clarithromycin 500 mg bid. When a flap is severely infiltrated and/or necrotic, it is hurting more than helping and removing it often helps the infection resolve. While infections after LASIK can be devastating, prompt attention and management can result in acceptable outcomes.

Take-Home Points

1. White "dots" in the flap interface are typically small bits of foreign material with a small sterile surrounding inflammatory reaction; however, they need to be differentiated from infectious infiltrates by history, examination, and close follow-up.
2. Suspicious infiltrates in the interface should be scraped for smears and cultures once the flap is lifted.
3. Aggressive antibiotic treatment and close follow-up is required when infection is suspected.

Self-Assessment Test

Anthony Cirino, M.D., Robert S. Feder, M.D., Lawrence Gans, M.D., Colman Kraff, M.D., Marian Macsai, M.D., Parag Majmudar, M.D., Christopher J. Rapuano, M.D., Michael Rosenberg, M.D., Steven Rosenfeld, M.D., Jonathan Rubenstein, M.D., and Michael Vrabec, M.D., F.A.C.S.

The following 50 multiple-choice questions are designed to help the reader assess acquired knowledge of LASIK surgery. Each question is followed by four short answers. Only one answer is correct. The answers and a short discussion are found in the next section (page **260**). Refer to the text for further study if a given topic is not well understood.

SELF-ASSESSMENT TEST

1. Which of the following statements about LASIK surgery is true?
   a. The need to leave a minimum of 250 μm of the stroma untouched has been proven.
   b. LASIK is always safer than PRK because Bowman's layer is not destroyed.
   c. LASEK is the same as LASIK only deeper.
   d. Entering the cycloplegic refraction into the VISX STAR S4 laser computer in a higher myope and performing LASIK may result in an overcorrection.

2. A 56-year-old patient is interested in refractive surgery. She is myopic and on initial screening was found to have a central corneal thickness of 635 μm. Which is the next step in the further evaluation of this patient?
   a. Perform video topography to evaluate corneal elevation.
   b. Perform specular microscopy.
   c. Obtain a diurnal curve.

d. Refuse to treat this patient because the corneas are too thick.

3. You are performing LASIK with a blade microkeratome on the second eye of a patient who is a high myope. You realize that you have lost suction and the flap is incomplete. What is the best choice on how to proceed?
   a. Place the flap back into position, abort the surgery, and recut a new flap after 6 months.
   b. Use a deeper plate to create a new thicker flap, then continue with the laser.
   c. Continue with the excimer laser ablation to finish the surgical plan.
   d. Convert to PRK since the flap is mostly epithelium.

4. The corneal flap will be thicker on the fellow eye if:
   a. the microkeratome blade is reused.
   b. the cornea is thin.
   c. the translation of a manual microkeratome head is faster.
   d. the plate thickness is increased.

5. Which of the following statements about residual stromal thickness (RST) is true?
   a. Leaving an RST of at least 250 μm guarantees that post-LASIK ectasia will not occur.
   b. RST can be accurately determined prior to surgery.
   c. Nomogram-adjusted ablation depth calculations should be used to determine RST.
   d. Ectasia can occur even when the RST is well above 250 μm.

6. The advantages of the low-vacuum setting on the Moria CB and M2 microkeratomes include:
   a. allows for cutting a thinner flap.
   b. affords greater protection to the optic nerve when cutting the LASIK flap.
   c. allows the surgeon to maintain control of the eye during laser ablation.
   d. less likely to cause postoperative dry eye syndrome.

7. The advantages of a manual microkeratome include:
   a. ability to vary the translation speed to create thinner or thicker flaps.
   b. creates a smoother stromal bed.
   c. less chance for LASIK flap complications.
   d. more reliable and reproducible flap thickness.

8. Which of the following statements regarding microkeratomes is true?
   a. Thicker corneas result in thinner flaps.
   b. Thinner corneas result in thinner flaps.
   c. Flatter corneas result in larger flaps for the same ring size.
   d. Steeper corneas result in smaller flaps for the same ring size.

9. When using the Nidek EC-5000 excimer laser, it is important to do which of the following prior to entering the treatment parameters into the laser?
   a. Verify that the patient's pupil has been dilated preoperatively.
   b. Verify which software version is present in the excimer laser system.
   c. Verify that the patient has punctal plugs in place.
   d. Obtain a WaveScan preparation for a CustomVue treatment.

10. Which of the following statements is true regarding the Nidek EC-5000 excimer laser system?
    a. The system has been approved for myopic, myopic/astigmatism, and hyperopic treatments with PRK.
    b. The laser has been FDA approved for LASIK treatments from −1.00 to −14.00 D without the correction of astigmatism.
    c. The laser has been FDA approved for LASIK treatments for the reduction of myopia with or without astigmatism ranging from −0.75 to −14.00 D with up to 4.00 D of cylinder.
    d. The laser does not have an FDA-approved tracking system.

11. Which of the following statements is true regarding single-piece microkeratomes?
    a. A single-piece microkeratome frequently results in a decreased overall time for intraocular pressure elevation during flap creation.
    b. A single-piece microkeratome can only be used for the creation of a nasal hinge.
    c. A single-piece microkeratome increases the risk of entrapping eyelashes or eyelid tissue when the LASIK flap is created.
    d. A single-piece microkeratome requires a higher intraocular pressure than a two- or three-piece microkeratome.

12. When the LASIK flap is created on the first eye and a small epithelial defect is noted, which of the following is the most appropriate course of action?
    a. The LASIK surgery should be terminated and the second eye canceled.
    b. A bandage contact lens should be placed on the eye after the LASIK flap is repositioned and prednisolone acetate drops should be initiated.
    c. No accommodations or changes in techniques are necessary when a small epithelial defect is noted on the flap.
    d. PRK should be performed on the second eye.

13. The recommended concentration of mitomycin-C for refractive surgery prophylaxis is:
    a. 0.2%
    b. 0.02%
    c. 0.02 mg/mL
    d. 2 mg/mL

14. Buttonhole flaps are more likely to occur in patients with:
    a. flat corneas.
    b. steep corneas.
    c. myopia.
    d. hyperopia.

15. The Orbscan topography device:
    a. uses Scheimpflug photography to measure the corneal contour.
    b. is not helpful in identifying early keratoconus suspects.
    c. cannot provide elevation data.

d. can provide a pachymetry map of the cornea.

16. The Zyoptix (Bausch & Lomb) system:
    a. can be used in patients with hyperopia.
    b. can be used to treat mixed astigmatism.
    c. is the system of choice for a patient with −8 D of myopia.
    d. can accurately correct refractive error less than −7 D of myopia and −3 D of astigmatism, with a maximum spherical equivalent of −7.5 D.

17. In the United States, the Bausch & Lomb Technolas 217 laser:
    a. utilizes an active eye tracker.
    b. has a customizable optical zone size with a customizable blend zone.
    c. has a cyclotorsional tracker.
    d. cannot treat hyperopia.

18. Mitomycin-C is:
    a. an anti-inflammatory agent.
    b. derived from a bacteria.
    c. an inhibitor of DNA synthesis.
    d. an antifungal agent.

19. PRK haze is:
    a. more common in low myopic ablations.
    b. never seen with LASEK.
    c. unpredictable, but more common in deeper ablations.
    d. not possible with modern excimer lasers.

20. DLK associated with the IntraLase can best be avoided by:
    a. use of topical steroids preoperatively.
    b. use of nonsteroidal eye drops preoperatively.
    c. assurance of the proper laser settings.
    d. use of doxycycline preoperatively.

21. Which of the following patients would be best suited to undergo LASIK with the Intralase rather than a blade microkeratome?
    a. a 55-year-old woman with a myopic refraction of −2.00 D
    b. a 32-year-old −12.00 D myope with preoperative keratometry values of 41.00 D
    c. a 22-year-old −2.00 D male
    d. a 35-year-old woman with Schirmer values of 0 and conjunctival staining

22. Explanations for the inability to obtain adequate suction for IntraLase flap creation include all of the following except:

a. small palpebral fissure.
b. boggy conjunctiva.
c. use of brimonidine preoperatively.
d. faulty suction cone.

23. The femtosecond laser creates a lamellar flap via the process of:
    a. thermal breakdown.
    b. plasma creation.
    c. carbon–nitrogen bond release.
    d. photodisruption.

24. The IntraLase can be used for all of the following procedures except:
    a. PRK.
    b. intrastromal ring segment (Intacs) insertion.
    c. penetrating keratoplasty.
    d. deep lamellar endothelial keratoplasty (DLEK).

25. A 42-year-old patient comes in for evaluation for refractive surgery. She wears toric soft contact lenses that she discontinued 3 days ago. Her manifest refraction (MR) shows 0.5 D of cylinder and her topography shows 1.25 D of cylinder. How do you plan her surgery?
    a. Treatment plan based on the MR.
    b. Treatment plan based on the topography.
    c. Ask the patient to stay out of her contact lenses for another week and then treat based on her repeat MR.
    d. Have the patient stay out of her contact lenses until the MR and topography are stable, repeatable, and consistent, no matter how long it takes.

26. A 26-year-old myope desires laser keratorefractive surgery:

Central corneal thickness = 595 μm OU

Scotopic pupil size = 6.0 mm OU

MR = −10.00 + 1.50 × 90 both eyes

CR = −9.50 + 1.50 × 90 both eyes

Keratometry = 42.00 D at 90° by 40.00 D at 180° OU

Pachymetry = 605 μm OU

Preoperative topography and elevation maps are normal OU

Is this patient a good candidate for LASIK?
a. No, because the CR differs too much from the MR.

b. No, because the average corneal power postoperatively will be too flat.

c. No, because of the risk of ectasia in this high myope.

d. No, because the amount of astigmatism on keratometry is greater than the amount of astigmatism on refraction.

27. A −3.00 D myope is determined to be a good candidate for LASIK. After the microkeratome pass, major sloughing of the corneal epithelium is noticed. The best course of action is to:

a. replace the flap and the epithelium as best as possible and do not perform the laser.

b. replace the flap and then perform PRK after debriding the epithelium.

c. perform the laser ablation as planned, reposition the flap, replace the epithelium as well as possible, and then apply a bandage contact lens.

d. amputate the flap and treat the bed with laser.

28. Which of the following is not a sign that adequate suction is being obtained with a mechanical microkeratome?

a. The patient reports dimming of vision.

b. Conjunctival vessels have blanched.

c. The Barraquer tonometer or pneumotonometer reads an IOP greater than 65 mmHg.

d. Pupil dilates and remains so.

29. Which statement regarding free caps is true?

a. They are thought to be less common in corneas with keratometry readings <40 D.

b. Excimer laser treatment to the stromal bed is contraindicated in the presence of a free cap.

c. Corneal ink marks make it difficult to manage a free cap.

d. A free cap can be lost or damaged as the microkeratome unit is removed from the eye and either prepared for the fellow eye or cleaned.

30. Which of the following is not considered a risk factor for epithelial loosening or an epithelial defect during LASIK?

a. anterior basement membrane dystrophy

b. age over 50 years

c. high astigmatism

d. epithelial shift or defect in the fellow eye

31. Proper management of epithelial loosening or defect during LASIK includes all of the following except:

a. the flap needs to be carefully examined to make certain the flap stroma is intact and the stromal bed examined to make sure it is uniform.

b. great care should be taken to replace the epithelium back in its original location.

c. if an epithelial defect occurs, the laser treatment should not be performed.

d. postoperatively, a bandage soft contact lens is often useful in management.

32. Risk factors for ectasia after LASIK include all of the following except:

a. central cornea that is thinner than the inferior periphery.

b. asymmetric inferior steepening on corneal topography.

c. keratometry readings greater than 47 D.

d. residual stromal bed less than 250 μm.

33. Proper management of DLK includes all the following except:

a. mild DLK (mild peripheral cellular infiltration) is treated with an increase in topical steroids and close follow-up.

b. moderate DLK (moderate peripheral and central cellular infiltration with an undulating pattern) is treated with an injection of steroid beneath the flap done at the slit lamp.

c. severe DLK (dense, undulating central and peripheral cellular infiltration, associated with decreased vision and photophobia) with a possible infiltrate should be treated with flap lift, scrapings to remove inflammatory material and for smears and cultures, interface antibiotics and steroids, postoperative steroids and antibiotics, and close follow-up.

d. oral steroids may be helpful in severe DLK.

34. Appropriate treatment options for epithelial ingrowth include all of the following except:

a. follow mild epithelial ingrowth not affecting vision.

b. lift the flap, remove epithelium from the stromal bed.

c. lift the flap, remove all of the interface epithelium, and suture the flap.

d. lift the flap, remove all of the interface epithelium, and apply fibrin glue to the flap margin.

35. Regarding intraocular pressure (IOP) and LASIK, all of the following are true except:
   a. the IOP should not be measured for at least 1 month after LASIK due to the risk of flap dislodgement.
   b. the measured applanation IOP is probably less than the true IOP after LASIK for myopia.
   c. the central applanation IOP measurement can be falsely low (e.g., 3 to 5 mmHg) if there is a fluid cleft between the stromal bed and the LASIK flap.
   d. elevated IOP after LASIK can appear identical to DLK at the slit lamp.

36. Proper management of ocular surface disease such as dry eyes and blepharitis in a LASIK patient includes all of the following except:
   a. patients with significant dry eye symptoms or epithelial punctate fluorescein staining should undergo further evaluation (e.g., with Schirmer test, tear break-up time) prior to LASIK.
   b. patients with dry eye signs and symptoms should be treated to decrease the signs and symptoms prior to final evaluation for LASIK.
   c. topical cyclosporine drops are often helpful pre- and postoperatively for dry eye signs and symptoms.
   d. dry eye symptoms are worse after LASIK for 3 to 6 months, but always return to baseline by 12 months.

37. Which of the following statements about glare, haloes, and night vision symptoms after LASIK is not true?
   a. Risk factors for glare, haloes, and night vision symptoms after LASIK are often considered to include high myopia, high astigmatism, and large pupils.
   b. Pupil size in normal and dim illumination should be measured prior to LASIK.
   c. Topical brimonidine and low-dose pilocarpine are helpful in reducing glare, haloes, and night vision symptoms in some patients.
   d. Patients with dim pupil diameters greater than 7 mm should not undergo LASIK.

38. A 46-year-old woman had bilateral LASIK for myopia 1 month ago. The preoperative refraction in the dominant OD was $-8.00 + 1.00 \times 90°$ and $-8.50 + 1.00 \times 90°$ OS. Postoperative visual acuity was 20/20 OD with an initial cycloplegic refraction of –0.25, and 20/40 OS with a cycloplegic refraction of $-1.50 + 1.25 \times 35°$. The patient is unhappy, complaining of difficulty seeing at distance and near when she covers her right eye. The most appropriate treatment would be:
   a. retreatment using laser following a flap relift.
   b. LRI.
   c. custom retreatment.
   d. nothing.

39. The patient from Question 38 returns 6 weeks later. The cycloplegic refraction is stable. The most appropriate retreatment would be:
   a. retreatment using the laser following a flap relift.
   b. LRI.
   c. custom retreatment.
   d. nothing.

40. A 30-year-old man had LASIK OD to correct a preoperative cycloplegic refraction of $-1.25 + 1.75 \times 160°$. His preoperative best-corrected visual acuity was 20/20. Postoperatively, his visual acuity was 20/25–. There were no microstriae, the flap was well centered, and there was no debris. Over the next 3 months, manifest and cycloplegic refraction varied by small amounts, but visual acuity could be corrected only to 20/25. Wavefront measurements showed a minimal spherical aberration, modest amounts of coma, and trefoil. Refraction over a gas-permeable contact lens improved the vision only slightly. The patient was adamant about doing something. The most appropriate retreatment would be:
   a. surface retreatment using custom treatment.
   b. surface retreatment with mitomycin.
   c. conventional laser retreatment.
   d. LASIK custom retreatment, if improvement with PreVue lens.

41. LASIK surgery is being planned OD for a patient with myopic astigmatism using

conventional excimer laser treatment on the VISX STAR S4 platform. The cycloplegic and manifest refractions are similar at $-4.00 + 2.00 \times 60°$ and are stable. The patient has a 7.0-mm pupil in dark illumination and corneal pachymetry of 558 µm. The examination is otherwise normal. A reasonable estimate of the ablation depth is:

a. 53 µm.
b. 45 µm.
c. 60 µm.
d. The ablation depth cannot be estimated until the nomogram adjustment is determined.

42. Which of the following can the surgeon change when designing a CustomVue treatment?
a. axis of astigmatism
b. magnitude of astigmatism
c. ±1.0 D sphere
d. ±10% nomogram adjustment

43. Which of the following is true?
a. The RMS value determines whether or not a patient is a candidate for CustomVue.
b. The percent preoperative HOA determines whether or not a patient is a candidate for CustomVue.
c. The RMS value is an overall assessment of the higher order aberrations.
d. Mixed astigmatism cannot be treated with the VISX CustomVue platform.

44. Which of the following statements is false?
a. Hyperopic treatments should result in a postoperative keratometry value of <49 D.
b. The lower limit keratometry value in a myopic treatment is 33 D.
c. Iris registration will passively track the cyclorotation of the eye during a CustomVue treatment.
d. The ablation zone can be enlarged out to 9.0 mm with CustomVue.

45. Which of the following statements best describes a patient who is not a good candidate for a CustomVue procedure?
a. The patient has an average keratometry reading of 40.5 D OU.
b. The patient has a high percent of vertical coma and spherical aberration on the preoperative WaveScan screening.

c. The patient is hyperopic and the cycloplegic refraction and WaveScan refraction correlate and indicate at least 1.5 D of latent hyperopia.
d. The scotopic pupil measures 8.5 mm.

46. A 52-year-old patient presents for LASIK consultation. His refraction is +5.00 D in both eyes with a BCVA of 20/20 in each eye. The anterior segment appears normal. Provided he understands the risks of surgery and the rest of the examination is normal, the potential surgical options include all of the following except:
a. hexagonal keratotomy.
b. phakic IOL.
c. clear lens exchange.
d. PRK.

47. Bioptics is a term that refers to:
a. a specialized multifocal implant.
b. a piggyback lens implant system in which one implant is placed in the ciliary sulcus and one is placed in the capsular bag.
c. the use of a long-lasting collagen contact lens after cataract surgery.
d. LASIK surgery performed some time after a phakic IOL has been implanted in order to refine the visual outcome.

48. Which of the following statements about Intacs is true?
a. Another name for Intacs is the "living contact lens."
b. Intacs can be used to treat ectasia after LASIK or PRK.
c. Intacs can be used to treat progressive effect after radial keratotomy.
d. Intacs are inserted at the limbus.

49. Conductive keratoplasty is a procedure performed with a(n):
a. holmium-YAG laser.
b. argon laser.
c. femtosecond laser.
d. radiofrequency probe.

50. The effect of the toric IOL is:
a. short lived.
b. dependent on accurate placement in the axis of the (+) cylinder in the refraction.
c. dependent on accurate placement in the axis of the (+) cylinder on keratometry.
d. dependent on accurate placement 90° away from the axis of the (+) cylinder in the refraction.

ANSWERS TO SELF-ASSESSMENT TEST

1. **Answer (d).** To obtain the correction corresponding to the cycloplegic refraction a nomogram-adjusted correction is entered into the VISX laser. The larger the myopic correction and the older the patient, the greater the reduction in the myopic power of the sphere. The 250-μm minimum is a rule of thumb only. It has not been proven and some patients may require a thicker residual bed to prevent ectasia. LASIK is not always safer than PRK. In the presence of epithelial basement dystrophy, PRK may be the preferred refractive procedure.

2. **Answer (b).** A central thickness of 635 μm is thicker than normal. However, the endothelium may be normal. A normal cell count, cell shape, and size as measured with specular microscopy would suggest that endothelial dysfunction is not the cause of the thicker-than-normal cornea. If the surgeon felt the thick cornea was due to endothelial dysfunction, the patient would not be a candidate for surgery. The other tests would not help evaluate the corneal endothelium.

3. **Answer (a).** It is best to abort the laser surgery at this point, because the full laser treatment cannot fit under the incomplete flap. It would be unwise to attempt to recut a deeper flap during the same surgery. PRK over a flap is associated with an increased risk of stromal haze.

4. **Answer (d).** Most microkeratomes have several microkeratome heads or spacer plates to insert to help create thinner or thicker flaps. Studies have also demonstrated that the faster the microkeratome pass, the thinner the flap that will be created. Other studies have shown that the average corneal flap is thinner in the second eye than the first eye, presumably due to the microkeratome blade getting duller after the first pass.

5. **Answer (d).** There are no published studies that can confirm the absolute safety of maintaining a residual stromal thickness (RST) of 250 μm. There are many published cases of ectasia in patients with an RST of >250 μm, and cases from the early days of LASIK surgery with <250 μm of RST that have not developed postoperative ectasia. The RST is more accurate when calculated using the non–nomogram-adjusted refraction and intraoperative pachymetry. It is believed that several factors might influence the development of ectasia including a subclinical keratoconus, wider ablation diameters, and individual patient healing factors. Please read the following excellent review article on this subject: Binder PS. Ectasia after laser *in situ* keratomileusis. *J Cataract Refract Surg.* 2003; 29: 2419–2429.

6. **Answer (c).** The Moria microkeratomes must utilize the high-vacuum setting during the actual creation of the LASIK flap. The period of high vacuum is when the optic nerve is most vulnerable to damage, especially if the patient has underlying glaucoma. The low-vacuum setting should not cause optic nerve damage. It is utilized for maintaining control of the globe during laser ablation. The low-vacuum setting does not have any effect on the flap thickness or postoperative dry eye syndrome.

7. **Answer (a).** The flap thickness varies with each microkeratome head, and even from patient to patient with the same head. Studies have demonstrated that there can be significant variability in flap thickness with each cut. The stromal beds are equally smooth with the manual and automated microkeratomes. Flap complications can occur with any type of microkeratome. One of the main advantages of the manual microkeratome is the ability to vary the translation speed and thereby create thinner or thicker flaps.

8. **Answer (b).** Thinner corneas result in thinner flaps. Thicker corneas result in thicker flaps. This was verified when six different microkeratomes were studied to determine the depth and size of the flap that is cut. A flatter cornea results in a smaller flap for the same size ring, and a steeper cornea results in a larger flap for the same size ring.

9. **Answer (b).** Prior to entering data into the Nidek EC-5000 laser for the desired refraction, it is necessary to verify if the software version is 2.25g or 2.25e. If it is 2.25e you will need to use the appropriate nomogram look-up table, which is supplied by Nidek, for entering the desired correction; then you must have the ability to utilize the nomogram to expand the optical zone and transition zone. With 2.25e you can expand the transition zone beyond 7.5 mm. With software version 2.25g you will not be able to expand the transition zone beyond 7.5 mm and it is not necessary to identify the desired correction on the look-up table because this software version does so automatically. WaveScan and CustomVue are available on the VISX STAR S4 laser. The Nidek laser has not been FDA approved for custom LASIK treatment.

10. **Answer (c).** The Nidek EC-5000 has been FDA approved for both PRK and LASIK for the treatment of myopia, with or without astigmatism, ranging from −0.75 to −14 D and astigmatism ranging from 0 to −4 D of cylinder. FDA trials for hyperopia and mixed astigmatism are currently under way.

11. **Answer (a).** A single-piece microkeratome does not require a higher elevation of intraocular pressure than a multiple-piece microkeratome. A single-piece microkeratome can offer the advantage of creating either a nasal or superior hinged flap without causing a prolonged period of elevation of intraocular pressure that can result from time necessary to assemble the microkeratome on the eye. With all microkeratomes the assembly must be verified and the intraocular pressure must be checked prior to creation of the corneal flap.

12. **Answer (b).** When a small epithelial defect is noted after the LASIK flap has been created on the first eye, it is not necessary to abort the LASIK procedure. The flap should be replaced after the laser treatment is performed and carefully repositioned. After an adequate period of time has transpired and the flap is in position, a bandage contact lens should be placed on the eye and topical prednisolone acetate should be started.

An intraoperative epithelial defect can result in DLK during the early postoperative period. It is important for the surgeon to recognize this potential complication and initiate topical prednisolone acetate early. Because the presence of a bandage contact lens and an epithelial defect put the patient at risk for possible bacterial keratitis, it is necessary to concomitantly treat the patient with a broad-spectrum antibiotic also.

For the second eye, care should be taken to avoid an epithelial defect. A methylcellulose-based lidocaine jelly can be placed on the cornea prior to placement of the microkeratome, and the microkeratome should be lubricated with a glycerin-based sterile artificial tear solution while it is advancing forward. After the microkeratome has advanced forward completely, suction can be released and the microkeratome can be gently removed, allowing the flap to slide out of the microkeratome without the epithelial trauma induced by reversal of the microkeratome head.

13. **Answer (b).** Extreme caution is advised in communicating the proper concentration and in accurate compounding of the MMC. The two concentrations of 0.02% and 0.2 mg/mL are equivalent.

14. **Answer (b).** Steep corneas, particularly with keratometry readings >47.00 D, are more likely to buckle centrally during the microkeratome pass, creating a buttonhole. Buttonholes can occur in corneas with keratometry readings <47.00 D, but are less likely. Do not proceed with the laser ablation if a buttonhole is detected in the ablation zone.

15. **Answer (d).** The Orbscan can provide a pachymetric map of the cornea. The values should not be used in calculating ablation depth. It provides elevation data and is useful in identifying early keratoconus. The Pentacam unit, a newly available topography system, uses Scheimpflug photography.

16. **Answer (d).** The Zyoptix (Bausch & Lomb) system for custom LASIK is not currently approved for treatment of

8

hyperopia, mixed astigmatism or myopic treatment above −7.00 D. It is approved for myopia with astigmatism where the astigmatic component is not greater than −3.00 D and the spherical equivalent does not exceed −7.50 D.

17. **Answer (a).** The Technolas 217 laser utilizes an active tracking system, but does not track cyclotorsional movements. While it has a customizable optical zone size, the blend zone size cannot be customized. The system is FDA approved for hyperopia with or without astigmatism.

18. **Answer (c).** Mitomycin-C inhibits scar formation because of its effect on DNA synthesis. It is derived from *Streptomyces caespitosus*, a fungus, and is not an anti-fungal or anti-inflammatory agent.

19. **Answer (c).** Haze associated with PRK is more common in deeper ablations. It is less likely to occur with modern lasers, but it is unpredictable. In general, it is less common in low myopic ablations, but the incidence is probably more closely related to ablation depth than to the degree of myopia. PRK haze can occur with LASEK.

20. **Answer (c).** Most cases of clinically significant DLK have been a result of laser settings that were too powerful, resulting in interface inflammation. While pretreatment with topical steroids is important, it is less important than making sure the raster energy and side cut energy are properly set. Nonsteroidal agents and doxycycline have not been shown to be important components in prevention of DLK.

21. **Answer (a).** Although it has been suggested that IntraLase causes fewer dry eye problems postoperatively, a patient with severe dry eye should not undergo LASIK. In those patients with moderate dryness, Restasis and punctal plugs may control the condition and allow for LASIK to be performed safely. Despite the ability of an IntraLase flap to create consistently thinner flaps than a blade microkeratome, the −12.00 D myope would not be a good candidate for LASIK with either technique—the cornea is too flat and the correction needed is too great.

A young healthy male has an excellent chance to have a good flap with a standard microkeratome. However, in a postmenopausal woman, the incidence of epithelial sliding with blade LASIK is much higher than with the IntraLase, and as such would be the preferred method of flap creation.

22. **Answer (c).** A small palpebral fissure can make it difficult to obtain proper suction. At times suction can be better acquired by not using a speculum. Multiple attempts at achieving suction may result in the conjunctiva becoming chemotic with adequate suction becoming impossible to obtain. An occasional faulty suction ring may need to be replaced. Brimonidine (e.g., Alphagan) drops may actually help obtain better suction because it can quiet the conjunctiva, but should be avoided nonetheless because of the increased risk of flap displacement postoperatively.

23. **Answer (d).** The IntraLase creates a lamellar flap via the process of photodisruption.

24. **Answer (a).** PRK (photorefractive keratectomy) cannot be performed with an Intralase. Stromal channels can be made with the laser for insertion of intrastromal ring segments. The laser has also been used experimentally for corneal trephination in penetrating keratoplasty and deep lamellar dissections for the DLEK procedure.

25. **Answer (d).** It is imperative that a patient refrain from contact lens use long enough for the cornea to return to its original shape. Although 1–2 week for a soft lens and 1 month for a gas-permeable contact lens is usually sufficient time for the cornea to resume its normal shape, this reversal of the contact lens effect can be quite variable. Therefore, the surgeon should wait until refractive and topographic stability can be documented before attempting refractive surgery.

26. **Answer (b).** It is not uncommon for the cycloplegic refraction (CR) to differ from the manifest refraction by 0.75 D in a 26-year-old myope. Although there is always a risk of ectasia in every LASIK patient, having an adequate corneal thickness and normal topography and

Orbscans probably portends a low risk of ectasia despite the high myopic correction needed. Astigmatism measured by keratometry is usually slightly greater in magnitude than astigmatism measured in a manifest refraction. The 0.50 D difference in this case is within the expected range. To fully correct this patient's myopia, approximately 9 D of refractive correction is needed. Each diopter of correction will flatten the cornea approximately 0.8 D. Therefore, this patient's cornea will be flattened approximately 7.25 D. Her average preop keratometry was 41.00 D, thus her postop keratometry will be 33.75 D, which is too flat. Corneas with an average corneal power less than 35 D have a degradation of vision due to the loss of the normal prolate corneal shape and this makes this patient a poor candidate for LASIK.

27. **Answer (c).** Loose epithelium after the microkeratome pass may mean that the patient has an occult corneal epithelial basement membrane dystrophy. This can lead to a number of postoperative problems, including DLK, epithelial ingrowth, delayed epithelialization of the cornea, and irregular astigmatism secondary to an irregular epithelial surface. Although the surgeon must anticipate these problems, continuing with the planned LASIK procedure and then applying a bandage contact lens is still the best treatment option. The chance for DLK and epithelial ingrowth exist once the flap is created whether the laser treatment is applied or not. Performing PRK over a freshly cut laser flap can lead to both DLK and intense corneal haze. Amputation of the flap is excessive and not necessary. Therefore, continuing with the planned ablation under the LASIK flap is the best option in this difficult situation. The ideal scenario would be to recognize the epithelial basement membrane abnormality preoperatively and treat the patient with photorefractive keratectomy (PRK) instead of LASIK.

28. **Answer (b).** Blanching of conjunctival vessels is not a sign of increased IOP. The surgeon should use all of the other clues to be certain adequate suction exists prior to creating the flap with the microkeratome. Some surgeons use finger tension instead of a tonometer, however, finger tension may not be as accurate. Surgeons should listen for a hissing sound, which indicates lack of proper suction. If the machine does not indicate adequate suction is achieved, it isn't. However, the converse is not true. Just because the machine indicates adequate suction, it may not actually exist. The suction port may be blocked by conjunctiva, causing the machine to indicate adequate suction without necessary IOP elevation. This scenario is termed *pseudosuction.*

29. **Answer (d).** Free caps need to be recognized immediately, prior to removing the microkeratome from the surgical field, to have the best chance of locating the free cap. In the event of a free cap, the cap needs to be found and stored in a safe place until it is needed. It can be placed epithelial side down on a moist 4 × 4 gauze pad or on the conjunctiva, ideally not hydrating the stroma. If the epithelial marks are fading, they can be augmented at this time. These marks are critical to correct orientation of the cap when it is replaced on the stromal bed. Once the cap is located, remarked if necessary, and safely stored, the surgeon needs to decide whether the laser ablation can proceed. Generally, if the stromal bed is uniform, well centered on the pupil, and large enough to accommodate the intended ablation, the laser treatment can proceed. The cap is then placed back on the stromal bed, being very careful to line up the epithelial marks. If the marks were placed asymmetrically, then the cap cannot be placed upside down. The interface is gently irrigated and the cap allowed to adhere. Some surgeons will place 1 to 4 interrupted sutures to secure the cap. Most will simply place a bandage soft contact lens on the eye. Corneas with keratometry readings flatter than approximately 40 D are thought to be at greater risk of a free cap. Larger suction rings should be used in eyes with lower keratometry readings.

The femtosecond laser may be advantageous in patients with flat corneas to reduce the risk of free cap.

30. **Answer (c).** Older patients, patients whose fellow eye has had an epithelial adherence issue, those with anterior basement membrane dystrophy, and those with a history of recurrent erosions are at greater risk for epithelial loosening or defects during LASIK. The type of refractive error probably plays no role.

31. **Answer (c).** Once an epithelial irregularity, such as a loosening or frank defect, is noted in the flap during LASIK, it is very important to determine the integrity of the flap stroma. If the flap stroma is normal and the bed is normal, then laser ablation can proceed in this eye. If a large epithelial irregularity is noted in the first eye, it is often best not to proceed with surgery on the fellow eye the same day. Fellow eyes have a similar tendency to epithelial irregularities. Prolonged visual rehabilitation may be required for eyes with epithelial abnormalities. A bandage soft contact lens is often used for comfort and to aid in epithelial healing in the presence of epithelial loosening or a defect. The lens is usually kept in for 3 to 7 days. Close follow-up is warranted in these patients because they are at higher risk for postoperative problems such as DLK and epithelial ingrowth. The Hansatome Zero Compression head or the femtosecond laser may both reduce the risk of epithelial damage during LASIK surgery.

32. **Answer (a).** Corneal thinning that is greater in the inferior periphery than in the center is indicative of an abnormal cornea and predisposes the refractive patient to ectasia. High keratometry readings, asymmetric inferior steepening, and thin residual stromal bed are all risk factors for ectasia after LASIK.

33. **Answer (b).** Mild DLK can be treated with increased topical steroids or close follow-up, so it can be treated promptly if it worsens. Moderate DLK is usually treated with increased topical steroids, for example, every 1 to 2 hours, and close follow-up. Severe DLK is usually treated with either hourly topical steroids or flap lift with or without scraping of the bed to remove inflammatory debris. If an infiltrate is present or suspected, the flap should be lifted, the bed scraped for smears and cultures, and the interface irrigated with antibiotics. Depending on the level of suspicion for infection, the eye should be treated with antibiotics and steroids and seen later the same day or the following day. Some doctors use a short tapering dose of oral steroids in moderate to severe cases of DLK. Injections of steroid are not generally used in the management of DLK.

34. **Answer (b).** Epithelial ingrowth can usually be followed unless it is affecting vision or the health of the flap. When removal is required, it needs to be removed from the stromal bed and the underside of the flap. A sharp blade (e.g., an Alcon 67 or Beaver #15) or a semisharp (e.g., Tooke) knife can be used to remove the epithelium. Care needs to be taken not to damage the flap when the epithelium is removed from its underside. In cases of primary epithelial ingrowth, flap lift and epithelial removal from both sides of the interface are probably adequate. In cases of recurrent epithelial ingrowth, simple flap lift and scrape can be performed, or sutures or fibrin glue can be used to secure the flap edge in attempt to prevent recurrent ingrowth.

35. **Answer (a).** The cornea can be gently applanated on postoperative day (POD) 1 if necessary. However, the IOP does not typically need to be measured on POD 1 and is typically deferred unless an abnormal IOP is suspected. Postoperative IOP measurements are routinely performed beginning at the 1-week visit. Thinner corneas tend to give falsely low applanation IOP measurements, and the thinner the cornea, the lower the measurement. Elevated IOP after LASIK, often a steroid response, can cause a DLK-like picture, which does not respond to steroids and is made worse by steroids. Elevated IOP can also cause a fluid cleft between the stromal bed and the flap. Applanation over this fluid cleft will give an extremely low IOP measurement masking the true

problem. Either a peripheral applanation or a peripheral TonoPen measurement will usually reveal the high IOP.

36. **Answer (d).** Many patients develop contact lens intolerance due to dry eyes and seek refractive surgery. Patients with dry eyes can have excellent results after LASIK, but they are at increased risk for slower visual rehabilitation and temporary to prolonged increased dry eye symptoms. Patients with signs and symptoms of ocular surface disease should be evaluated preoperatively for conditions such as dry eyes and blepharitis with tests such as Schirmer test, tear break-up time, and lissamine green or rose bengal staining. They should be treated for any existing conditions to optimize the ocular surface prior to LASIK. A healthier surface should improve the accuracy of the refraction and aid in postoperative healing. Artificial tears, topical cyclosporine 0.05%, and punctal occlusion can be helpful in many patients both pre- and postoperatively. While most patients are troubled by worse dry eye–type symptoms for a maximum of 3 to 6 months after LASIK, some patients are bothered for years. Surface ablation, such as PRK, tends to induce fewer dry eye–type symptoms than LASIK.

37. **Answer (d).** While the exact relationship of pupil size and glare, haloes, and night vision symptoms is not known, many surgeons believe that large pupils increase the risk, at least in some patients. Consequently, pupil size should be measured preoperatively, and if the pupils are large (generally considered to be greater than about 6.5 mm in the dark), patients should be counseled that they may be at increased risk for increased glare, haloes, and night vision symptoms compared to preoperatively. This is also true for patients with high myopia and/or high astigmatism. All patients should be told that they could have worse glare, haloes, and night vision symptoms after LASIK surgery. Most surgeons do not have an absolute cutoff for pupil size. Topical brimonidine (e.g., Alphagan) and low-dose pilocarpine (1/2 to 1/32%) can be helpful in reducing glare, haloes, and night vision symptoms. It can be used several times a day or just before driving home in the evening.

38. **Answer (d).** This patient had a large correction. No retreatment should be planned until at least 3 months to allow adequate time for full recovery. In addition, no retreatment should be performed until two cycloplegic refractions, at least 1 month apart, are the same.

39. **Answer (b).** This patient is in the presbyopic age group, and the complaints are in the nondominant eye. She has a spherical equivalent of about −1.00. An LRI would eliminate the oblique astigmatism and convert her to monovision at little risk. If she continued to be unhappy, a laser retreatment could still be performed. One could argue that a trial fit with a contact lens would determine whether she would like monovision, but a conventional soft lens would not give her good enough vision to make a good decision.

40. **Answer (d).** In this case, the inability to improve vision with a contact lens in a patient with a normal cornea indicates that surface irregularities were not likely a cause of the decreased vision. Under this circumstance, a surface treatment would be of questionable visual value with a potential for haze, regardless of whether mitomycin was used. Conventional retreatment under the flap would also be of questionable value because simple refraction did not improve the vision. A wavefront measurement was taken with the VISX WaveScan analyzer and can be used to cut a PreVue lens. The PreVue lens allows the doctor and the patient to reasonably decide whether custom retreatment would be potentially beneficial. In the absence of clear subjective improvement with the PreVue lens, the best course would be continued observation.

41. **Answer (a).** Given the pupil size of 7.0 mm, a 6.5-mm treatment zone with a blend zone would be used. The per-diopter ablation depth for a 6.5-mm treatment zone is 15 μm/D. The spherical equivalent of the cycloplegic refraction is 3 D. So the ablation depth would be 45 μm plus an additional 8 μm for the blend for a total estimate of

53 μm. Always use the non–nomogram-adjusted refraction to estimate ablation depth. The laser computer should not be used for the estimate if a nomogram-adjusted treatment is entered into the computer.

42. **Answer (d).** The software allows for a 10% nomogram adjustment. The axis of the cylinder cannot be changed, nor can the magnitude of the cylinder. When the nomogram adjustment is changed, this changes the entire treatment by whatever percent is entered. The software also gives the surgeon the ability to change the magnitude of the sphere by ±0.75 D.

43. **Answer (c).** The RMS value is a number that is calculated to determine the overall HOA of the eye. This number is not used to determine treatment. It can be used to observe the net result of HOA changes, which occur as a result of surgery. VISX is FDA approved for custom treatment of mixed astigmatism.

44. **Answer (b).** The postoperative keratometry value should be kept at 35 or above in myopic treatments. The surgeon should attempt to calculate this by multiplying the total spherical equivalent to be treated by 0.7 or 0.8 and subtract that value from the preoperative keratometry value. This will give the surgeon a rough estimate of the final keratometry.

45. **Answer (c).** When there is a significant difference in the manifest and the cycloplegic refractions in hyperopic patients, these patients can be difficult to treat with or without CustomVue. The significant amount of latent hyperopia makes it hard to determine the correct refractive error to treat. An attempt should be made to see if the patient can relax into the increased amount of hyperopia with either spectacles or contact lenses. If they can tolerate the increased amount of hyperopia and the WaveScan refraction is consistent with the latent amount, then a WaveScan treatment can be performed. If the WaveScan is more consistent with the refractive error that does not reflect the latency, then a WaveScan treatment should not be performed.

46. **Answer (a).** Hexagonal keratotomy has been abandoned due to lack of predictability and safety. Provided the anterior chamber is deep enough, a phakic IOL could be considered. Clear lens exchange is an option even if the anterior chamber angle is somewhat shallow, because the surgery will lessen the risk of angle closure by deepening the anterior chamber. A multifocal or accommodating IOL should be considered to preserve accommodation. Of the keratorefractive techniques, PRK is a better option than LASIK because there is less regression after PRK; therefore, the treatment will not need to exceed approved levels. The accuracy of keratorefractive surgery falls off at this level of hyperopia, and the patient should be warned of the potential loss of BCVA.

47. **Answer (d).** Bioptics has come to mean the combination of refractive surgery techniques in order to maximize the visual function. Bioptics extends the limits of refractive surgery without excessive treatment in the cornea.

48. **Answer (b).** Intacs can be used to treat low myopia. They can improve BCVA and improve contact lens tolerance in some keratoconus patients; and they can also be used to treat ectasia after LASIK or PRK. They cannot be used to treat hyperopia, which is the consequence of progressive effect. They are not inserted at the limbus, but within a 7-mm-diameter ring around fixation. The "living contact lens" refers to epikeratoplasty.

49. **Answer (d).** Conductive keratoplasty is performed with a radiofrequency probe that causes shrinkage of tissue even in the deep stroma. The femtosecond laser is used to create a LASIK flap. The holmium-YAG laser has been used in a contact and non-contact device for hyperopic treatment, but the results were transient. The argon laser is not used to correct hyperopia.

50. **Answer (c).** The effect of the toric IOL is permanent provided the lens does not rotate. It is dependent on accurate placement in the axis of the plus cylinder on keratometry. Because the refraction is based in part on lens-induced astigmatism, it should not be used in the calculation or alignment of the lens.

8

Conclusion

LASIK involves continuing education. Experience is a great teacher, and surgeons should routinely learn from the cases they perform. It is important to refine continually surgical technique and surgical planning, as well as patient management skills. Embrace change, because the field of refractive surgery is rapidly changing. Integrate new technology and techniques into your practice. Seek information from respected colleagues, journals, and meetings; and share what you learn with others. Safe and successful surgery not only helps your patients, but through word of mouth, it serves to widen patient interest in LASIK. Be sensitive to patient complaints after surgery and address problems promptly. There is a remedy for most postoperative problems, and appropriate treatment can often quickly reverse a patient's attitude about surgery.

We hope this handbook has increased your knowledge about the LASIK technique and patient management. We also hope that you will continue to refer to the relevant cases discussed herein as you encounter challenging preoperative, intraoperative, and postoperative issues. It is hoped that the handbook will serve as an able consultant always at the ready to assist you in the decision-making process.

Contact Information

Additions Technology, Inc.
950 Lee Street, Suite 210
Des Plaines, IL 60016
888-8INTACS
888-846-8227
www.keratoconussolutions.com
intacs@additiontechinc.com

Alcon Surgical
6201 South Freeway
Fort Worth, TX 76134-2099
800-757-9195
www.alconlabs.com

AMO Advanced Medical Optics, Inc.
1700 East St. Andrew Place
P.O. Box 25162
Santa Ana, CA 92799-5162
800-366-6554
For Amadeus: 714-247-8200
www.amo-inc.com

Anamed, Inc.
25651 Atlantic Ocean Drive, Suite A1
Lake Forest, CA 92630-8835
949-707-2740
www.anamedinc.com

ASICO Ophthalmic Surgical Instruments
26 Plaza Drive
Westmont, IL 60559
800-628-2879
630-986-8032
Fax: 630-986-0065
www.asico.com
info@asico.com

Bausch & Lomb, Inc.
1 Bausch & Lomb Place
Rochester, NY 14604
585-338-6000
For Hansatome/Zyoptix XP: 800-338-2020
www.bausch.com

Becton Dickinson
For K-4000: 800-237-2174
www.bd.com

Carl Zeiss Meditec
5160 Hacienda Drive
Dublin, CA 94568
877-486-7473
www.meditec.zeiss.com

Eyeonics, Inc.
6 Journey, Suite 125
Aliso Viejo, CA 92656
866-393-6642
www.eyeonics.com

Ferrara Ophthalmics Ltda.
Avenue do Contorno, 4747, Suite 615
30110 100 - Funcionários
Belo Horizonte - MG - Brazil
55 (31) 3223-3108
www.ferraraing.com.br

Moria
For Moria M2: 800-441-1314
For CB: 49(0)6027/508-0
http://www.moria-surgical.com

Nidek
47651 Westinghouse Drive
Fremont, CA 94539
510-226-5700
800-223-9044 (U.S. only)
Fax: 510-226-5750
www.usa.nidek.com
info@nidek.com

Refractec, Inc.
5 Jenner, Suite 150
Irvine, CA 92618
800-752-9544
www.refractec.com

STAAR Surgical
1911 Walker Avenue
Monrovia, CA 91016
626-303-7902
www.staar.com

Storz Instrument Company
See Bausch & Lomb entry
800-338-2020
www.bausch.com
www.storz.com

Summit Technology
For SKB microkeratome: 800-757-9195
www.alconlabs.com

VISX
See AMO entry
www.visx.com
www.amo-inc.com

Index

Figures are indicated by page numbers followed by *f*; tables are indicated by page numbers followed by *t*